Encyclopedia of Metaphysical Medicine

By the same author:

Beyond the Body: The Human Double and the Astral Planes
Encyclopedia of Esoteric Man

Encyclopedia of Metaphysical Medicine

Benjamin Walker

ROUTLEDGE & KEGAN PAUL
LONDON AND HENLEY

First published in 1978
by Routledge & Kegan Paul Ltd
39 Store Street,
London WC1E 7DD and
Broadway House,
Newtown Road,
Henley-on-Thames,
Oxon RG9 1EN
Set in IBM Press Roman by
Express Litho Service (Oxford)
and printed in Great Britain by
Redwood Burn Ltd
Trowbridge and Esher

British Library Cataloguing in Publication Data

Walker, Benjamin

Encyclopedia of metaphysical medicine.
1. Pathology
I. Title
616   RB111

ISBN 0 7100 8781 0

Contents

Introduction	*page* ix	depression	*page* 60
abulia	1	diagnosis	61
acupuncture	3	diet	63
aetiology	6	disease	65
allopathy	8	drug therapy	67
anaphrodisiacs	9	dysgenics	72
angst	10	eccentricity	76
anxiety	11	electrotherapy	78
aphrodisiacs	13	embryonics	80
aromatherapy	15	epidemics	83
ars moriendi	18	epilepsy	87
artificial generation	20	erotomania	92
art therapy	24	etherosis	94
asylums	25	ethics and healing	98
aversion therapy	28	eugenics	101
behaviour therapy	29	exorcism	102
biomagnetic therapy	30	experimental medicine	104
biotelemetry	33	fear	107
bleeding	35	fever	108
borboric therapy	36	floritherapy	111
cancer	39	furor	113
catalepsy	41	genius	114
cataplexy	42	geotherapy	118
chromotherapy	44	group therapy	121
constipation	45	herbalism	126
convulsions	48	homoeopathy	127
cupping	51	hormone therapy	129
cyclothymia	52	hydropathy	132
death diagnostics	53	hypnosis	134
degeneration	56	hysteria	137
depersonalization	58	iatrogenics	140

Contents

incubation	*page* 143	physiotherapy	*page* 214
infection	145	phytotherapy	215
infertility	148	placebo	216
influenza	150	pneumopathy	217
kinesiotherapy	154	possession	220
leprosy	156	primitive medicine	223
magnetotherapy	158	psychiatry	227
mania	159	psychic surgery	229
massage	160	psychic vampirism	230
mass hysteria	161	psychodiagnostics	231
medical materialism	164	psychodrama	234
melancholy	165	psychogenic death	235
mental illness	168	psychopathy	237
menticide	170	psychosomatics	239
metallotherapy	171	psychotherapy	240
microbes	173	quackery	242
migraine	175	rejuvenation	245
mind cure	177	religious therapy	249
molecular biology	179	scatotherapy	250
monomania	181	schizophrenia	254
multiple personality	185	sexophobia	256
music therapy	186	sex therapy	258
naturopathy	190	shunamism	260
necrophilia	191	sleep therapy	262
neurosis	192	sociopsychosis	264
nightmare	194	somnambulism	268
obsession	196	spiritual healing	269
occupational therapy	198	stigmata	272
opposites	199	stress	273
organotherapy	202	suicide	275
osteopractic	203	syphilis	277
pain	205	thanatomania	280
pain therapy	207	thanatophilia	281
paraesthesia	209	theomania	283
patient	212	therapy	285

thermosomatics	285	urinoscopy	293
touch healing	288	xenophrenia	294
transference	289	zone therapy	295
tuberculosis	291	**Index**	299

Introduction

Much of the material for this volume has been assembled from areas that lie outside the boundaries demarcated by modern orthodox medicine, and is therefore beyond the pale of scientific respectability. An attempt has been made here to provide a concise account of the whole dimension of pathology and therapy which might roughly be classed as occult, spiritual, fringe, out-of-the-way, off-beat, and, for want of a more comprehensive term, metaphysical.

The term metaphysical medicine as used here covers various shades of meaning. It is applied to the causes and treatment of disease believed to arise from pathologies of what is known in occultism as the second body, or the non-material substratum of the human organism. It covers arcane medical theory and abstract speculation, orthodox and unorthodox, relating to the effects of sickness on the mind, the association between disease and genius, and the role of disease in history. It is also extended to include the ethical principles that underlie medical practice, and all aspects of medical morality, ancient and modern.

However far we have advanced in our scientific culture, we are still short of an understanding of ourselves if we have not graduated to a stage above the materialistic. In the sphere of medicine, we know that the deeper problems of health and healing are not wholly solved by attending exclusively to the mechanics and chemistry of the body. The human being functions on several levels, somatic and psychosomatic, psychological and parapsychological, physical and metaphysical, which constantly interact to make an individual what he is, and sickness is a predicament in which all these levels often become involved.

Perhaps in no other field has the experience of the human race been so uniformly concentrated for so long a period of time, as in the art of healing. This art reached a surprising degree of sophistication and subtlety in the early stages of human civilization. We know that the psychological and indeed spiritual insight of ancient and primitive societies was quite remarkable, and many physical and mental ills were effectively dealt with by methods well established long before modern scientific techniques came into use. The fact that this experience, some of it dating from preliterate times, has survived to this day, and finds contemporary sponsors and exponents, is a tribute to its enduring value.

We cannot dismiss as superstitious all those methods and traditions that have helped human groups from sickness to health for countless millennia, nor can we brand as credulous those who today believe that certain of these ancient principles and remedies are worth examining afresh in the light of present knowledge.

It has now been established that almost anything can be pathogenic, or disease-producing, and almost anything can be therapeutic, or healing. The range of therapies is therefore a wide one, and a realization of this fact has

Introduction

created a renewal of interest in remedies and prophylactics that are found in the simple elements immediately at our disposal: water, sunlight, fresh air, natural sleep, herbs, fasting; and has also created increasing misgivings about technological treatment, and synthetic drugs of high potency.

The material presented in this volume will not be found in the usual medical encyclopedias, nor in the usual books dealing with fringe medicine. The object of this compilation is to make a brief survey of the whole field, and not to suggest cures. It should therefore be made clear that this is not a handbook of home medicine, and is not intended to provide remedies for self-treatment.

I have benefited greatly from information supplied by the practitioners of some of these therapies; and of course owe an immense debt of gratitude, which I gratefully acknowledge, to the authors of the many books on the subject that I have had the opportunity to read. Most of these have been listed in the bibliographies, which have been compiled from material currently accessible, and will be of use to those who wish to pursue the subject in greater detail. As in my earlier works of reference, an asterisk after a word indicates that there is a separate article on that subject.

B.W.
Teddington

ABULIA

(Gk. *a*, 'non'; *boule*, 'will'), or aboulia, the inability to make up one's mind or to act on a decision, a mental condition often found in depression, melancholia, dementia, epilepsy, and in certain neurotic conditions like psychasthenia. The term has broader implications which suggest a state of apathy, indifference and helplessness, stemming from a lack of faith or interest in oneself and in others.

Abulia is to be distinguished from another privative concept, that of ataraxia (Gk. 'non-agitation'), greatly esteemed by the Stoical philosophers of classical antiquity, who regarded it as an eminently desirable state of mind, and an ideal to be attained. Ataraxia implied not apathy, but an attitude of philosophical calm in the face both of adversity and triumph, joy and sorrow, success and failure. A Greek citizen of Pergamum in Asia Minor, beset by troubles and sorely harassed by a shrewish wife who nagged him more than Xanthippe did Socrates, when asked to name his newborn son, named him Galen (from the Greek word for 'calm'), because he wished the boy to have, above all other virtues, the quality of ataraxia. The boy Galen was destined to become one of the most famous physicians of all time.

A medieval variant was acedia (Gk. *akēdeō*, 'non-caring'), in the sense of 'not being involved'; and its derivative accidie, meant spiritual apathy, feelinglessness or lack of concern. The latter was sometimes translated 'sloth', one of the seven deadly sins, and more evil than all the others. This sloth did not imply laziness, but indifference and tepidity, an absence of ardour and enthusiasm for matters of human concern. It was the only one of the sins that could outweigh the seven virtues put together.

Abulia is primarily a condition of spiritual emptiness. Nothing exists in the life of the abulic to excite his affections or stimulate his will. The absence of direction in his life makes every effort meaningless. In the Bible, God's message to the prophet at Patmos for the Laodiceans makes clear the penalty for such an attitude: 'I know thy works, that thou art neither cold nor hot: I would thou wert cold or hot. So then because thou art lukewarm, and neither cold nor hot, I will spue thee out of my mouth' (Rev. 3:16).

Abulia is related to, yet distinct from, another concept, known as anomie (Gk. *nomos*, 'rule'), or the absence of standards, originally applied to those who, owing to lack of physical or mental energy, were unable or unwilling to adjust to circumstances. Old people, hermits, eccentrics, are prone to anomie. Here again the term is also used in a more extended sense to include all those whose standards of behaviour are unclear, or in conflict with the prevailing norm. They are alienated from their own traditions, lack a sense of continuity with their past, and consequently drift into a state of disorganization and disorientation. Émile Durkheim (d. 1917) the French sociologist

1

believed that a breakdown of personal or social standards inevitably leads to delinquency and crime, and not infrequently to suicide. Not only individuals, but social institutions can degenerate into an anomic state, as we find in the sphere of sociopsychosis*.

Translating the ancient concept of abulia into modern terms psychologists today speak of men being afflicted with the meaninglessness of their lives. A general sense of abulia and intellectual malaise is often experienced by those whose lives lack a deeper purpose or motivation. It is experienced when even successful people suddenly begin to wonder what their work is all about, and feel disenchanted with their fame and prosperity. Life, they feel, has somehow passed them by, and their attainments are so much Dead Sea fruit that has turned to ashes in their mouth, and nothing has really been worth the effort.

With abulia both idealism and hope are lost. If the world has any significance it is not apparent and not worth bothering about, for nothing really matters. Students of the modern crisis point out that for all the material progress of modern civilization, Western man is afflicted with boredom and lack of purpose. Many people lose their reason because they lose their faith. Carl Gustav Jung (d. 1961) wrote that a large proportion of his patients were suffering from a sense of emptiness in what they were doing, because life had become devoid of meaning.

Existentialist psychologists lay great emphasis on the need for reappraising philosophical and religious issues like values, meanings and purposes, without which there is an existential vacuum, leading to a vacuum neurosis in all sections of society. Where parents and teachers lack definite principles, the children grow up disturbed. Young people become oppressed with a sense of pointlessness and futility, a lack of clear values, and an absence of purpose, and are unable to organize their lives. Many demand a credo by which they can restore a sense of direction to their existence.

In the view of some existentialists a meaningful life cannot be without its ordeals. To think that the elimination of suffering is the highest goal of man is to open up a prospect of bitter disappointment. Although suffering is best avoided, if possible, it is inevitable and indeed necessary, and all religions teach the value of its discipline. Its real effects on us are generally hidden and widely different from what we imagine at the time, and its value is only realized when seen in retrospect. The suffering over, it is often found to have brought an expansion of the personality, and greater maturity of spirit.

Viktor Frankl (b. 1905), Austrian psychologist, who spent many months as a prisoner in Auschwitz concentration camp, thinks we need a better understanding of the positive aspects of life as well as of suffering and death. In his view the sexual frustration of Freud's day has given place to the current existential frustration. He contrasted Freud's will to pleasure and Adler's will to power with his own will to meaning. Frankl created a system of existential analysis which he called logotherapy, a 'logos of existence'. The term 'logos' primarily signifies meaning, and logotherapy is meant to help the patient develop a set of values based on a wider world-view and to put meaning back into life.

Books

Bakan, David, *Disease, Pain and Sacrifice: Towards a Psychology of Suffering*, Beacon Press, Boston, 1971.

Bettelheim, Bruno, *The Informed Heart*, Thames & Hudson, London, 1961.

Frankl, Viktor, *The Will to Meaning: Foundations and Applications of Logotherapy*, World Publishing Co., New York, 1969.

Jung, C. G., *Modern Man in Search of a Soul*, Routledge & Kegan Paul, London, 1945.

Ledermann, E. K., *Existential Neurosis*, Butterworth, London, 1972.

May, Rollo *et al.*, *Existence: a New Dimension in Psychiatry and Psychology*, Basic Books, New York, 1958.

Sykes, Gerald, *The Cool Millennium*, Prentice-Hall, New Jersey, 1968.

ACUPUNCTURE

(Lat. *acus*, 'needle'), a method of relieving pain and curing ailments by pricking a part of the body with a needle. The point punctured is not the organ affected and not even necessarily near the source of the trouble, but may be in another part of the body altogether. Thus, the little toe may be pricked to cure a pain in the shoulder.

This system of therapy first originated in China, where it is said to have been practised since the Bronze Age. The earliest treatise was reputedly compiled by Huang-ti (*c.* 2500 BC), the Yellow Emperor. This work is lost but a Chinese manual called *N'ei Ching*, written about 150 BC, is believed to record all the acupuncture theory and practice up to that time. Subsequently the art was greatly altered in taoist treatises especially as an aid to sex magic. From China acupuncture spread to Japan, Korea, Tibet, Nepal and other countries in the East.

In Chinese medical theory the vital, bipolar *yang–yin* energy that is everywhere diffused in the universe, flows in a free rhythm through the human body, where it is called *ch'i*, 'breath'. It permeates every part of the body and, in the normal, healthy organism, circulates freely and continuously, carrying the subtle potencies of breath, blood, the nutritive elements and the life-force through the physical frame. The vehicle that actually conveys this energy is a ramifying network of invisible 'subtle arteries' known as meridians.

The Chinese distinguish 14 major meridians running longitudinally down the length of the body, from the scalp to the toes, along which the vitalic force is distributed; and some 800 tiny points or nodes on the body's surface which are directly linked by a system of lesser branching channels to the limbs, head, trunk and the internal areas and organs. Of the main meridians, 5 connect with the 5 *fou* organs, which are yang and hollow and concerned with food, namely, stomach, small intestine, large intestine, gall-bladder and bladder; and 5 connect with the 5 *tsang* organs which are yin and solid and concerned with breath and blood, namely, heart, lungs, spleen, kidneys and liver. Two other meridians control reproduction and vitality; and still 2 others are diffused as yang and yin potencies, making 14 meridians in all.

A precise knowledge of the 'map' of the meridians and nodes is essential for the practice of acupuncture. For the use of the Chinese Imperial College two life-size bronze statues were cast in about AD 775, perforated with over

800 holes to indicate the nodal points, and these remained the standard guide for many centuries. But the ordinary physician did not depend on such models to locate them. More commonly he used charts based on traditional diagrams which only approximately marked the nodal position. Ordinarily only about 365 nodes are listed, but seldom are more than 100 used by any one practitioner.

The theory underlying acupuncture is that if any part of the body is diseased or any organ not functioning properly, it is because the flow of the vital current in the corresponding meridian is impeded. Disease results from sluggishness in the circulation of the life-force and an imbalance in its distribution, which manifests in a morbid condition of one of the vital organs, and it becomes the doctor's business to find out where the deficiency is and to treat it by stimulation in order to restore the lost balance.

Diagnosis is made in the usual way, by examining the tongue, eyes, pulse, and so on. Since all the meridian lines pass either directly or as subsidiary channels through the chest and abdomen, examination, diagnosis and treatment are frequently effected by light digital pressure in certain places in these areas. The shape, size, hardness and 'fluidity' in and around the areas are all noted, and the centre of the trouble located in this manner.

Treatment, which may be both preventive and curative, consists in regulating the rhythm and restoring the yang-yin balance, and thus remedying any derangement in the circulation of the ch'i energy. This can be done in one of several ways. The nodes can either be toned up (stimulated) or toned down (sedated), so as to achieve the correct volume of the flowing energy. As already indicated the nodes are not necessarily near the site of the organ it is desired to heal, and it makes no difference how deep-seated or inaccessible the organ may be. Thus, for affections of the head certain points in the foot may be treated; for pain in the back the knee may be treated. Trouble on the right side calls for treatment on the left side, and pain in the front calls for treatment in the rear.

The usual method in acupuncture consists in pricking the appropriate nodal point with fine needles made of gold, silver, steel or copper. They may be pushed in direct, or given a clockwise or anti-clockwise turn, or vibrated gently after insertion, depending on the nature of the disease. The needles are stuck far enough into the flesh to stay in position and not drop off, but in some cases they are pushed in rather deeper. They are left in the flesh for a few minutes and then removed. The method of withdrawal also varies.

Often the relevant node is subjected to a deep and firm pressure of the fingertips or finger-nails, held at right angles to the flesh, and then stimulated by a gentle to and fro or circular, boring movement. The finger must be moved with the tissue beneath it, and not just rubbed over the skin. The duration of this treatment may take anywhere between thirty seconds to three minutes. The movement is rather brisk if the organ is to be toned up, and gentle if soothing action is required.

Yet another method is known as *moxabustion*, in which the nodal points of the body are heated, blistered or scorched, by burning a roll of dried moxa, a downy material from the leaves of a certain kind of wormwood. Modern Western practitioners use a small moxa hammer, which is heated over a spirit lamp for a few seconds and then applied to the nodes, the pointed end for toning, the rounded end for soothing.

Chinese practitioners claim that acupuncture will cure most human ailments, including sciatica, neuritis, bronchitis, asthma, diabetes, malaria, tonsillitis, beriberi and infantile paralysis. Thousands of patients from all over the world have testified that acupuncture has cured chronic complaints where all the resources of Western medicine have failed. Acupuncture gives anaesthesia, and major surgery has been performed on kidneys, lungs, liver, brain, ovaries and other internal organs, on patients who are anaesthetized after two or more needles are inserted at selected sites; in some cases an electric current is passed through the needles for about twenty minutes. This numbs one part of the body but leaves the patient conscious and talking throughout the operation.

Since the end of the Second World War acupuncture has become more generally known and practised in the West. There are over 30 acupuncture clinics in Britain alone. Russian scientists tracing high-frequency electrical fields in man, have found that the human bioflux can be tapped at hundreds of points on the skin surface, which are connected with organs deep within the body. These points correspond exactly with the Chinese acupuncture nodes. A special instrument, the tobiscope, developed in the USSR, can locate these points. In Japan, Dr Hiroshi Motoyama of Tokyo, has apparently established a correlation between the *nadi* circuitry of yoga, and the acupuncture meridians.

The efficacy of acupuncture is ascribed to the fact that it might stimulate the production of antibodies in the blood, or that it perhaps excites the pituitary or adrenal glands. It is known that when the skin is pricked a sudden biochemical change is effected in the system, and there might be some therapeutic value in a sharp and stinging pain.

Eastern experts maintain that a number of the 800 nodes are vital crosspoints and that it is possible to interrupt the flow of energy through them, and so produce paralysis or death. Exponents of certain forms of Chinese and Japanese physical culture claim that by touching one of these nodes or 'holes' in a certain way, an expert can cause the effects to manifest themselves only after some hours, days or even months, at the end of which time the victim becomes paralysed or dies. This 'delayed death-touch' is known to the masters of *shorinji kempo*, a kind of Japanese boxing.

Books

Austin, Mary, *Acupuncture Therapy*, Asi Publishers, New York, 1972.
Barclay, Glen, *Mind Over Matter,* Arthur Barker, London, 1973.
Lavier, J., *Points of Chinese Acupuncture*, Health Science Press, London, 1965.
Loung, Ti Sang, *Akupunktur und Räuchern mit Moxa*, Munich, 1954.
Mann, Felix, *The Treatment of Disease by Acupuncture*, 3rd edn, Heinemann, London, 1974.
Morant, G. S. de, *L'Accuponcture chinoise*, 2 vols, Paris, 1939–41.
Motoyama, Hiroshi, *Chakra and Nadi of Yoga and Meridians and Points of Acupuncture*, Institute of Religious Psychology, Tokyo, 1972.
Ostrander, Sheila and Schroeder, Lynn, *PSI: Psychic Discoveries Behind the Iron Curtain*, Sphere Books, London, 1973.

Stanley, Krippner and Rubin, Daniel, *Galaxies of Life: the Human Aura in Acupuncture and Kirlian Photography*, Interface, New York, 1973.
Veith, Ilza, *The Yellow Emperor's Classic of Internal Medicine*, William & Wilkins, Baltimore, 1949.

AETIOLOGY

(Gk. *aitia*, 'cause'), the study of causes, specifically with regard to the origins of disease. Physicians look for symptoms in their patients, and from these symptoms make their diagnosis*. The cause of the disease may then become apparent, but this is by no means always the case; quite often the actual cause remains unknown. All causes are broadly classifiable into two categories: *exogenous*, or originating from outside, and *endogenous*, or originating from within. In general the ancient aetiologies stressed the external factors, witchcraft, demons, environment; and modern aetiology stresses internal factors, like hormones, stress, anxiety.

In ancient times the study of causes was undertaken in far greater detail, since it was held that the apparent symptoms did not always reveal the underlying malaise, which could only be understood against the background of the total self, for many obscure factors militate against a person's health and .welfare. A combined catalogue of the principal theories, past and present, including all likely causes would cover almost every possible contingency.

Thus, in primitive societies diseases are often attributed to a demoniacal cause: evil spirits possess the body and have to be exorcized*. Disease may also result from the loss or displacement of the soul, and it becomes the physician's job to find and restore the soul. Disease may come from wilful *maleficia*, that is, witchcraft and sorcery. It may arise from a breach of taboo or failure to observe a religious or social rite. It may be caused by the intrusion of some disease-object, such as a piece of bone, pebble, splinter or worm, which must be removed, usually by the witch-doctor sucking it out. In more advanced societies disease is sometimes ascribed a divine causation, and is then regarded as a form of chastisement sent from above.

Again, astrological factors, the position of the planets and constellations, are believed to predispose one to certain diseases, and render one prone to weakness of certain parts or organs of the body. In addition to these there are the various cosmobiological factors that are thought to have a direct bearing on a person's health: sunspots, lunar cycles, seasonal changes, time of day or night, atmospheric phenomena, the weather, all of which play their part. Aretaeus (fl. AD 100), Greek physician of Cappadocia, laid great emphasis on the effect of climate in the aetiology of disease. Ecological or environmental factors are also to be taken into account, including the nature of the soil (*see* geotherapy), water, air, topology.

Hereditary factors take in the physical and psychical tendencies inherited by the individual, including the racial background of his parents and ancestors. This complex of causes is known as diathesis, which is the hereditary or constitutional predisposition of an individual to a particular disease. According to the circular definition that is implicit in diathesis, the cause of migraine, or rheumatoid arthritis, for instance, is the inbuilt constitutional liability of the person to get these ailments. It is the diathesis not the disease that is inherited.

Equally, the social and domestic circumstances from which the individual has emerged and in which he is placed can play a significant part in causing disease. In particular, the mental and physical health, moral conduct and social behaviour of the mother during pregnancy, as well as the circumstances attending the birth of the child, for example, foetal disease or birth injury. Reincarnationists attribute all disease to *karma*, or the deeds done in a previous existence, whose consequences are carried over into this life.

According to yet another theory, many illnesses are due to a pathological condition of the etheric body, which according to sensitives can be diagnosed from an examination of the patient's aura or bioplasmic emanation.

Sickness may further emerge from the wider sphere of sociopsychosis*, or disease of society itself, which infects the individual. Also from progress and technological advancement, and the accompanying angst* of modern civilization. Psychosomatic factors or emotional causes, especially sorrow, fear, anxiety, hatred, envy, jealousy, loss of love or some traumatic mental shock, play a major contributory role. So do lack of friends, lack of support for the ego from family or peers, discouragement and disappointment, and a hostile environment. In modern life many of the factors causing stress* lead to disease. Some sicknesses again are said to be iatrogenic*, that is, brought on by doctors themselves, and the hospitalization, drugs and other treatment prescribed by them.

Physiological causes, according to the older pathologies, may depend on the *crasis* (Gk. 'mixing') of the four 'humours' in the body: *eucrasis* is a proper balance, *dyscrasis* an imbalance of these humours. In modern terms this is equivalent to a hormonal disturbance due to malfunctioning of the endocrine glands, or other chemical imbalance. Also overindulgence in food, drink, smoking, sex, drugs, sleeping and exercise. Conversely the lack of some of the above, such as undernourishment and insomnia, will lead to deterioration in health.

Microbes and viruses are of course the more obvious cause of many illnesses, but these often operate in strange ways, causing infection only when circumstances are favourable. Most disease germs are carried by everyone all the time, but stress or weakness empowers and activates them. Lastly, accidents and injury directly affect the body.

Today as in the ancient past there is a tendency towards polyaetiology, that is, finding more than one causative factor in disease, with all the causes interlocked. Hereditary (genetic), constitutional (diathetic), environmental (sociological), individual (idiosyncratic) and other factors are all taken into account to form a composite picture.

In the esoteric view, both predisposing causes (for example, heredity) and provoking causes (for example, excessive eating or accident) are ultimately always occult in origin, prompted by far-reaching concatenations of circumstances.

Books

Benivieni, A., *The Hidden Causes of Disease*, Springfield, Illinois, 1954.
Clements, F. E., *Primitive Concepts of Disease*, Berkeley, California, 1932.
Guirdham, A., *Cosmic Factors in Disease*, Duckworth, London, 1963.
Paracelsus, *The Occult Causes of Diseases*, trans. by Agnes Blake, London, 1930.
Theosophical Research Centre, *Some Unrecognized Factors in Medicine*, 2nd edn, Theosophical Publishing House, London, 1949.
Wolfram, E., *Occult Causes of Diseases*, Rider, London, 1940.

ALLOPATHY

(Gk. *allos*, 'different'), a system of healing traceable to the physician Galen (d. AD 201), whose therapy rested on the principle of *contraria contrariis curantur*, 'opposites are cured by opposites'. 'Hot' diseases are cured by 'cold' remedies and cold diet; wet by dry, and so on.

It became fashionable with Galen's followers to prescribe a combination of drugs: one drug was the active agent to attack a manifest symptom; another an antidote to counteract any ill-effects of the first drug; an adjuvant to help the active agent; a drug to restore the bowel function; yet another to cure the debility resulting from the ailment, and many others, all mixed with an inert vehicle, either water or chalk. Physicians thought that medicines should have as many substances as possible, and prescriptions with 50 ingredients were not unknown. This was known as polypharmacy, or multidrugging.

Associated with this was the system of polypragmacy (Gk. *pragma*, 'action' or 'treatment'), or the multiplicity of treatments. The patient was subjected at one and the same time to a complex régime of starvation, sweating, emetics, purgatives, enemas, bleeding, slashing the flesh and burning with hot irons. This produced what was termed a syncrisis (or in more stubborn cases, metasyncrisis) which brought the patient to a state of collapse, after which he was left to recover.

These drastic methods, used by many eminent physicians in Rome and Asia Minor, were adopted by certain members of the Arabian school, and were standard practice in medieval Europe. Paracelsus (d. 1541), who once burned the books of Galen and Avicenna before starting one of his lectures, was a violent opponent of the system. But his advocacy had no effect on the practice of healing. Louis XIII (d. 1643) of France was given 213 purgatives, 212 enemas and 47 bleedings, all in one year, and many like him suffered a similar fate. The next great name in the battle against polypharmacy was Samuel Hahnemann (d. 1843) who first used the term 'allopathy', in contrast to his own system of homoeopathy*.

Today the name allopathy is generally given to all forms of therapy opposed to such naturopathic* régimes as herbalism, diet, simple remedies and natural sleep. The tendency of modern allopathic practice is a reversion to the old doctrines of polypharmacy and polypragmacy. We have today a mechanistic concept of the body and an engineering concept of healing, since the patient is the same everywhere, and the tendency is to treat a disease by eliminating its symptoms.

In both mental and physical illnesses we have a multiplication of therapies where several cures are tried simultaneously, and a general 'riding madly in all directions'. These include surgery, including the removal of troublesome limbs and organs; electric and other forms of shock; behavioural conditioning; encounter groups; psychotherapy; and above all, powerful combative drugs. The average medicine-cabinet contains at least 25 drugs, some of them taken regularly. Even those who are perfectly healthy tend to dose themselves. Pregnant women are given drugs at various stages of pregnancy. The dying and those in intensive care are a medicine-cabinet in themselves, and a testimony to the durability of the Galenic ideal.

Books

Ackerknecht, Erwin, *Therapeutics: From the Primitives to the Twentieth Century*, Hafner, New York, 1973.
Inglis, Brian, *Fringe Medicine*, Faber & Faber, London, 1964.
Sigerist, H. E., *A History of Medicine*, Oxford University Press, 1961.
Singer, C. and Underwood, E. A., *A Short History of Medicine*, Clarendon Press, Oxford, 1962.

ANAPHRODISIACS

Anaphrodisiacs have an effect opposite to that of aphrodisiacs*, tending to reduce sexual desire or causing temporary or permanent sterility. Their study is important both for those who desire to improve their virile power, since they learn what to avoid; and for those who wish to get their sexual appetite out of the way so that they can get on with what they consider to be more important matters.

Many drugs act as anaphrodisiacs. A number that initially stimulate sexual passion ultimately reduce desire, and if continued, kill it altogether. Cocaine, banisterine (caapi), myristica (nutmeg), LSD and others, which increase the pleasures of intercourse and orgasm, end up by weakening one or more of the triggering processes that bring about erection and ejaculation in the first place.

Also possessing anaphrodisiac properties are salicylic acid, quinine, camphor, menthol, the bromides, valerian and the solanaceous drugs. Among the foods, lettuce, cucumber and dried coriander are sexually depressing. Among drinks, coffee and tea in excess reduce the erectile powers, as do all acid drinks such as lemon and orange juice, and vinegar. Soda water is also a sexual depressant. It is said that an infusion of white water-lily (*Nymphea alba*) taken for 12 days will make a man incapable for one year; taken for 40 days it will permanently extinguish all sexual desire.

In ancient and medieval folklore numerous scatological substances figure among the anaphrodisiacs. According to Pliny (d. AD 79) a lizard drowned in urine has an anti-aphrodisiac effect on the man whose urine it is. Pigeon dung and snail excrement taken with oil or wine have the same effect. A man in love with a woman or bewitched by her, can be cured by placing some of the woman's ordure in his shoe and wearing it. This strange superstition was once very widespread in Europe.

Both tobacco and snuff are anti-aphrodisiac. Indeed, it has been said that there is a latent antagonism in the male body between tobacco and women, so that a taste for one diminishes the taste and capacity for the other. For this reason most true Lotharios eschew smoking. A famous physician said, 'Any man who smokes cigars and drinks soda water can sleep with my wife', so sure was he that such a man would be impotent.

One's way of life also affects one's sexual capacity. Silk clothing enfeebles the erectile powers by engendering and then dissipating bodily warmth. Most modern man-made fabrics are harmful for the same reason. There is no substitute for cotton and woollen clothing for preserving one's sexual ability.

Both cold and heat are harmful. Cold feet hinder successful performance. Too much warmth, especially around the genitals, is equally detrimental. So is too tight a constriction of the organs. The tight pants of youthful fashion which exert a constant pressure on the crotch reduce potency. The same applies to sitting for long periods, whether on a chair, or in a car; and riding, especially horse riding. Hippocrates (d. 359 BC) wrote that the Scythians had great difficulty in erecting as a result of long periods spent in the saddle, and the Scythian race died out as a consequence.

Any excess of eating, drinking, sleeping, hard physical labour or exercise can also produce an anaphrodisiac effect. One exception is walking, best done at a moderate pace. Walking is supposed to have a wonderful effect on the vitalic plexus at the crotch, which sitting interferes with. Anyone wishing to reduce his potency should avoid walking.

All ascetic practices, especially prolonged abstinence and disuse of the sexual apparatus, erode erotic potency. Finally, worry, fear, anxiety, all actively inhibit desire. So does brainwork, especially mathematics, which is highly detrimental to the amorous instinct. A prostitute once told J.-J. Rousseau (d. 1778), 'Leave women alone and study mathematics.'

Books

See under aphrodisiacs

ANGST

A German term meaning dread, apprehensiveness, uncertainty, whose implications extend beyond psychology into philosophy and religion. In its most elementary form angst is expressed in instinctual animal fear.

But fear* provides only an intimation of true angst, which actually belongs to a different order of feeling altogether. The related French word *angoisse*, and the English word *anguish*, come from the Latin *angor*, which means 'strangling' and 'suffocation'. Angst we are told arises from a civilized and sophisticated environment and is common to every such milieu. Though ours has been called the age of anxiety*, angst was already old when Buddha (d. 483 BC) first defined the concept in religious terms, and explained it as arising from desire. It appears in the writings of the ancient Egyptians, Chinese and Hebrews.

Much of the phrenetic activity of mankind today, both in seeking political solutions to problems, and trying to find solace in progress and prosperity and in new and more exciting ways of living, is prompted by the same instinct that makes a man panic, run faster and in circles when he has lost his way.

Angst is a malaise that cannot be cured by affluence, psychology or pills. Good health, security from financial worry, the fulfilment of every material, social and sexual need, do not render one immune to its profound and bewildering melancholy. Our new freedom from the older anxieties that beset mankind, often seems to bring even deeper anxieties in its train. For some reason, in the midst of his pleasure and prosperity modern man is both bored and frightened. He has a deep-seated dread that something basic to his essential individuality is threatened. He is frustrated, and becomes afflicted with a sense of guilt, sin, self-pity and unworthiness. He has a nostalgic yearning for something that is gone.

According to Søren Kierkegaard (d. 1855) and other existentialists, angst stems from an intimation of the *mysterium tremendum*, the overwhelming unknown that lies hidden in even the most commonplace events, an awareness of which fills the mind with a profound dread. In a sense angst finds expression in *Weltschmerz*, 'world ache', a general despair over the whole human predicament, the vastness of the universe, man's loneliness and the immense ignorance about the ultimate nature of things. This dominates the deepest stratum of human thought and feeling and is reflected in modern art, literature, music, poetry and philosophy. It is an expression of the modern sociopsychosis*.

Certain psychologists hold that angst is fundamentally associated with the suffering soul that has not discovered the purpose of life (*see* abulia). Men are overcome by the feeling that their existence is futile and without meaning. They are not at the centre of things any more, have somehow missed the point of the ultimate significance of life. It is as though man has an unappeased hunger for the holy, a deep instinct for God and religion, that a purely material or intellectual life cannot satisfy. Man has acquired knowledge and lost reverence. He has gained the world and lost his soul.

Books

Brunner, Emil, *The Theology of Crisis*, London, 1939.
Dodds, E. R., *Pagan and Christian in an Age of Anxiety*, Cambridge University Press, 1965.
Field, M. J., *Search for Security*, Faber & Faber, London, 1960.
Frankl, Viktor, *Man's Search for Meaning*, Beacon Press, Boston, 1962.
Kierkegaard, Søren, *The Concept of Dread*, Princeton University Press, 1944.
Odier, Charles, *L'Angoisse et la pensée magique*, Neuchâtel, 1947.

ANXIETY

A mental condition of uneasiness and apprehension, different from and to be distinguished from fear*. Anxiety has been defined as a state of mild, prolonged fear, or dread of something still unknown. Fear is a response to an external threat or danger which is perceived; anxiety is primarily internal in origin, arising in the mind, and the reason is often unrelated to anything specific. In general we show fear of an object, and anxiety about a situation.

In its milder phases anxiety is quite common, and is useful in survival and success. Mild attacks (nervousness, stage-fright) provide an added impetus to our activity. But when anxiety becomes morbid or constant, it is a sign of nervous or mental disorder.

Its causes and physiological concomitants resemble those of stress*, including loss of appetite, sleep and sexual drive, often leading in a vicious circle back to anxiety about such loss. In the Freudian view anxiety arises as a result of repressed sexual tension.

Basically most anxiety springs from situations arising out of uncertainty. The unknown is a constant menace, for it presents a threat of sudden changes and a possibly unpleasant future. Life is full of disruptions occasioned by quarrels, accidents, failure, births, deaths and change. Adjustment to a new situation often causes anxiety. Some writers list the condition under such self-explanatory names as separation anxiety, castration anxiety, persecutory anxiety, examination anxiety, station anxiety, and so on. The latter term was once specifically applied to the violent onrush of unease that afflicts people on the point of departing from or arriving at a place. It includes the fear of missing the means of travel. Sigmund Freud (d. 1939) himself suffered from station fears and used to reach a station an hour or more beforehand so anxious was he about travelling.

Today the term is used more generally to cover most forms of anxiety, the 'station' referring to any transitional stage. Station fears include all anxieties arising from a dread of any kind of change; the forebodings that beset one on departure from a familiar place; separation from loved ones; arrival at a new place; meeting new, perhaps hostile, people; finding that things will not be the same when one returns; missing something during one's absence.

Some psychologists are of the opinion that anxiety represents part of a wider sociopsychosis*. It reflects a spiritual illness, and is in fact only a lesser version of existentialist angst*.

Books

Basowitz, H. *et al.*, *Anxiety and Stress,* McGraw-Hill, New York, 1955.

Cattell, R. B. and Scheier, I. H., *The Meaning and Measurement of Neuroticism and Anxiety*, Ronald, New York, 1961.

Dodds, E. R., *Christian and Pagan in an Age of Anxiety*, Cambridge University Press, 1965.

Freud, S., *The Problem of Anxiety*, Norton, New York, 1936.

Goldstein, M. J. and Palmer, J. O., *The Experience of Anxiety*, Oxford University Press, New York, 1963.

Hiltner, S. and Menninger, K., *Constructive Aspects of Anxiety*, Abingdon, New York, 1963.

Hoch, P. H. and Zubin, J. (eds), *Anxiety*, Grune & Stratton, New York, 1950.

Levitt, Eugene E., *The Psychology of Anxiety*, Bobbs-Merrill, Indianapolis, 1967.

May, R., *The Meaning of Anxiety*, Ronald Press, New York, 1950.

Rycroft, Charles, *Anxiety and Neurosis*, Allen Lane/The Penguin Press, London, 1958.

Sarason, S. B. *et al.*, *Anxiety in Elementary School Children*, Wiley, New York, 1960.

Spielberger, C. (ed.), *Anxiety and Behavior*, Academic Press, New York, 1966.

Wittenborn, J. R., *The Clinical Psychopharmacology of Anxiety*, Thomas, Springfield, Illinois, 1966.

APHRODISIACS

Aphrodisiacs (from Aphrodite, or Venus, goddess of love) stimulate sexual desire. In a specific sense the term is applied to any means, natural or artificial, that is used to draw a flow of blood down to the genitals, resulting, in the case of the man, in the erection of the penis, coupled with a desire for intromission and ejaculation; and in the case of the woman, a desire to have a man make love to and penetrate her, and to reach a climax in orgasm. In a more general sense it also applies to any means that will remove sterility and barrenness in woman, impotence in man, strengthen his erectile powers, improve his capacity to emit seed, increase the seed and thicken it. Conversely, means and measures used to diminish these conditions are known as anaphrodisiacs*.

A great many things and a wide variety of activities can lead to the arousal of sexual feelings. Pornographic art and literature; the sight of attractive members of the opposite sex; travel, the motion of a train, the excitement of a journey; certain kinds of pain, for instance, flagellation on the buttocks. Even rest, boredom and idleness can be aphrodisiacs. In Latin, *Venus otia amat*, 'Venus loves idleness'.

More particularly the term refers to a drug or food that directly stimulates an erection or desire for intercourse. The use of drugs, some of which are poisons and irritants, can be extremely dangerous: while causing a violent stimulation, they inhibit natural desire, so that the arousal is not necessarily connected with a normal sexual relationship, but merely an uncontrollable urge to achieve orgasm. In most cases such strong aphrodisiacs provoke a temporary excitation that at the same time destroys the very roots of potency. They act directly on the nervous system so that after continued use further stimulation, natural or unnatural, becomes ineffectual.

Furthermore, some aphrodisiacs can kill. The great Roman general Lucullus (d. 57 BC), a member of the first triumvirate, having been given too potent a love philtre by his freedman who desired to win his affection, went insane and died. The Roman poet and philosopher Lucretius (d. 51 BC) killed himself in a frenzy brought on by a love potion offered him by his wife Lucilia. The excesses of the Roman emperor Caligula (d. AD 41) were said to be partly attributable to a too violent aphrodisiac administered by his wife Caesonia, which drove him out of his mind. Ferdinand of Castile (d. 1516) died as a result of an overdose of cantharides.

Many aphrodisiacs found in the plant kingdom work on the principle of analogy, signature and sympathy. They include poisons like the deadly nightshade (belladonna), *nux vomica* (strychnine), thorn apple (datura), cannabis, cocaine, hashish, the South American turnera plant (damiana) and sabal (the saw palmetto).

Bulbs and roots include eryngo (sea holly), garlic, horseradish, the leek, onion, parsnip, radish, carrot, turnip, chive and shallot.

The more exotic plants used specifically for aphrodisiac purposes include the yohimbe, widely employed in Africa; the quebracho of South America; the muiracitin of Brazil; the bamboo shoots of China. From the male-shaped root of a member of the ivy family growing in China and Korea, comes the oily extraction called ginseng, which is believed to restore virility.

Medieval writers mentioned the lycopodium, with its claw-like roots; the mandrake, which is phallic in shape; the satyrion, a kind of orchid; the pyrethron, which kindles the flame of love; the mushroom, shaped like a penis; the truffle.

Among vegetables: artichoke, spinach, asparagus, beans, capsicum (paprika, red pepper and chillies), celery, cabbage, especially the wild variety known as rocket which grows on the Mediterranean shores. Among seeds and berries: anise, caperberry, caraway, coriander, cubeb, cummin, juniper, mistletoe and colorine (the seed of the Mexican red bean). Among nuts: the chestnut, pistachio and almond. Among fruits: the fig, pomegranate, quince and dates. Among herbs: cress, darnel, dill, fennel, gilly-flower, mint, parsley, tarragon, thyme, valerian. Among flowers: the extracts of petals and stems of the rose, verbena, elecampane, yarrow, vanilla and certain orchids. Among grains and cereals: rice, barley, wheat and lentils. Spices, effective because they set up an irritation in the bladder, kidneys and rectum, include cardamom, cinnamon, cloves, nutmeg, pepper, saffron, turmeric, ginger and mustard.

Many vegetables, particularly those that create flatulence can promote an erection. Martial (d. AD 104) the Latin poet said, 'If your wife is old and your members languid, these vegetables do more than fill your belly.' In some parts of Germany men eat flatulent foods like beans, peas, lentils and radishes in the expectation that the accumulated gas will help them to attain more powerful erections.

Sea foods are popularly believed to have excellent aphrodisiac properties because of their alleged phosphoric content. They include many varieties of fish such as the carp, salmon, trout, anchovy, cod and red mullet. The roe or eggs of fish, especially cod roe, and caviare (the roe of the sturgeon) are also highly valued. So are all shellfish and molluscs, like crabs, crayfish, lobsters, prawns, shrimps, oysters, scallops, cockles, mussels, clams, periwinkles and snails. Eels and the eel-like pseudo-fish, the lamprey, reputedly increase seminal fluid. Also various kinds of jellyfish, notably the ribbon-like cestus, called Venus' girdle.

Some species of insects and insect products are aphrodisiac: ants, especially the winged variety, and also black ants. Spanish fly, a type of beetle, is the source from which the highly potent cantharides is made. Honey, from the honey bee, used both as a food and drink, is regarded as a superlative sex invigorator, especially if mixed with pepper.

Among reptiles, the flesh of snakes is very popular in the East. The lizard, especially the variety known as the skink, is boiled in oil and the oil applied to the male organ to give it strength. The skink can also be dried, powdered, mixed with milk, and drunk. The Arab physician Avicenna (d. 1037) recommended 'milk of chameleon', whatever that may be.

Birds and game also figure on the menu of those seeking sexual vigour. Exotic dishes include dove's brain, goose tongue, goose liver (*pâté de foie gras*). Eggs, especially the yolk, and more especially of birds like the plover, are very good.

All kinds of animal flesh is eaten 'to inspire lust', such as beef, venison, mutton, veal, and their brain, liver, marrow, testicles. The ancient Greeks spoke of the highly aphrodisiac properties of *hippomanes*, now unidentifiable, but described sometimes as a herb, sometimes as a black fleshy excrescence as large as a fig found on the forehead of a newborn foal, and sometimes as the thick jelly-like substance that exudes from the private parts of mares on heat. The pulverized horn of a rhinoceros or the antlers of deer also yield good results.

Milk and milk products like butter and cheese are excellent. Goat's milk is particularly potent. All manner of liquids are imbibed for their aphrodisiac properties. The juice of certain herbs and plants, notably those that exude a white sap, 'virgin's milk', or a red sap, 'dragon's blood'. Soups, particularly onion, fish, cheese, mushroom, lentil. Also bird's nest soup, made of seaweed stuck together with fish spawn.

Alcohol in all its forms has strong aphrodisiac properties, but only if taken in moderation. This includes spirits (brandy, whisky, rum), beers (ale, cider, stout), wine (champagne, hock, moselle, vermouth), and liqueurs (benedictine, absinth, chartreuse). Alcohol sweetened with sugar, once a popular restorative, was favoured by Louis XIV (d. 1715) to revive his flagging ardour.

Other tonic drinks were galenia, attributed to Galen (d. AD 201), made of crushed almonds, pine seeds, ginger, mixed with honey. Also hippocras, attributed to Hippocrates (d. 359 BC), a mulled wine spiced with crushed ginger, cinnamon, cloves, vanilla and sugar. Bitters, or decoctions made from bitter herbs, roots and other substances, were prescribed as a general tonic. Such were bitters of gentian, quinine and cusparia (the chief ingredient of angostura bitters).

Finally, many aphrodisiacs are derived from scatological substances, such as the bodily exudations of men and animals. Some of the most famous love philtres and love potions contain such materials. Among them were dried and powdered human flesh, powdered bones, especially of the human skull, animal horns and teeth, human and animal excrement, urine, blood, gall, secundines (after-birth), sweat, semen and menses.

Books

Belham, George, *The Virility Diet*, Corgi Books, London, 1967.
Davenport, John, *Aphrodisiacs and Anti-Aphrodisiacs*, London, 1869.
Douglas, Norman, *Venus in the Kitchen*, Heinemann, London, 1952.
Leyel, C. F., *Elixirs of Life*, London, 1948.
Lowenstein, J., *The Treatment of Impotence*, Hamish Hamilton, London, 1947.
Walton, A. H., *Love Recipes Old and New*, London, 1956.
Wedeck, H. E., *Dictionary of Aphrodisiacs*, Peter Owen, London, 1962.

AROMATHERAPY

A branch of pneumopathy* based on smell, since odour is believed to play a very important part in healing. Its study is the province of osphresiology (Gk. *osphresis*, 'smell') which deals with odours and olfactory reactions.

Aromatherapy is concerned more specifically with the effects of pleasant smells as found in flowers, fruit, spices, herbs, perfumes and aromatic substances. The natural fragrance arising from living plants, as well as the aromas from compounded ingredients are equally efficacious in aromatherapy, but each kind of odour has its particular virtue, and sets up its own kind of magnetic vibrations.

Scents, perfumes and essences are prepared in many ways. They may be made by bruising flower petals, leaves, twigs, roots and other ingredients that go into the making of the material required. The whole may be dried and ground into a powder or paste and blended with other aromatic substances. These may be used as spices in cooking to give flavour to food; or mixed with oils for massaging the body or rubbing into the hands; or used in the preparation of soaps, cosmetics, unguents, pastilles and suppositories.

They can also be moulded into incense sticks, or sprinkled on the thurible or temple brazier, or even the domestic hearth. Burning incense helps to create a devotional frame of mind, but occultists warn against its use without a precise knowledge of the ingredients it contains and the purpose for which it was made. Some incense sticks, especially those made for use in certain Eastern cults, have hallucinogenic properties, which give rise to fantasies of sight and sound, and cause bad dreams. Some fumes produce a soothing drowsiness, as did the sleep-inducing gums and laurel leaves of the oracles. They can also inspire the prophetic mood and promote clairvoyance.

The therapeutic value of aromas was widely studied in ancient times, but the knowledge is now largely lost. It was believed that the sense of smell affords a direct channel to the etheric body and through it to the interior psyche. Michel de Montaigne (d. 1592) suggested that physicians might make greater use of perfumes since their effect on human mood and physical condition is beyond dispute. Apart from flowers (*see* floritherapy) the fragrance of fruit is also said to have healing virtues, apples, oranges and lemons being the most frequently prescribed. In the past those entering a diseased house or passing through a crowd, used to hold a 'scent apple' to their nose as a safeguard against infection.

A wide variety of crushed herbs, tree bark, spices of different kinds were inhaled for sundry ailments. After the introduction of tobacco into Europe, sniffing tobacco was held to be efficacious against the plague. Snuffs in general are aromatic, as well as being nasal irritants. It is to be noted that unpleasant and strong odours were also regarded as having therapeutic value, though this more properly forms the subject of pneumopathy.

The most elaborate class of substances used in aromatherapy are undoubtedly the manufactured perfumes. Plato (d. 347 BC) in his *Republic* puts perfumes on the same level as spiritual pleasures, a view followed later by Thomas More (d. 1535) in his *Utopia*. But this applied only to certain kinds of perfume, which experience has shown to be conducive to sublime religious moods and elevated thoughts.

At the other end of the scale, scents and sweet-smelling lotions and creams are part of every woman's repertory for luring the opposite sex. Certain perfumes provoke strong erotic reactions. They have an obscure but quite perceptible effect on the erection centres, and are as effective as any aphrodisiac in stimulating the sexual appetite of the male.

All the sophisticated civilizations of the ancient world knew the secrets of aromatherapy, and a vast assortment of aromatic substances was applied to the body to emit health-giving odours and create a pleasing atmosphere. Egypt, it seems, led the field in the manufacture of the finest perfumes. The scent of the incenses, spices and balms used in the pharaonic tombs has survived to this day after two, three, and even four thousand years.

The choicest among these was *merhu*, which the Greeks called *khyphi* (or chypre), a product famous throughout the ancient world. From its Egyptian name comes the Hebrew *mor*, from which we get such words as myrrh (an aromatic gum), myrtle (with its fragrant flowers), myrobalan (a sweet balsam), myristica (the nutmeg), myrica (the tamarisk plant) and many others. There were said to be several varieties of khyphi, which contained not only pleasant ingredients like myrrh, frankincense, mace, aloes, cuscus (an aromatic rush), galangal (of the ginger family), cinnamon, cloves and nard, but also camel urine, extract of civet, and an unknown ingredient called tchet oil, described as 'semen of the gods'.

The Jews followed the Egyptian fashion. It has been said that all the great seduction scenes in the Bible were enacted in an aura of perfume. Ruth came anointed with perfume to Boaz (Ruth 3:3). Judith anointed herself with rich perfume to captivate Holophernes (Judith 10:3). Esther rubbed herself with myrrh and sweet oils for a period of twelve months (Esth. 2:12) before she went to Ahasuerus. The Song of Solomon is 'saturated with perfume'.

The Greeks were no less sensitive to the subtle role of perfumes, both in the chamber of healing and in the chamber of love. Hippocrates (d. 359 BC) recommended introducing myrrh and other aromatic substances into the vagina to increase sexual excitement in both men and women. Two great centres of the perfume industry in ancient Greece were Corinth, near Athens, and Paphos in Cyprus.

In Roman times spices and aromatics were imported from as far afield as Persia and India, and the traffic annually depleted the Roman treasury of millions. A perfume called seplasium, named after Seplasia, the scent market of Capua, was almost as famous as chypre. Roman aristocrats maintained private perfumers with fully equipped laboratories in their own houses, and many perfumes were named after favourite mistresses: nicerotiana after Nicerotas, foliatum after Folia. The general populace bought their requirements from the myropola and aromatarii, or perfumers.

The Roman aromatic arts persisted into the Middle Ages and were imported from Italy into France. The Marquise de Pompadour (d. 1764) spent more than half a million livres annually on perfumes; and the Comtesse du Barry (d. 1793) took great care to perfume her genitals to please Louis XV. Because of the almost irresistible lure of perfume and its strong sexual and 'sinful' associations, its use was often condemned by the church as a form of sorcery. It is of interest to note that the modern apothecary, or pharmacist, is a direct descendant of the medieval specialists in perfume.

Modern experts claim to have recovered some of the secrets of this ancient art. The magician Aleister Crowley (d. 1947), for instance, claimed to make perfumes each with its own peculiar potency: to give nightmares, cause the bowels to loosen, attract the opposite sex, trigger orgasm, produce drowsiness and even kill.

The influence of scents and smells is almost always present around us. All things have their aroma. According to medieval writings, angels are delicately perfumed; devils come and go in a smell of sulphur. Saints and sinners give off distinctive odours, which form part of their aura. Sensitive people are reputedly able to distinguish good individuals from bad by the smell-aura surrounding them, and in the case of evil-doers can even tell the nature of their sin, whether adultery, theft, murder or covetousness.

In general, the character and disposition of a person can be determined by the perfume he likes. Men are said to be more sensitive to agreeable odours, and women to noxious ones. Similarly one's mood and temper can be altered by exposing one to the right perfume, so that a frivolous and irreverent mood can be changed to a meditative and prayerful one. Thus: ambergris creates a mood of eroticism; cloves arouse suspicion and slander; bergamot induces meditation and piety; musk, sensuality; eau-de-cologne, purity; patchouli, depraved thoughts (*see also* floritherapy).

Books

Bedichek, Roy, *The Sense of Smell*, Michael Joseph, London, 1960.
Bloch, Iwan, *Odoratus Sexualis: A Study of Sexual Scents and Erotic Perfumes*, Panurge Press, New York, 1934.
Claremont, Lewis de, *Legends of Incense, Herb and Oil Magic*, New York, 1938.
France, Hector, *Musk, Hashish and Blood*, Walpole Press, London, 1900.
McCord, C. P. and Witheridge, W. N., *Odours, Physiology and Control*, New York, 1949.
Macht, D. I., *The Holy Incense*, Baltimore, 1938.
McKenzie, D., *Aromatics and the Soul*, Heinemann, London, 1923.
Moncrieff, R. W., *Odour Preferences*, Leonard Hill, London, 1966.
Piesse, G. W. S., *The Art of Perfumery*, 4th edn, Philadelphia, 1880.
Redgrove, H. S., *Scent and All About It*, Heinemann, London, 1928.
Tardif, E., *Odours and Perfumes*, New York, 1919.
Thompson, C. J. S., *The Mystery and Lure of Perfume*, John Lane, London, 1926.

ARS MORIENDI

The 'art of dying', a traditional body of belief and practice connected with the last moments of a person on his death-bed. The art was developed by the ancient civilizations of Egypt, Babylonia, Greece, Rome, India, China, Tibet and others, and formed the basis of their dying, death, burial, mourning and post-mortem canons.

Fundamentally all rites pertaining to the *ars moriendi* are separation rites, based on the belief that the dead need help to be liberated from their terrestrial frame, from loved ones and earthly associations, and that provision must be made for the smooth passage of the soul to the next world. It was primarily an aid to overcoming the terrors of a final transition, from this world to an unknown one.

Death is hedged in by fears. There is the fear of the actual physical pain of dying, for oneself as well as for those one loves; the fear of losing what has been acquired on earth as a result of hard work, inheritance and good fortune; the fear of losing wisdom, health and sensual delights; the fear of continuing in poverty, or carrying on disease and disablement; the fear of punishment for evil done on earth; the fear of the unknown, of the prospect of entering upon a new pilgrimage or entering a new kind of life with a new set of values; the fear of extinction.

The *ars moriendi* underlies most initiation ceremonies, and is the background of most religions. It is found embodied in the Egyptian *Book of the Dead*, in the Orphic *Descent into Hades*, in the Tibetan *Bardo Thodol*, in Hindu texts like the *Garuda Purana*. It formed a central part of the Greek mysteries, which gave one an astral experience of death: in his *Metamorphosis* Apuleius (d. AD 170) says, 'I drew near the confines of death; I trod the threshold of the goddess of death; I was borne through all the elements; and I returned to earth.' The medieval handbook *De Arte Moriendi* epitomizes the Christian idea of the dying moments.

Certain religions like the Tibetan assume a great responsibility for those who are passing away, and by chants and hymns address a flow of exhortations to the dying during the transition period. Whether it is desirable for a living person to instruct the soul on the point of passing over or presume to guide it with specific directions along its journey to the next world, and to undertake to launch it successfully in its new life, is questionable. It is generally felt that such practice is definitely injurious, being a form of 'post-mortem suggestion' that might have harmful consequences. It is far better to pray direct to the divine power that is in charge 'over there', and leave the transition in the hands of the guardian entities. A true *ars moriendi* should be a religious therapeutic for the last moments, consoling the dying and fortifying his spirit by prayers. Among Roman Catholics the last rites include the sacrament of extreme unction, when the eyes, ears, nostrils, lips, hands and feet of the dying person are anointed, and a prayer offered that God in His own most tender mercy may pardon whatever offences he has committed.

To the mystic, life itself is essentially an education in the art of dying, and it is expedient that man should constantly keep before him the fact that he is mortal and will one day have to face death. Herodotus (d. 425 BC) who visited Egypt in the fifth century BC describes how during the Egyptian banquets a model of a mummy, or a skeleton painted red, used to be taken around the festive hall to remind the revellers of their ultimate fate: 'As you drink and feast, remember that you too will die and be as one of these.' Such a *memento mori*, 'reminder of death', was presented in different guises all over the world on festive occasions. A victorious Roman general at the height of his fame, when being taken on his triumph through the city, had a slave standing beside him in his chariot who whispered at intervals into his ear, reminding him that his glory would pass and that he was only mortal. The death dance of the Middle Ages, enacted by a 'skeleton' in fluttering shrouds, was a corresponding 'mummy at the feast', a similar reminder of the end of life.

The philosopher believes that one should give considerable thought to an understanding of what death is about, so that at the moment of death it might be faced calmly and stoically, if possible transcending bodily suffering and infirmity, without recourse to stupefying drugs. It has been the purpose of many religious doctrines to teach that the body is a tomb, as the Orphics had it, or a chrysalis according to the Chinese, and that death is a release of the spirit from a heavy encumbrance. The sufis taught that life was a night spent at a caravanserai, a halt on the road home, and that death was the next morning, the beginning of the next stage in the soul's journey.

Christian mystics speak of life as an episode, an incident, leading to a glorious destination. Life on earth is a preparation for another life, infinitely more real than this. Human existence is a divine privilege and death a necessary experience in the understanding of our destiny. Bodies are given us to afford us a chance to acquire knowledge on the material plane, to perfect our souls by self-sacrifice, to temper the emotions by love and patience. To accept the fact of death is to accept life here as a phase in a broader process of 'becoming', and to know that the human situation, whatever its limitations, can be transcended.

Books

Birrell, F. F. L. and Lucas, F. L., *The Art of Dying: an Anthology,* Hogarth Press, London, 1930.
Budge, E. A. Wallis, *The Book of the Dead*, Routledge & Kegan Paul, London, 1950.
Evans-Wentz, W. Y., *The Tibetan Book of the Dead*, Oxford University Press, 1951.
Kubler-Ross, Elisabeth, *On Death and Dying,* Tavistock Publications, London, 1970.
O'Connor, Mary, *The Art of Dying Well: the Development of the Ars Moriendi*, AMS Press, New York, 1966.
Raglan, Lord, *Death and Rebirth*, London, 1934.

ARTIFICIAL GENERATION

The fertilization and development of a new living entity by artificial means. Although it has been practised for ages in stock-breeding and agriculture, the term is used more specifically for techniques applied to human beings. It deals with artificial insemination and artificial fertilization, usually because of the sterility of either partner, or the malfunctioning of the sexual apparatus; and with the development of the foetus outside the natural environment of the womb. Because this involves growth outside the womb, the more advanced forms of artificial generation are known as ectogenesis (Gk. *ektos*, 'outside'), resulting in the so-called test-tube baby. Such growth in an artificial laboratory environment is said to be growth *in vitro* (Lat. 'in glass'), as distinguished from natural growth *in vivo* (Lat. 'in the living' womb).

The consecutive stages in all forms of generation involve the following factors: (a) *sperm*, which may be taken from the husband, or from a donor, either of whom may be living or dead at the time the generative process is started; (b) *ovum*, which may be taken from the wife, or from a non-wife, either of whom may be living or dead at the time the process begins; (c) *insemination*, or the depositing of sperm to meet the ovum, which may be by intercourse with the woman, or by syringe; (d) *fertilization*, or conception, the union of sperm and ovum, which may be in the womb of the woman, or in a dish in the laboratory; (e) *impregnation*, or the implanting of the fertilized egg in the natural womb, or in a plastic or other artificial womb in the laboratory; (f) *development*, which is a continuation of the process in (e) above, until the organism grows to full maturity.

If the sperm used belongs to the husband the operation is known as AIH (artificial insemination by husband); if it belongs to a male who is not the husband it is called AID (artificial insemination by donor). The sperm may be used immediately after the sample is given, or it can be stored till required. There are commercial sperm banks in the USA which store the sperm of eligible young men whose family histories have been ascertained and whose health is checked by clinical tests. Sometimes a husband decides to store his sperm as a safeguard before an operation for vasectomy, so that if he should later decide to have a child his sperm could be retrieved and used.

Sperm storage is now a standard process. The man retires to a small laboratory cubicle with an armchair and some pornographic magazines, masturbates and deposits the sperm in a dish or tube. The sperm is diluted with a glycerol preservative and frozen. In this frozen state human sperm can be stored for years at the temperature of liquid nitrogen, $-196°C$.

Next comes the fertilization of the ovum. By means of a syringe the sperm is deposited near the cervix at the time of the woman's ovulation. Scientists envisage the day when there will be banks of deep-frozen sperm and ova (ova can also be removed and stored in the same way) for free use on demand by anyone who needs it. A woman could be impregnated with a fertilized organism created from defrozen egg and sperm of donors long dead.

Scientists have had only partial success in the creation of test-tube babies. The technique of making one woman's egg grow in another woman's womb involves the following: (a) the woman (wife) is treated with gonadotropin, a pituitary hormone which acts on her sex glands, causing the ovary to produce several ova simultaneously. (b) Then comes the investigation known as laparoscopy, in which a gas is introduced into the abdomen to separate the organs, for purposes of identification. (c) Under general anaesthesia a minor surgical operation is performed and the ova removed from the ovary. (d) In a specially developed medium the wife's ova and the husband's sperm are separately induced to continue the process of maturing exactly as in the natural environment within the body. (e) At the same time the hormone interactions are artificially induced in the other woman (the non-wife) to simulate conditions of a woman who is one week into pregnancy. (f) Egg and sperm are then brought together in a dish for fertilization, and after two or three days the blastocyst or fertilized egg is introduced into the womb of the non-wife. (g) If the blastocyst attaches (implants) itself onto the wall of the uterus, the non-wife becomes pregnant and can bear the child.

So far scientists have been able to grow an embryo *in vitro* up to the blastocyst stage (up to about seven days). But they have not succeeded in implanting the week-old blastocyst in a woman's womb for further development. The reason for this is not clearly understood, but is thought to be due to the difficulty of timing the ovulation cycle of the recipient. Her hormone balance must correspond exactly with that of a pregnant woman carrying a blastocyst at that stage of development, otherwise it will not attach itself to her uterine wall.

Scientists hope they will eventually overcome this hurdle. Not only do they expect to be able to cause a blastocyst fertilized outside the womb to grow normally thereafter in another womb, but also to grow it outside the body of a woman, *in vitro* in the laboratory, to full maturity.

The idea of ectogenesis was discussed by many early writers from the time of Aristotle (d. 322 BC), largely based on the belief in spontaneous generation. But it was only in recent times that it began to be considered a scientific possibility. It was first predicted by the English biologist J. B. S. Haldane (d. 1964) in his *Daedalus* in 1924, and the theme was further developed by his friend Aldous Huxley in his *Brave New World* (1932).

An Italian surgeon Daniele Petrucci claimed to have been the first to fertilize human ova with human sperm in a plastic womb. Nutrition was provided by plasma taken from a number of pregnant women, and the embryo allegedly grew for two months. Other investigators, however, were unable to duplicate his experiments and many scientists are sceptical about them.

Experiments in artificial generation have, of course, been successfully performed with animals. As long ago as 1890 Walter Heape of Cambridge University transferred a fertilized egg from a female rabbit to a female hare, from which young were born.

Since then the process has been successfully carried out with other animals. Techniques have been evolved for transferring the fertilized eggs of large farm animals into small temporary foster animals (or even storing them in a vacuum flask), and shipping these carriers to another part of the world where the eggs are transferred to an animal of the original breed for normal development till birth.

For example, by administering the appropriate drugs to a cow, super-ovulation or overproduction of ripened eggs can be induced, and by artificial insemination 100 or more eggs can be fertilized. But before the rudimentary embryos can attach themselves to the wall of the womb they are flushed out and implanted into the uteri of 100 rabbits. These rabbits are then transported anywhere in the world for implantation of the eggs into 100 cows. Fertilization of eggs *in vitro* would make the cost of production and transport even cheaper.

There are apparently still further possibilities in artificial generation. Scientists are now considering the prospect of what is called cloning, and also of producing progeny from either sex.

As every cell of the body (and not the reproductive cell alone) contains the entire genetic code of the individual, it might be possible to create new individuals (clones) from cells taken from any part of the body. A clone (Gk. *klōn*, 'twig') is one of a number of organisms produced asexually from a single ancestor by the normal process of cell division. The products are genetically identical individuals. A clone is a true replica of its single parent, all the clones being derived from the same adult cell. As plants are propagated by grafting a twig on to a tree, so human beings could be cloned by similar 'cuttings' or 'vegetable breeding'.

Biologists have already been able to produce clones of frogs. A cell is taken from a frog embryo and its nucleus injected into an unfertilized egg, which has been previously emptied of its nucleus. From this, adult animals are obtained. The cloning of animals like prize bulls or racehorses, or of animals with superior intelligence for replacing human labour, or even of human beings with exceptional qualities, has not yet been attempted but is within the bounds of possibility.

One-parent progeny is another likely candidate for scientific experiment in the future. The parent may be either male or female. Parthenogenesis (Gk. *parthenos*, 'girl') or 'virgin birth', involves artificially stimulating the ovum extracted from a girl, so that it develops into a complete organism, without normal fertilization by male sperm. The female is thus the only parent of parthenogenetic progeny. Parthenogenetic reproduction has been successfully carried out on rabbits.

Androgenesis (Gk. *andros*, 'man') involves the removal of the nuclear material of the ovum and the introduction in its place of a spermatozoon, which provides the genetic material. The cell thus altered begins to divide until it develops into a complete organism. Here, the male is the only parent of androgenetic progeny.

Several ethical, legal and social questions arise in any consideration of artificial generation. Artificial insemination may mean that the father does not know the woman he has impregnated, or who his offspring is. Similarly the woman does not know the man who has impregnated her, nor in some cases the identity of her offspring, who may be born in the womb of another woman. The donor is still further removed from all the vital consequences of his masturbatory act. Does the insemination of a woman by the sperm of a man who is not her husband constitute a form of adultery, even if it has the consent of the husband? Does the incapacity of a couple for generation by normal means suggest that they might be unfitted by nature to propagate their kind? Is it right to use artificial methods of reproduction in such cases and thus perpetuate possible dysgenic* traits in future generations? In view of the growing overpopulation of the world, should the infertile couple not adopt rather than undertake such methods of having a child? In any event, how can we tell whether the artificial transfer of sperm and ovum and the artificial fertilization of the ovum will not result in a defective child being produced?

Will not the artificial generation of human beings lead to the dehumanization of the procreative process, and make a mockery of marriage, and of human and social relationships? How will the child cope with the thought of having been born in such a manner, contrary to the methods imposed by nature and sanctioned by religion, and of being alienated like a monstrosity from the normal processes that have engendered all the rest of the human family?

Books

CIBA Foundation, *Law and the Ethics of AID and Embryo Transfer*, Elsevier, Amsterdam, 1973.

De Ropp, Robert, *The New Prometheans: Creative and Destructive Forces in Modern Science*, Jonathan Cape, London, 1972.

Etzioni, Amitai, *Genetic Fix*, Macmillan, London, 1973.

Fuller, Watson (ed.), *The Social Impact of Modern Biology*, Routledge & Kegan Paul, London, 1971.

Hamilton, Michael (ed.), *The New Genetics and the Future of Man*, Eerdmans, Grand Rapids, Michigan, 1972.

Harrington, Alan, *The Immortalist*, Panther Books, London, 1973.

Jones, Alun and Bodmer, Walter, *Our Future Inheritance: Choice or Chance?*, Oxford University Press, London, 1974.

Leach, Gerald, *The Biocrats*, Jonathan Cape, London, 1970.

Ramsey, Paul, *Fabricated Man: the Ethics of Genetic Control*, Yale University Press, 1970.

Rosenfeld, Albert, *The Second Genesis*, Arena Books, New York, 1972.

Taylor, G. Rattray, *The Biological Time-Bomb*, Thames & Hudson, London, 1969.

ART THERAPY

Through the medium of drawing, painting and, less commonly, sculpture and modelling, art therapy is sometimes treated as a branch of occupational therapy*. Here, the patient is not given any special lessons in technique, but just instructed on how to use his material, and he then proceeds to draw or paint, without guidance as to subject or method.

The work thus spontaneously produced by the mentally ill differs from the work of the professional artist, since intellectual and technical excellence and the intrusion of the conscious mind impede art therapy, which is why it is not successful with the trained artist.

To be effective the patient must allow himself to drift into a kind of automatism, or free association with pen and brush, so that material from the unconscious has a chance to rise to the surface. Art in these unrehearsed conditions reveals symptoms extremely helpful in psychodiagnosis. It enables the therapist to analyse and interpret the patient's work, trace the sources of the trouble, and suggest a course of treatment, which might even be a continuation of the artistic work.

This type of therapy is believed to have great curative value. As a form of self-expression it fulfils a deep inner urge, providing a means for the release of the creative faculty. Material from the unconscious is brought out in symbolic form, colour and shape. By establishing contact with the unknown side of himself the patient finds an outlet for his repressed thoughts, wishes and fears. He exteriorizes the sources of conflict within himself and thus starts a healing process, becoming his own therapist. As he reconciles the inner and the outer, the unknown and the familiar, a process of integration, or curative reconciliation, takes place.

Neurotic art is a kind of objectified and projected dream, a script of the psyche, a page from the diary of the inner life. What is depicted in spontaneous art comes from deep within, a fact often recognized by patients, who are reluctant to show their work to anyone since they feel they are giving away some personal secret. Like music therapy, art therapy provides an outlet for the impulsive side of the mind, and reinforces the imaginative faculty. It is, therefore, not usually recommended for schizophrenia*.

The paintings of mental patients frequently resemble those of children and primitives. They are a projection of untrammelled fantasy. Often they take on curiously symbolic forms, so that abstract themes, geometrical

24

designs, arabesques and mandalas are quite common among psychotics. The strange association between neurotic art and modern painting is often very startling. Modern artists who reject form and realism produce work that is very like neurotic art: non-representational, dissonant, fragmented. It seems that where the art of the psychotic reflects his own illness, the work of the modern artist reflects the illness of society.

Art critics visiting exhibitions of the mentally ill are often perplexed and disturbed by what they see. As one critic queried, 'Are all these people artists, or are all modern artists crazy?' Others object to such exhibitions, since they upset one's ideas of art, of madness, of anthropology, and of philosophy (Lyddiatt, 1970, p. 130).

Books

Kellog, Rhoda, *What Children Scribble and Why*, N.-P. Publications, California, 1955.

Kris, E., *Psychoanalytic Explorations in Art*, International Universities Press, New York, 1952.

Lyddiatt, E. M., *Spontaneous Painting and Modelling: a Practical Approach in Therapy*, Constable, London, 1970.

Meares, Ainslie, *The Door of Serenity: a Study in the Therapeutic Uses of Symbolic Painting*, Faber & Faber, London, 1965.

Naumberg, Margaret, *Schizophrenic Art: Its Meaning in Psychotherapy,* Grune & Stratton, New York, 1950.

Naumberg, Margaret, *Psychoneurotic Art: Its Function in Psychotherapy*, Grune & Stratton, New York, 1953.

Phillips, W. *et al.*, *Art and Psychoanalysis,* New York, 1957.

Plokker, J. H., *Artistic Self-Expression in Mental Disease*, Skilton, London, 1964.

Westman, H., *The Springs of Creativity*, Atheneum, New York, 1961.

ASYLUMS

Asylums or mental hospitals have generally had a bad record through the ages. In ancient and medieval times the insane were regarded as being possessed by demons, and were flogged in an effort to drive the invaders out. Even so eminent a humanist as Sir Thomas More (d. 1535) advocated the whipping of lunatics from time to time.

Towards the end of the sixteenth century Bedlam (Bethlem Hospital, London) was reported to be too loathsome for any man to enter. In the seventeenth century the diarist John Evelyn (d. 1706) found no improvement. In the eighteenth century the pictures of William Hogarth (d. 1764) show it no better. In Germany in the same century patients used to be lowered into a snake-pit to drive them through fits of terror back to sanity. In England at the suggestion of Erasmus Darwin (d. 1802), grandfather of Charles Darwin, the whirling bed and gyrating chair were installed in some mental hospitals. Patients were rapidly rotated in these contraptions until the blood came out of their mouth, nose and ears.

The French physician Philippe Pinel (d. 1826) was the first to break through this benighted attitude and to introduce radical reforms to relieve the plight of the insane. But despite several improvements made in asylum care by him and others, the situation of patients has only marginally been mitigated in the contemporary scene. Thomas Szasz draws parallels between institutional psychiatry and the Spanish Inquisition. Gregory Zilboorg says that the notorious witch manual *Malleus Maleficarum* (1486) could, with slight emendations and with the substitution of 'patient' for 'witch', serve as a modern textbook of descriptive clinical psychiatry. Albert Deutsch, speaking of the conditions in some of the mental hospitals in the early 1940s, even in the wealthier states of the USA, says that the scenes in some of the wards rivalled the horrors of the Nazi concentration camps.

The treatment 'meted out' to the insane has all the marks of punishment somewhat reminiscent of the snake-pits of old. Like the medieval cure of possession by half-suffocating and half-drowning the victim, the patient today is 'brought to his senses' by subjecting him to the distressing procedures of insulin coma, or by sending powerful electric currents through his body to produce epileptic-like convulsions.

Most commonly the hapless sufferer is given massive injections of extreme potency that virtually paralyse most of his mental functions. The 'armamentarium' of modern psychiatrists (the term is their own) includes a gun specifically designed to fire a drug-filled syringe at psychotic patients.

Even worse than the pharmacological assault is the physical violence of brain surgery such as leucotomy and lobotomy, for schizophrenia and manic depression, when the nerve connections in the prefrontal lobes of the brain are severed. This operation was introduced in 1935 by the Portuguese neurologist Egas Moniz (d. 1958) who in 1947 received the Nobel Prize for his work.

Recent psychosurgery has added further refinements such as hemispherectomy, gyrectomy, amygdalotomy, thalamotomy and cordotomy, which sever the nerves of the brain and spinal cord. The result is to convert a troublesome patient into a docile vegetable who ceases to bother the hospital doctors and staff, and also ceases thereafter to participate in his own existence. This, say the critics, is the practical application of the satirical principle: 'If your head aches, cut it off.' Some of these methods have now been discontinued, or are in disrepute, but other no less barbarous methods of mind control are being tried.

Besides the specific forms of treatment, the general milieu of the mental hospital still leaves much to be desired. The denizens form part of a lost world. The stigma of having a relation in an asylum tends to make people forget about them. Many families are only too glad to abandon their care to the obscurity of a mental institution.

It has been said that mental hospitals often perpetuate mental illness. Conditions in many of them are more destructive of self-respect and self-identity than a jail. The wards are cluttered up with bored patients who sit around aimlessly, or wander through the corridors with nothing to do, nothing to interest or stimulate them. They become demoralized and helpless. They develop what has been called an institutional neurosis, the lethargy that binds patients to the place where they are maintained and makes them irrecoverably dependent. Few are capable of autonomous existence after even a few months' stay in such an institution. There is apathy, lack of initiative, and deterioration in personal habits. Through despair and frustration over their lot many retreat into depression.

Because of the low priority of mental care there are fewer mental hospitals than needed. They are consequently overcrowded. The number of trained personnel who wish to work in asylums is limited. Staff are put off by the conditions of work and the general aspect of degradation they see around them, hence there arises the problem of understaffing. The attendants form a tyrannical NCO cadre of their own. Physical violence by the staff is not unusual. Patients are forced into abject submission. Recalcitrants and unamenables are sometimes strait-jacketed and kept in solitary confinement for long periods. The whole environment tends to foster brutality in staff and insensitivity in nurses.

A very high proportion of mental patients are females: there are over thirty women to every male in English mental asylums. Complaints about persecution, physical ill treatment, sexual assault, are often ignored by doctors and staff, or 'interpreted' to the patient's detriment. Chesler points out that prostitution, rape, and sexual molestation of female children by adults are commonplace in American state asylums.

Psychiatrists who take up hospital work tend to adopt a doctrinaire approach to their patients. Perhaps a sense of their own inadequacy in the face of the immense and growing problems confronting them makes them fall too easily in line with the general situation they find. Because of indifference on the part of authorities to such institutions, experimental medication and surgery are practised with comparative freedom from interference and control.

It is well known that with good administration, an atmosphere of trust and freedom, the preservation of personal identity, and the provision of proper interests to keep patients employed, the need for sedative drugs and supervision is considerably reduced, and the general morale in asylums raised all round.

Books

Barton, Russell, *Institutional Neuroses*, John Wright, Bristol, 1959.

Caudill, W. A., *The Psychiatric Hospital as a Small Society*, Harvard University Press, 1958.

Chesler, P., *Women and Madness*, Allen Lane, London, 1974.

Deutsch, Albert, *The Mentally Ill in America: A History of their Care and Treatment from Colonial Times*, 2nd edn, Columbia University Press, 1952.

Freeman, H. L. and Farndale, J. (eds), *New Aspects of the Mental Health Service*, Pergamon Press, Oxford, 1967.

Freeman, W. and Watts, J. W., *Psychosurgery in the Treatment of Mental Disorders and Intractable Pain*, Thomas, Springfield, Illinois, 1950.

Goffman, Erving, *Asylums*, Penguin Books, Harmondsworth, 1970.

Jones, K. and Sidebotham, B., *Mental Hospitals at Work*, Routledge & Kegan Paul, London, 1962.

Stanton, A. M. *et al.*, *The Mental Hospitals*, Basic Books, New York, 1954.

Szasz, Thomas S., *The Manufacture of Madness*, Routledge & Kegan Paul, London, 1971.

Zilboorg, Gregory, *The Medical Man and the Witch During the Renaissance*, Johns Hopkins Press, Baltimore, 1935.

AVERSION THERAPY

A form of treatment that helps a person to overcome certain bad habits or to alter undesirable patterns of conduct. Its methods have grown out of behaviour therapy*, derived from the experimental techniques of Pavlov and Watson, with additional material from the learning theories of animal ethologists.

It is mainly applied to the cure of such problems as enuresis (bed-wetting), fetishism, homosexuality, transvestism, gambling, and addiction to alcohol, smoking and drugs. Aversion is usually established by associating the undesirable habit with an unpleasant or painful reaction, so as to condition the patient against the habit. It thus progressively reduces the inclination to resort to that line of activity.

Mild suffocation, the inducing of nausea (by administering apomorphine), electric shocks, the use of disagreeable chemical substances, are among the devices employed. Thus, a smoker might be given tablets containing ferrous sulphate and alum, which create a bad taste in the mouth whenever he smokes. Or the tongue is brushed over with a silver nitrate stick and then rolled around the palate. When a cigarette is smoked this again produces an unpleasant taste. But the latter can be dangerous as it may result in silver poisoning.

Similarly an alcoholic might be given emetics, or Antabuse (disulfiram), which causes vomiting, vertigo and headaches, leading eventually to a distaste for alcohol. Like other chemical aids in aversion therapy it has its dangers, since it occasionally produces impotence and peripheral neuritis.

Aversion therapy is a new name for an age-old method, used by parents and by society in general for weaning a recalcitrant from an undesirable trait. We find it codified in the injunction: 'Spare the rod and spoil the child', based on a Biblical text (Prov. 13:24). The corporal punishment of a disobedient child; the instilling of tribal taboos at initiation ceremonies; the disciplinary regulations imposed by schools and military establishments; disapproval by one's peers and colleagues; the arousal of one's sense of shame; the creation of guilt feelings; the threat of pain and punishment; the expression of public outrage at any tilting at established standards, are all time-tested forms of this therapy.

Books

Bancroft, J. H. J., *Aversion Therapy*, University of London, 1966.

Eysenck, H. J., *Behaviour Therapy and the Neuroses*, Pergamon Press, Oxford, 1960.

Franks, C. M., *Conditioning Techniques in Clinical Practice and Research*, Tavistock Publications, London, 1965.

Leitenberg, H. (ed.), *Handbook in Behavior Modification,* Appleton-Century-Crofts, New York, 1974.

Lovibond, S. H., *Conditioning and Enuresis*, Pergamon Press, Oxford, 1964.

Rachman, S. and Teasdale, J., *Aversion Therapy and Behaviour Disorders,* Routledge & Kegan Paul, London, 1969.

B

BEHAVIOUR THERAPY

Behaviour therapy is concerned principally with observable behaviour and its expression, control and alteration. It has a materialistic basis, ignoring such abstractions as mind, consciousness and introspection, and because it is chiefly experimental and disdains subjective impressions, claims to be scientific and objective.

Its earliest exponent was Ivan Pavlov (d. 1936) the Russian physiologist, whose work on the salivary reflexes of dogs led to his theory of the conditioned reflex. Pavlovian reflexology is the foundation of behaviourist theory. The American apostles of behaviourism are John Broadus Watson (d. 1958) and Burrhus F. Skinner (b. 1904).

Since it is based on experimental psychology, behaviourism is largely confined to laboratory methods, aimed at arriving at a workable table of responses and adaptations to given stimuli. Its findings were established after studies with monkeys, dogs, rats, pigeons, geese and worms. It has had great success in animal training.

Basically two broad streams of conditioning are used. In classical or Pavlovian conditioning, the subject is passive, and the experimenter does things to the animal, and makes it respond. In operant or instrumental conditioning, the animal has to be active, press buttons, pull levers and depress keys, in order to modify the situation and obtain rewards or avoid unpleasant consequences (the older carrot and stick). In the process the animal may be subjected to electric shocks, starvation, mutilation and sleeplessness.

Behaviour therapy is said to be very successful with children, for the manipulation of mood, temperament and action, by a system of rewards and punishments, along with programmed instruction. Much stress is laid on early programming, both of animals and children, because of the tenacity and irreversibility of imprinting, or the impressions received during the sensitive, critical periods of life, especially very early life.

Essentially, then, it is a method of total conditioning, which includes deconditioning, counterconditioning, reconditioning, desensitization and other devices. The cause of delinquent, antisocial, undesirable behaviour, is believed to be due to lack of conditioning, to deficient conditioning, to inadequate conditioning, or malconditioning. It is claimed as practical, quick and effective. Conditioning procedures have had some success with phobias, sexual deviation, alcoholism and rehabilitation, as well as with neurotic symptoms, psychopathy, bad habits, unsocial or undesirable behaviour.

Deconditioning entails the unlearning and extinguishing of maladaptive early conditioning, often by a series of painful situations created each time the undesirable trait or behaviour pattern comes to the fore, in order to inhibit the original response. This is exemplified in aversion therapy*. Reconditioning

29

entails building up and reinforcing the conditioned responses of the kind considered desirable, usually by rewards each time the desired activity is manifested.

Desensitization is used in the treatment of physical, mental or emotional oversensitivity, as found in allergies, fears, phobias or traumas. The patient is made to relax, and is then very gradually re-exposed to the stimuli to which he is sensitive, until the anxiety decreases and disappears. Thus, a child afraid of noise is gradually exposed to sounds of increasing loudness, each sound being associated with a pleasant idea or situation. An asthmatic, sensitive to a particular allergen, will be injected with minute doses of that allergen, and the dose of the allergen gradually increased until a tolerance is built up.

Implosive or implosion therapy, also called flooding, is the opposite of desensitization, and is used in overcoming deep-seated avoidance responses. Here the patient is exposed to his particular phobic situations as vividly as possible without giving him a chance to escape, until he is unable to feel the fear any longer. 'Implosion' implies a bursting from within, and suggests the onslaught of the phobia and the eventual collapse of the fear symptoms.

In essence, behaviour therapy is mechanistic and deterministic, a technology rather than a psychology. It is concerned with outward manifestations, and does not seek to trace a condition to its source, or to deal with causes. It has been labelled 'muscle-twitch psychology', because it is concerned principally with S-R, or stimulus-and-response, and explains all mental operations in terms of muscular, glandular, neural and reactive reflexes. An eminent behaviourist has even suggested that thinking takes place in the vocal cords because they vibrate when people think. Behaviourist methods are highly suggestive of brainwashing and menticide*, and its techniques are in fact commonplace in totalitarian states both of the extreme left and the extreme right.

Books

Bandura, A., *Principles of Behavior Modification*, New York, 1969.
Eysenck, H. J. (ed.), *Experiments in Behaviour Therapy*, Pergamon Press, Oxford, 1964.
Franks, C. M., *Conditioning Techniques in Clinical Practice and Research*, Tavistock Publications, London, 1965.
Harlow, H. F. and Woolsey, C. N. (eds), *Biological and Biochemical Bases of Behavior*, University of Wisconsin Press, 1958.
Hull, C. L., *Principles of Behavior*, New York, 1943.
Meyer, V. and Chesser, E., *Behaviour Therapy in Clinical Psychiatry*, Allen Lane/The Penguin Press, London, 1970.
Paul, G. L., *Insight versus Desensitization in Psychotherapy*, Stanford University Press, 1966.
Skinner, B. F., *Science and Human Behavior*, New York, 1953.
Yates, A. J., *Behavior Therapy*, Wiley, New York, 1970.

BIOMAGNETIC THERAPY

A method of healing by what was earlier known as animal magnetism, the universally diffused energy that was thought to be localized in special concentration in all living things in the form of biomagnetism or bioflux. Life, activity, breathing, all create magnetic fields. It is now scientifically established that even protoplasm exhibits biomagnetic properties; living cells have north and south poles. In fact all animal species possess the properties of magnetism, polarity and vibration. It is suggested that the very air breathed out has north polar magnetism, after the south polar magnetism has been inhaled.

This biomagnetic energy is found in the human body as an invisible 'fluidum', which in certain circumstances becomes strongly charged. Soviet scientists experimenting on subjects with psychic gifts like ESP and PK, have found that such subjects can cause the electromagnetic fields around them to vibrate.

Certain people normally have an abundance of personal magnetism, and by the force of their emanations are able to exert their influence over others. In this sense we still speak of a person having a 'magnetic' personality. Strong personalities carry the fiery magnetism in their brain, breathe it from their lungs, shed it from their hands, and send it vibrating forth when they function in their special spheres. The king on his throne, the officiating priest, the great orator on the platform, all radiate biomagnetism in a high degree.

Some persons again, consciously or unconsciously, act as psychic sponges, drawing into themselves the strength of those around them, and so enervate and drain anyone with whom they come into contact (*see* psychic vampirism). Others, by their silent presence, give out soothing and harmonious impulses. Especially endowed individuals, formerly called 'magnetizers', were believed to draw out sickness from the sick and neutralize it, especially disorders of the nervous system, and through the nerves, other diseases as well.

It was further believed that the biomagnetic 'fluid' could be stored in the body, and augmented by breathing exercises. It could be communicated to others through the eyes, voice and hands. It could also be transferred by concentration and manual passes to inanimate objects, to render them talismanic. Such objects could then be worn close to the skin to pass their healing emanations into the system. A glass of water could be 'magnetized' with healing intent, and if this were drunk could effect a cure. Conversely, if magnetized with vicious intent it could poison and kill.

Belief in biomagnetism has its roots deep in the past. The Ebers Papyrus (*c.* 1630 BC) of ancient Egypt instructs the healer: 'Place thy hand upon the patient to calm the pain, and say that the pain shall depart from him.' Greek medical literature contains references to a similar faculty. Hippocrates (d. 359 BC) said: 'It hath oft appeared that I could draw from the afflicted parts of my patients, aches and impurities by laying my hands or moving them over the area concerned, as if my hands possessed some strange healing power.'

There have been a number of ardent supporters of the belief in such an emanative and curative energy. Paracelsus (d. 1541) held that the human body possessed the properties of a magnet. Robert Fludd (d. 1637) believed that epilepsy and hysteria could be cured by making hand-passes over the sufferer; also that sympathy and antipathy between two people depended on their magnetic radiations. Jean Baptiste van Helmont (d. 1644) propounded the theory of the *magnale magnum*, a magnetic force universally diffused which could be drawn down and directed by the operation of the will.

But the theory of a fluidic force within the body found its greatest prophet in Franz Anton Mesmer (d. 1815), who first named it 'animal magnetism', and after whom the treatment was known for a time as 'mesmerism', the true forerunner of hypnotism*. In order to treat the large number of patients who came to him, Mesmer built an oak tub which he filled with iron filings and bottles of magnetized water; from the tub bent iron rods projected outwards, which the patients, sitting around the tub, applied to the affected parts of their bodies.

Mesmer's pupil, Jacques de Chastenet, Marquis de Puységur (d. 1825), went a step further. He magnetized an elm tree by appropriate passes and hung cords from it, which patients held to receive the magnetic effluvium. Jean Philippe François Deleuze (d. 1835) equated animal magnetism with nerve-force, and first demonstrated the reality of post-hypnotic suggestion. Alexandre Bertrand (d. 1831) denied the existence of any magnetic fluid but established the genuineness of *somnambulisme*, or 'magnetic sleep' (i.e. deep hypnosis) and rapport, which he said were achieved by suggestion.

In England a well-known case of magnetic healing was that of Miss Harriet Martineau (d. 1876), a Birmingham author whose books on theology, philosophy, sociology and travel brought her immense fame. She became a chronic invalid in 1839 and had been treated without success by the best physicians. In 1844 a travelling magnetizer named Spencer Hall treated her for three days by magnetic passes, with astonishing success, so that she was able to eat and sleep comfortably for the first time in five years. Thereafter the treatment was continued by her maid. Her published account of her marvellous recovery lost her many friends.

Subsequently, John Elliotson (d. 1868) was dismissed from his post as professor of medicine at London University because of his attempts to introduce curative magnetism into medical practice. He founded a mesmeric hospital and pressed the claims of mesmerism for over a decade. James Esdaile (d. 1859), a Scottish surgeon, performed major operations on patients under hypnosis, without the aid of anaesthetics. Another Scotsman, James Braid (d. 1850), like Bertrand, rejected the idea of a magnetic fluid passing from hypnotist to subject, but found that suggestion alone could make a person go into a trance. It was he who coined the term 'hypnotism'.

The French physician Auguste Ambroise Liébeault (d. 1904) of Nancy, agreed with Braid. The so-called Nancy School which he founded was continued by his friend and disciple Hippolyte Bernheim (d. 1919), who hypnotized some 10,000 patients, and collected data on a massive scale. He concluded that most of our social and religious behaviour patterns are influenced by suggestion. It was while watching Bernheim at work that Freud learned of the existence of the unconscious mind. By this time the theory of animal magnetism had been almost completely abandoned, and hypnosis, based on suggestion, took its place. The whole field of modern depth psychology owes its rise to the studies of these early pioneers.

Also famous in the history of animal magnetism is the school of Salpêtrière, named after the hospital for the insane in Paris. Here it was that Philippe Pinel (d. 1826) took the insane out of their dungeons and gave them sunny rooms and pleasant grounds for exercise. His reforms were continued by his pupil Jean Esquirol (d. 1840). But it was Jean Charcot (d. 1893) of the same school who gave hypnotism a scientific status, with numerous experiments, including a series to ascertain the influence of magnets on hysterical patients. He considered hypnosis to be a pathological state, akin to hysteria. His most notable pupils were Pierre Janet (d. 1947), noted chiefly for his studies on hysteria, and Sigmund Freud (d. 1939), founder of psychoanalysis.

Books

Barnothy, Madeleine F. (ed.), *Biological Effects of Magnetic Fields*, Plenum Books, New York, 1964.

Binet, A. and Féré, C., *Animal Magnetism*, Kegan Paul, London, 1887.

De la Warr, George and Baker, Douglas, *Biomagnetism*, Delawarr Laboratories, Oxford, 1967.

Ellenberger, Henri, *The History of the Unconscious*, Allen Lane, London, 1970.

Halacy, Daniel S., *Radiation, Magnetism and Living Things*, Holiday House, New York, 1966.

Lee, E., *Animal Magnetism and Homoeopathy*, London, 1838.

Ostrander, S. and Schroeder, L., *PSI: Psychic Discoveries Behind the Iron Curtain*, Sphere Books, London, 1973.

Podmore, Frank, *From Mesmer to Christian Science*, Methuen, London, 1963.

Pressman, A. S. *Electromagnetic Fields and Life*, Plenum Press, New York, 1972.

Rochas, E. A. de, *Le Fluide des magnétiseurs*, Paris, 1891.

Thompson, Sylvanus, *Magnetism and Growth*, Frowde, London, 1902.

Walker, Benjamin, *Encyclopedia of Esoteric Man*, Routledge & Kegan Paul, London and Stein & Day, New York, 1977.

White, George Starr, *The Finer Forces of Life*, Health Research, Mokelumne Hill, California, 1969.

BIOTELEMETRY

Biotelemetry studies the living body by means of highly sensitive apparatus such as electrodes, microphones and photoelectric devices, which can measure and record the biosignals or physiological fluctuations taking place at any time. The study has made important contributions towards unravelling the many secret processes that occur in the human body, both during normal and xenophrenic* states, including sleep, dreams, drunkenness, trance, hypnosis, and so on. The suffix '-graph' stands for the apparatus; and '-gram' for the tape, paper or other record.

Pulse beats are registered by the sphygmograph; arterial blood pressure by the sphygmomanometer; heart beats by the cardiotachometer; electrical variations during heart contractions by the electrocardiograph (ECG); respiration by the pneumograph; respiratory volume or lung capacity by the spirograph; electrical activity during eye movements by the electro-oculograph (EOG); pupillary reflexes by the pupillograph; auditory acuity by the phonometer; hearing thresholds by the acoumeter or audiometer; involuntary movements of the larynx during thought by the laryngograph; lip movements during apparently silent reading by the labiograph; skin temperature by the thermistor; tremors of the body by the tromometer or tremograph, used for tracing the involuntary tremors of the hand during thought; muscular activity to determine freshness and fatigue, by the ergograph; changes in the muscle potential by the electromyograph (EMG). Psychogalvanic reflexes (PGR), also called galvanic skin response (GSR), or fluctuations in skin resistance, are registered by the GSR machine, which monitors by means of electrodes attached to the fingers the changes in the electrical conductivity of the skin, and the variations in the level of neural activity as they affect the amount of sweat on the fingertips. Volume variations in the blood vessels in different parts of the body are recorded by the plethysmograph, for example, for registering the changes in the size of the penis during dreams. Gastrointestinal motility is registered by the electrogastrograph. Perhaps the most interesting of the telemetrical devices is the electroencephalograph (EEG), which measures 'brain waves', or the electrical activity of the brain.

Early graphic records of physiological and psychological processes were obtained on the kymograph (Gk. *kyma*, 'wave'), a rotating drum usually covered with smoked paper on which the fluctuations were recorded. Today multiple machines are frequently used, with separate channels recording several items on one chart. For example, the polygraph, one version of which is popularly known as the lie-detector, may be a combination of the GSR machine, the sphygmomanometer, the pneumograph and other devices for recording reactions in different parts of the body. Some multiple machines are complicated electronic and computerized devices with as many as thirty amplifiers and monitoring systems with automatic data processing.

Among the more curious applications of biotelemetry have been the investigations, notably by Dr William Masters and Mrs Virginia Johnson, into the physiological responses of men and women during sexual activity. The wrists, temples, phallus, vagina and anus of the respective subjects are wired for the record and they are put through their paces either with volunteer partners or singly with artificial aids. For women, a plastic phallus is provided, which she can control for length, weight, stiffness, thickness, and rate and depth of thrust, according to vaginal development, mood or desire. The tensions of the internal tissues, the point at which lubrication commences, the various phases leading up to the climax, are automatically recorded on telemetric graphs or colour film.

In spite of the information gained, the degree of reliance that can be placed on biotelemetry, in gauging the psychological or even the physiological state of the person under examination, is open to question. Where emotional factors intrude a device cannot be regarded as infallible, since it may provide misleading information. Today lie-detectors are no longer regarded as dependable. 'Love technology' of the Masters and Johnson variety has only a marginal relationship to happiness in married life, which continues to deteriorate at an accelerated pace all over the western world, and not for want of sexual knowledge. Biotelemetric gadgets used in medicine have been known to give varying recordings. Certain states of mind, either of the scientist or his subject seem to throw the apparatus out of kilter.

This has also been noticed in experiments with people of strong extrasensory powers, and often occurs without their knowledge or intention. Research workers investigating psychic phenomena often report inexplicable interference with their apparatus and the failure of equipment at critical times. Thus, there have been repeated breakdowns in lighting during the filming of psychic surgery. It would appear that psychics and their activities can exert an uncanny and unaccountable effect on laboratory equipment. Cameras are put out of action; tape recordings and video systems become inoperative and useless; there is interference with gauss meters (for measuring increase and decrease in magnetic fields) and similar instruments. In some cases material is asported, only to reappear when the experiment is halted. Witnesses of psychic surgery report that samples of diseased organs taken for analysis have vanished without any possible explanation. Such psi-matter gaps, between psi-conditions and material apparatus cannot at present be accounted for.

Books

Brown, C. C. (ed.), *Methods in Psychophysiology*, Baltimore, 1967.
Carlson, Rick J. (ed.), *Frontiers of Science and Medicine*, Wildwood House, London, 1975.
Hammond, David, *The Search for Psychic Power*, Scientific Book Club, London, 1976.
Masters, W. and Johnson, V., *Human Sexual Response*, Little, Brown, Boston, 1966.
Payne, L. C., *An Introduction to Medical Automation*, Pitman, London, 1966.
Tomlinson, H., *The Divination of Disease*, Health Science Press, London, 1953.
Tromp, S. W., *Psychical Physics*, Elsevier, New York, 1949.
Venables, P. H. and Martin, I. (ed.), *Manual of Psychophysiological Methods*, Amsterdam, 1967.

BLEEDING

Bleeding, or causing the blood to flow from a living person, as an act of propitiation, sacrifice or healing. All forms of blood sacrifice from beheading to finger-lopping, imply bleeding, but the term is more specifically used for those forms not involving the loss of life or limb. In all parts of the world from Bengal to Peru bleeding has been used as a means of placating the deities so that they might send down rain, remove a blight, heal sickness or bestow the blessings of fertility.

In a secular context bleeding or blood-letting was mainly a therapeutic practice. It was believed that just as a blockage of the intestinal canal due to an excess of food could cause all manner of digestive disorders, so blockage of the blood vessels due to a plethora or excess of blood could block the veins and inflame the blood, causing all kinds of blood diseases. In order to relieve the excess, blood-letting was necessary.

This was done in a number of ways. The use of leeches was common from very early times wherever they were available. These blood-sucking worms were applied to various parts of the body until they became engorged with blood and dropped off on their own, each taking about half an ounce of blood with it. The easiest way was simply to make a small incision in the flesh, or rub the skin with pumice stone, or cut a vein. This latter was known as phlebotomy or venesection, both words meaning 'vein cutting'. Cupping* was another related device used for relieving congestion caused by excess of blood.

The history of bleeding goes back to earliest antiquity. The Egyptians were said to have got the idea from the hippopotamus, which has a habit of casting itself among the sharp rocks and stones near the shore of a river, and wounding itself to be relieved of the pressure of blood that accumulates in its system from time to time. The Greeks too were familiar with it, and it was supposed to have been popularized in Greek medicine by Erasistratus (d. 260 BC), grandson of Aristotle.

The practice, common throughout Europe, survived as a standard treatment till the end of the last century, and indeed in some places till our own day. In the Middle Ages there were special phlebotomy tables showing when the blood was to be let, in which part of the body and in what quantity. This was determined by such factors as the season of the year, the position of the planets and the time of day. It was used to calm down an overexcited patient, drive out sickness, fever and malaise, remove bad humours from the system, and purge any deleterious substances sheltering in the blood. Large amounts of blood, sometimes a litre at a time, were drawn off, either direct from the affected area or from the side of the body opposite the diseased area.

It is said that Frederick the Great (d. 1786) had his veins opened before battles to calm his nerves. George Washington (d. 1799) during his last illness was frequently administered the same treatment. Among his physicians was Benjamin Rush (d. 1813), one of the signatories to the Declaration of Independence, who was a staunch advocate of bleeding, and it is said that his reliance on this method dispatched Washington before his time. The celebrated Canadian physician Sir William Osler (d. 1919) continued to recommend blood-letting for pneumonia until the first decade of the present century. When Joseph Stalin (d. 1953) lay dying his physicians used every possible method to effect his recovery. While some physicians used the newest scientific gadgetry and administered the latest drugs, others were simultaneously applying leeches to the dictator's head and neck.

Bleeding is still used in certain diseases. For instance, where there is an excess of red blood cells the condition known as polycythaemia results, which is the opposite of anaemia. The blood sometimes becomes so thick that it cannot flow properly, and blood-letting becomes necessary. Again, in some kinds of heart failure, the load on the circulation may be relieved by blood-letting. Bleeding is also used in certain forms of rejuvenation* therapy.

Books

Brockbank, William, *Ancient Therapeutic Arts*, London, 1954.
Clements, H., *Magic, Myth and Medicine*, London, 1955.
Dawson, W. R., *Magician and Leech*, Methuen, London, 1929.
Gordon, B. L., *Medicine Throughout Antiquity*, Philadelphia, 1949.
L'Étang, Hugh, *The Pathology of Leadership*, Heinemann, London, 1969.
Smith, Anthony, *The Body*, Allen & Unwin, London, 1968.

BORBORIC THERAPY

(Gk. *borboros,* 'dirt, mire, mud'), or healing by the application or ingestion of dirt or filth, has been practised in all communities from earliest times. The ingredients used include mud and soil, chalk, decaying vegetable matter, mildew, moulds of all kinds, ferments of honey, broth, bread, but excluding substances discharged from the bodies of men and animals, like dung, saliva, urine, and semen, which forms the subject of scatotherapy*.

The eating of earth was particularly widespread in antiquity. The best variety was said to be obtained from the Aegean island of Lemnos, where it was found in the natural state in the shape of small round pellets, each tiny bole suitable for swallowing. It was known as *terra sigillata*, 'sealed earth', because the clay was believed to bear the sacred seal of the goddess Diana. This lemnian clay, held in wide esteem all over Western Europe, was included in the pharmacopoeia till 1848, as a specific for sore eyes, haemorrhage, excessive menstruation and the plague.

Various kinds of edible earth can still be bought in Java, India, Thailand, North Africa, Mexico and Central America. In the USA a certain William Windsor (*c.* 1880) founded a sect of earth-eaters who used to dig some four to five feet deep into the soil and eat the earth. They claimed that this was healthy and vitalizing (*see* geotherapy).

Filth-eating, as distinguished from mud-eating is often symptomatic of mental illness. What is known as *allotriophagy* (Gk. *allotrios*, 'strange'; *phagein*, 'to eat'), or swallowing and later vomiting up strange objects, appears to be a common feature of certain kinds of mental derangement, hysteria and 'possession', usually among adolescents. In allotriophagy unpleasant, injurious and even painful things are swallowed. They include dirt and dung, masses of stinking filth, repulsive fluids, crooked pins and nails, small bones, gravel, cinders, balls of hair, feathers, egg-shells, pieces of wood, parchment, fragments of cloth, wood shavings, bits of glass and porcelain.

Literally hundreds of allotriophagy cases are recorded in the annals of witchcraft, sorcery and madness in the sixteenth, seventeenth and eighteenth centuries. Among the numerous theories advanced to account for it, one medieval explanation held that this unnatural hunger was due to an invading spirit who demanded foul and unwholesome things to eat. (It has been found in our own times that worshippers possessed by the *loa*, or spirit of the Voodoo cult, bring up pins and pieces of sharp metal.) Modern explanations include: a hysterical impulse to ingest unpalatable or revolting objects: a desperate need to lacerate the insides for some hidden sin, the chief sin of adolescence being masturbation; an urge to commit suicide, for the same reason; or vitamin and mineral deficiency in diet, which creates an unhealthy appetite for nasty substances.

More specifically, dirt therapy is applied to the use of dirty and unpleasant substances for genuinely healing purposes. Anthropologists, when they first came across these remedies in the nineteenth century among tribal peoples, referred to them as 'sewage pharmacology' (German, *Dreckapotheke*, 'filth pharmacy'), but subsequent, more serious investigation, and the study of records on these methods of therapy as used by the peoples of antiquity, has shown that the 'filth' frequently worked wonders. Moulds were prescribed for internal troubles, chest complaints, eye diseases, open sores, and the casualties among those to whom such treatment was given were no higher than among the patients in modern hospitals.

The Egyptians recommended the lees of beer for digestive disorders, as well as for swellings, tumours and ulcers. Today their curative value has been confirmed, since lees are known to be rich in minerals and yeast. The Egyptians also ate mould-covered bread for diseases of the kidneys and bladder, and applied it externally to suppurating wounds. The efficacy of moulds in therapy is now a proven fact. Similarly cobwebs, which were applied to deep cuts, are now known to contain a substance that clots blood.

In Greek legend we find Nestor making a poultice of cheese, onion and meal, mixed with wine, for the wounds of Machaon. Many ancient peoples used the products from ferments of all kinds in treating open wounds and bruises. To this day Negroes on the coast of Guinea, Peruvians, tribal communities in India and Australasia universally use soil in their therapy. In many parts of Brazil peasants will put field-mould on cuts and wounds, and in rural Ukraine, Greece and Yugoslavia, country-folk smear the fungoid growth from mouldy bread over septic wounds.

Mud and moulds were employed all over Europe till the eighteenth century for both internal and external use. For some hundreds of years soldiers on the battlefield were applying mouldy bread to their wounds, until well into the nineteenth century. In England the moss on dead men's skulls was a standard ingredient in many salves and ointments, and was recommended by the most eminent physicians. Urine, dung, saliva and semen, the bones and flesh of animals, so called 'unicorn horn', feathers, egg-shells, toadstools, viper's blood, 'mummy powder', the scum found in ponds, mud from graveyards, were all made up into pastes, ointments or mixtures, to be rubbed on or swallowed by the ailing. In Europe till the early years of the present century, cow dung was often smeared on sores.

It is only within the last few decades that some of these healing properties of dirt have come to be scientifically recognized. All mud and soil are known to produce different kinds of antibiotic substances. In 1946, after examining thousands of soil cultures, Professor Selman A. Waksman discovered the antibiotic streptomycin, now used in the cure of tuberculosis. Dr Benjamin Duggar and his colleagues, having analysed some 30,000 soil specimens, discovered a type of soil near cemeteries that yielded the material from which the wonder-drug aureomycin was extracted.

Again, the waste products that result from fermentation and the metabolism of certain moulds are today known to inhibit the growth of bacteria. The use of moulds eventually came into its own as proper therapeutic practice after Alexander Fleming (d. 1955) discovered penicillin.

Books

Böttcher, Helmuth, *Wunderdrogen,* Cologne, 1959.
Bourke, J. G., *Scatologic Rites of All Nations,* Lowdermilk, Washington, DC, 1891.
Derrey, François, *The Earth is Alive,* Arlington, London, 1968.
Gordon, B. L., *Medicine Throughout Antiquity,* Philadelphia, 1949.
Thompson, C. J. S., 'Terra Sigillata, a Famous Medicament of Ancient Times', *Proc. of 17th International Congress of Medical Sciences,* London, 23, 1913, 433–44.
Thorwald, J., *Science and Secrets of Early Medicine,* Thames & Hudson, London, 1962.
Zilboorg, G., *The Medical Man and the Witch During the Renaissance,* Johns Hopkins Press, Baltimore, 1935.

C

CANCER

(Gk. *karkinos*, 'a crab'), a malignant growth resulting from the degeneration and mutation of the body cells, which causes them to multiply furiously and abnormally, invading adjacent tissue and so spreading in the form of secondary growths to other parts. The disease was so named by Hippocrates (d. 359 BC), because he thought of it as spreading out its claws in all directions like a crab. Cancer occurs both in plants and animals, but man is more prone to it than any other species.

No certain cure has been found for it yet. It strikes down the healthy, the young, the strong, without discrimination, and the chances of complete cure, though somewhat improved, are still slender. There are many varieties of the disease, and medical treatment that can alleviate one variety may be useless against another. Most cancers are non-infective, and a few are hereditary. In the past seventy years the incidence of cancer in civilized countries has risen more than six times. It is the disease civilized people dread most.

The ultimate cause of cancer (if there is a single cause) has not yet been established, but a number of factors are definitely known to contribute to it. Some forms arise from chronic irritation; some are due to glandular maladjustment; many are caused by carcinogenic (cancer-generating) substances, the list of which is constantly multiplying to include many ordinary household items. Certain cancers are caused direct by a virus, but there are some viruses that although not carcinogenic themselves, produce changes in the cell structure and render them vulnerable to substances which trigger off the cancer process. No one is immune to cancer, and we are all hosts to cancer cells.

The reproductive glands and organs are known to be closely connected with cancer, and it would appear that attempts to prolong the period of sexual activity beyond the 'normal' age tend to accelerate the chances of cancer attack. Prostatic cancer in men is slowed down by the administration of female sex hormones, and breast cancer in women regressed by giving male sex hormones. But whether these hormones can be supplied by sexual intercourse or whether excessive sex brings on cancer is a point debated by two schools of thought.

On the other hand, spirit-healer Harry Edwards (d. 1976) suggested the primary cause of cancer was psychosomatic, rather than a virus infection. John Pfeiffer quotes from a work by an early nineteenth-century

French physician entitled *Medicine of the Passions*, in which the latter states that certain cancers are caused by 'jealousy, hatred and chagrin'. Other researchers concur that cancer in certain areas of the body indicates the emotional origin of the disease. Thus, breast cancer is due to continued frustration of sexual desire, which upsets the balance of the mammary glands, causing them to become rebellious, intensely unhappy and finally 'insane'. As eminent cancer specialist, Sir Heneage Ogilvie, said, 'A happy man never gets cancer' (Edwards, 1965, p. 80). According to the findings of Dr Joost Meerloo, a Columbia University psychiatrist, 'Stress, mental shock or maladjustment may be a causative factor in cancer' (Edwards, 1965, p. 89).

A case has also been made for linking the incidence of cancer to the mineral balance of the soil. At the end of the last century Dr Alfred Haviland, concluding an extensive study on the relationship of disease to geological factors said, 'Those who have reason to dread cancer should live in high, dry districts characterized by either limestone or chalk formations.' Another expert, Dr Lakhovsky, believed that clay, marl, alluvial deposits, carboniferous strata, mineral ores, which are impermeable to cosmic rays, are associated with a high incidence of cancer; whereas soils such as sand, sandstone and gravel are associated with a low incidence of cancer (Lakhovsky, 1951, p. 28).

Following this lead other authorities have referred to the existence not only of cancer districts, but even of cancer villages, cancer streets and cancer houses. According to one theory cancer occurs in those houses where people have been exposed for many years to a strong 'dowsing' area, so that houses built above clay or marl (good conductors) have more than the average number of cancer cases, as compared with those built on sandy soil.

Occultists believe that besides psychosomatic factors, besides the influence of cosmic rays and soil radiations, cancer has another far more subtle cause. However careful the diagnosis and therapeutics, however deep the doctors penetrate to the physical causes of the disease, they will find that cancer in many of its forms recedes still further and further from their understanding. This is because cancer, although it manifests in the somatic system, is fundamentally not a disease of the physical body, but a malignancy of the etheric double.

Among the many curious folk-remedies prescribed for cancer was eating toads and frogs, for these 'suck the poison of cancer' from the system. John Wesley (d. 1791) recommended an infusion of horse-spurs (the callosities that form on the inner side of a horse's legs), dried and powdered in warm milk and ale.

Books

Ash, Michael, *Health, Radiation and Healing*, Darton, Longman & Todd, London, 1962.
Edwards, Harry, *The Healing Intelligence,* Herbert Jenkins, London, 1965.
Fortune, Dion, *Psychic Self-Defence*, Aquarian Press, London, 1952.
Haviland, Alfred, *The Geographical Distribution of Disease in Britain*, London, 1892.
Lakhovsky, Georges, *The Secret of Life: Cosmic Rays and Radiations of Living Beings*, 2nd edn, True Health Publishing Co., London, 1951.
Pfeiffer, John, *The Human Brain*, Gollancz, London, 1955.
Shannon, J. W., *Cancer and Water*, San Diego, California, 1917.

Steiner, P. E., *Cancer, Race and Geography*, Baltimore, 1954.
Tromp, S. W., *Psychical Physics,* Elsevier, New York, 1949.
Voisin, André, *Soil, Grass and Cancer*, Crosby Lockwood, London, 1959.

CATALEPSY

A deep trance characterized by more or less complete anaesthesia or insensibility to pain, and catatonia, which is a statue-like rigidity of limbs and muscles. In catalepsy a person is unconscious, and this should be distinguished from cataplexy*, where the person remains conscious.

In catalepsy the limbs are sometimes movable but will retain the position in which they are placed, a condition described as *flexibilitas cerea*, 'waxen flexibility', like the limbs of a wax doll. Usually associated with nervous disorders, catalepsy is characteristic of hysteria* and certain forms of schizophrenia*, and can also result from great emotional shock.

In the cataleptic state, which may last for several days, the vital functions may be reduced to a minimum and a death-like condition prevails. According to experts on astral projection, when a person is physically cataleptic, he is in that condition because he is astrally cataleptic, the astral double being within a few feet of his physical, or within 'cord range', but the process of discoincidence is not quite completed.

Catalepsy can be produced by hypnosis*. Theatrical demonstrations are often seen where a subject is hypnotized into a cataleptic state and supported horizontally with his head and his heels resting on the backs of two chairs, with more rarely, a stone slab placed in the middle of his body and smashed with a hammer. Psychologists ascribe the genesis of this extraordinary increase in muscular tension to the latent hysteria of epilepsy*.

Catalepsy can also be artificially induced by pressure on certain arteries, especially the carotids along the neck. In Egypt certain Coptic cults of great antiquity practise cataleptic trance as part of their regular ritual. It can be induced voluntarily by occult techniques acquired after long training, as well as by the use of drugs. Eastern wonder-workers are able to bring it on by an effort of will, and achieve a state of suspended animation before allowing themselves to be buried alive for several hours at a time.

Suspended animation is a condition of the living body in which all the activities that characterize life, such as movement, respiration and the beating of the heart, are temporarily suspended, giving the appearance of death according to clinical diagnosis. Certain animals have the habit of aestivation (Lat. *aestas*, 'summer'), remaining dormant during the hot season to avoid the rigours of heat and drought. Others go into hibernation (Lat. *hibernus*, 'winter'), remaining dormant throughout the winter against cold and the lack of food.

During the coma of catalepsy the breathing and heart rate are almost normal. In suspended animation the coma is accompanied by drastically decelerated heart action and respiration. The hamster, a small rodent, may lie inert for months and its breath rate fall to as little as 1 per cent of normal.

The bat hibernates easily, and its heartbeat drops from 180 to an astonishing 3 beats a minute, and its breathing from 8 breaths a second to 8 a minute.

During the Arctic winters certain Alaskan and Siberian insects undergo a stage when their metabolic processes are not only reduced, but apparently cease altogether, and they remain in a lifeless state, frozen solid, until late spring when they revive. Scientists refer to this kind of suspended animation as *anabiosis*, and have experimented to see whether larger, warm-blooded animals could be made to 'die' by instantaneous freezing, and then be revived by warmth in the same manner. If so, they envision a time when an astronaut on prolonged journeys through space, if frozen by the same process, would be saved the boredom and emotional stress of flights lasting many decades, and would survive without food, water, or atmosphere, going through the experience without ageing, to be restored to life by automatic heating devices as he neared his destination. These studies are connected with the subject of thermosomatics*.

There are well-attested cases of people in a state of coma and suspended animation exhibiting all the symptoms of death, who after a trance of several hours, sometimes days, suddenly 'come to life'. Because of a failure in death diagnostics*, some of these unfortunates are buried before they are actually dead.

Books

Cannon, Alexander, *The Power Within*, Rider, London, 1950.
Christopher, M., *Seers, Psychics and ESP*, Cassell, London, 1971.
Hull, C. L., *Hypnosis and Suggestibility*, Appleton-Century, New York, 1933.
Muldoon, C. and Carrington, H., *The Projection of the Astral Body*, Rider, London, 1929.
Oswald, John, *Suspended Animal Life*, London, 1901.
Rawcliffe, D. H., *The Psychology of the Occult*, London, 1952.
Temkin, O., *The Falling Sickness*, 2nd rev. edn, Johns Hopkins Press, Baltimore, 1971.

CATAPLEXY

The state of total immobility, rigidity and powerlessness into which a human being or animal is thrown as a result of a sudden deafening noise, blinding light, shock or fright. It is briefly defined as fright hypnosis. An animal may become rigid, and feign death, when it is threatened and feels it cannot escape. During cataplexy, consciousness is retained, and the term is therefore used in contradistinction from catalepsy*, which is accompanied by unconsciousness.

The study of cataplexy in animals has taught psychologists a great deal about human reactions in similar situations. Many birds and animals can be rendered immobile if one covers their eyes. Constriction also seems to produce a catatonic response in animals, which may perhaps account for the comparative stillness of babies wrapped in swaddling-clothes. The snake-charmer's grip on the back of a cobra's neck reduces it to instant and sometimes rigid immobility.

Light taps on the head serve a similar purpose with birds. The cock seems to put the hen into a cataplectic state during copulation by first pecking her on the head and back of the neck, and seizing her by the comb. The hen offers no resistance, remaining motionless during the act and for some moments thereafter. After her trance she shakes herself and cackles noisily.

Rubbing, stroking and rhythmic movements in general, are common methods of inducing cataplexy in animals. Many animals become immobile simply by laying them on their backs, or standing them on their heads. A frog can be put into a trance if it is turned over on its back and its belly given a few light taps.

Athanasius Kircher (d. 1680), a learned Jesuit of wide-ranging interests, described the old method of 'fascinating' a cock. The bird is placed on the ground with his beak firmly held down to a chalked line. When released the cock becomes immobile in a ridiculous manner as if secured by his beak to the chalk mark, until he is disturbed by something else. Similarly, putting a piece of white putty at the end of a pigeon's beak will hypnotize it.

Zoologists tend to dismiss the idea that animals can transfix their prey by some sort of hypnosis, though some experts believe that it does happen. Snakes are said to fascinate frogs, birds and rabbits. Cats can fascinate snakes. Many animals cannot bear the steady gaze of human beings. The sudden roar and rush of a beast of prey immobilizes its victim.

David Livingstone (d. 1873), the celebrated missionary and explorer of the African continent, described how when he was in Mabotsa, a wounded lion sprang upon him and grabbed him by the shoulder. The horrible roar of the beast and the speed and shock of the attack, he says, produced a stupor similar to that which might be felt by a mouse when seized and shaken by a cat. It brought a sort of dreaminess and numbness in which there was no sense of pain or feeling of terror, although he was quite conscious of all that was happening to him. The shaking banished fear and paralysed sensation, and he felt no horror as he looked round at the beast. When the lion let go for a moment, Livingstone recovered and managed to get away.

Cataplexy, or consciousness without response, may occur in cases where a person is somehow immune to the full effects of an anaesthetic, so that he is paralysed but conscious, and an operation can be performed on him while he is aware of what is being done, though he is incapable of making this fact known, even when he is in great pain. Such cases with certain kinds of paralysant drugs, do occur, but are fortunately extremely rare. In a related condition we have the boxed-in syndrome, as it is called, where a person is conscious but inarticulate or unable to communicate his feelings. Very senile and very sick people may perhaps be in this situation, though we have no means of telling. The person who is being buried alive and is aware of it might be in some such state of panic immobilization.

To a limited degree cataplexy is found in the everyday life of men and women in civilized societies, and even in common parlance we speak of a person being frozen with terror or paralysed by fear. All stress* situations trigger reactions that resemble the numbing symptoms of cataplexy.

Books

Fabre, I. M. and Kafka, G., *Einführung in die Tierpsychologie*, Barth, Leipzig, 1913.
Hempelmann, F., *Tierpsychologie*, Leipzig, 1926.
Kenny, A. J. P. *et al.*, *The Nature of Mind*, Edinburgh Univeristy Press, 1972.
Livingstone, David, *Missionary Travels and Researches in Southern Africa*, Murray, London, 1865.
Sudre, R., *Treatise on Parapsychology*, Allen & Unwin, London, 1960.
Voelgyesi, F. A., *Hypnosis in Man and Animals*, Ballière, London, 1966.

CHROMOTHERAPY

Chromotherapy (Gk. *chrōma*, 'colour'), or healing by colour, an extension of the doctrine of signatures, is of very ancient lineage. Pythagoras (d. 500 BC) taught that certain diseases could be healed by exposing the sight to harmonious patterns of colour. Where beauty in an atmosphere of restful colours purifies the nature, the contemplation of ugliness in an environment of lurid colours stimulates to violence and crime.

Recent research has confirmed that colour does in fact affect the brain, muscle tension, nerves and the viscera generally. In particular, colours are known to exert a definite influence on mental conditions. The radiations of the colour spectrum are vibrations of varying frequencies and wavelengths that have a measurable effect on health and thought. Industrial organizations today fully recognize the value of the right colour schemes that make for efficiency in workshop, factory and office, and prevent fatigue and so reduce accidents.

The stimulating colours are red, orange and bright yellow. They make for action and excitement. Patients in mental hospitals are adversely affected by red and orange decorations. The soothing colours are cream, pale blue, green. They make for coolness and restfulness. In 1868 an exponent of chromotherapy, Augustus Pleasanton, so lauded the curative virtues of sunlight shining through blue glass, that for several months thousands of panes of blue glass were being sold and fitted into windows all over the country.

It has been found that manic depressives prefer warm colours like red; schizophrenics prefer cool colours like blue or green. Brown is the colour of paranoia. Excessive sensitivity to colour may point to a neurotic or psychotic condition. Colour response is also heightened in epilepsy*.

Primitive and intellectually undeveloped people like strong and bright colours. Children like reds, oranges and luminous colours; elderly people, blues and greens; aggressive people prefer deep colours. Cultured people choose pastel shades; while fussy, arty and 'queer' people go in for the in-between subtle shades. A growing consciousness of colour, and a desire to surround oneself with vivid, garish and bright tones often betrays the degenerate, like the love of loud and cacophonous music.

Colours stimulate the sexual instincts, increase muscular tension, affect one's mood and concentration, influence one's sense of space, time and movement. Each colour has its occult vibration. *Black* is melancholic, the colour of mystery and secret power; recommended for cancer*, paralysis and epilepsy.

Blue is cold, intellectual, loyal; it stimulates the pituitary and is recommended for skin and respiratory diseases, nervousness and anxiety. *Brown* is passive and neutral; recommended for liver and stomach complaints. *Green* is tranquil; recommended for circulatory and heart diseases, and shock. *Orange* is proud and sensitive; stimulates the pancreas; recommended for diseases of the lower abdomen. *Pink* is timid and retiring; recommended for rheumatism and lumbago. *Purple* is spiritual and regal; it stimulates the pineal gland; recommended for depression. *Red* is violent and aggressive; stimulates the adrenal glands, increases the pulse rate, respiration and blood pressure; recommended for lymphatic ailments and smallpox. *Yellow* is intuitive and changeable; recommended for asthma, migraine and eye-disease. *White* represents potentiality, purity and barrenness; stimulates the thymus; recommended for aggression and violence.

Books

Birren, Faber, *Color in Your World,* Collier Macmillan, New York, 1966.
Bopst, H., *Colour and Personality*, New York, 1962.
Brunler, Oscar, *The Influence of Colours on Mind and Health*, London, 1945.
Cheskin, L., *Colors: What They Do For You,* Liveright, New York, 1947.
Hessey, J. D., *Colour in the Treatment of Disease*, Rider, London, 1939.
Hunt, Roland, *Seven Keys to Colour Healing*, Daniel, London, 1963.
Iredell, C. E., *Colour and Cancer*, Lewis, London, 1940.
Mayer, G., *Colour and the Human Soul*, London, 1930.
Whitten, I. B., *What Colour Means to You*, London, 1948.

CONSTIPATION

The failure to have regular and satisfactory bowel motions; it has been the source of a prolific tradition both in psychology and the occult. During the costive state there is a feeling of uneasiness, pressure in the lower bowel, palpitations, perhaps a sense of suffocation. Medically, constipation causes a mild toxaemia (poisoning) of the system, with certain side-effects, and the resultant 'auto-intoxication' may account for some of the delusions of witches, and the hallucinations of neurotics. Although constipation was never deliberately employed as a technique in mysticism, it may have made its contribution to the visionary states of ascetics living on a sparse and inadequate diet.

During and after the process of evacuation, distinct physiological changes take place. Breathing, circulation and cerebral processes are all affected. There is a feeling of lightness, exhilaration and relief, at times of exaltation. Indeed there are people who aver that the pleasurable sensations accompanying evacuation exceed those of sexual intercourse. Many have confessed that their best ideas and highest inspirations have come to them during their brief sojourn in the water closet. In his theory of drama Aristotle (d. 322 BC) did not feel it out of place to speak of great tragedy as a cathartic, purging the mind of the emotions of pity and terror and thereby purifying and refining the passions.

The ancients paid great attention to their bowel functions, and took every care to avoid constipation. Herodotus (d. 425 BC), writing of the Egyptians, said that 'they take purges for three days in succession every month, seeking to preserve health by emetics and enemas, for they believe that all diseases proceed from the residue of the food they consume'. The court official who administered the enema to the pharaoh was given the title, Shepherd of the Royal Anus. In Canaan and other communities along the eastern Mediterranean littoral, there were deities dedicated to the scatological egesta, including dung, who were worshipped with offerings, to ensure regular evacuation, for which gratitude was due to the deity.

In many parts of the world it was believed that demons lurked in the bowels, and that excrement was as much a devilish as a human product. Throughout the Middle Ages and right up to the eighteenth century in Europe, the enema or clyster was part of the treatment of 'possession', in order to evict the invading entity which was thought to have taken up residence inside the victim. The devil took his departure along with the passing of stool. Even today, those who practise psychic healing have observed that at the critical stage of the illness, the patient often has a heavy rectal discharge and passes out an unusually offensive quantity of faeces, as though some alien and intrusive substance had been dislodged and sent forth from the body.

Constipation was commonly thought to be responsible for many sexual deviations. Towards the end of the last century a group of doctors began practising 'orificial surgery', or surgical interference with the sexual and anal orifices, which they believed were subject to irritation in adolescence owing to pressure on the rectum, and thereby inhibited the moral and religious aspirations of youth. They performed circumcision and clitoridectomy to check masturbation in boys and girls, and forcibly dilated the anus to ease the expulsion of faeces. By these means, it was thought, youth would be 'released from every fetter that binds, and the spirit directed Godward'.

However grossly they might have perverted the idea, these physicians are thought to have been correct in one respect: they recognized the close connection between costiveness and erethism. In our own day Sigmund Freud (d. 1939) wrote, 'The retention of fecal matter, with the intention of using it as masturbatory stimulus of the anal zone is one of the most common causes of constipation.'

Because of the importance attached to evacuation, all its concomitant paraphernalia, the purgatives, enemas and laxatives, often assumed special significance in social life. It is said that the ancient Egyptians regarded the ibis as a sacred bird because it was from this creature's habit of drawing water into its long beak and squirting it into its rectum, that they got the idea of the clyster. In some countries the enema became an actual cult implement. In southern Africa, for instance, there are Negro sects with whom colonic lavage forms part of the baptismal rite.

Similarly the place where the process of evacuation took place, ranging from any convenient spot of ground, to the domestic hearth or the precincts of a sacred shrine, has a long and interesting history, which can be traced from the beginnings of civilization. Among the earliest civilized accessories of the function was the chamberpot, which figures in Egyptian, Greek and Roman literature, and can be seen in temple frescoes and vase paintings.

Purgatives and laxatives were often invested with near-sacred properties, and played a prominent and lucrative part in commerce. Alexander the Great (d. 323 BC) was said to have left a colony of Greeks on the island of Socotra in the Indian Ocean to ensure regular shipments of the bitter aloes which grew there, and whose medicinal properties included a strong purgative action. The Spaniards of the West Indies called the castor-oil plant the *palma christi*, 'the palm-tree of Christ', while the Indians of northern California prepared a cathartic from the bark of a tree which they named *cascara sagrada*, 'sacred bark'.

As a valuable cathartic, antimony also has a history going back to ancient times. It figured in medieval European alchemy and was the subject of a famous work by a German alchemist, Basil Valentine (d. 1460). Antimony irritates the intestinal tract, causing loose motions, and was usually taken in the form of pills. The pill itself passed out unaltered and was recovered from the pot. Such 'perpetual pills' were passed down in families as precious heirlooms.

Nor have artists found the subject beneath their notice. In his *L'Attente du Clystère* the painter François Boucher (d. 1770) produced what Aldous Huxley called 'the most terrific pin-up girl of the century, perhaps of all time'.

Sigmund Freud was the first to highlight the importance of toilet-training in infancy, and point out the likely consequences of neglecting this aspect of the infant's education. In the beginning a child's libido or erotic sensations are centred first on the mouth, and this oral phase lasts for a year or two. After this period the child moves on to the sensations associated with the anus, and gets erotic pleasure from the action of emptying its bowels or holding back the faeces. If this anal phase is not passed, we find that the child becomes anal fixated, and remains preoccupied with various forms of anal activity.

As a rule parents are aware of the importance of regular bowel motions in the child's life, and the parental anxiety is communicated to the child, and implants in the child's mind the seeds of ownership. This can lead at times to a virtual 'battle of the chamberpot'. Faeces becomes the child's earliest property, obviously a valuable possession, and every act of evacuation is regarded as a kind of donation which he bestows in exchange for approval, praise or love, and which he withholds when he wants to show disapproval or annoyance. The German expression for the bowel movement of the child is *Bescherung*, which means 'bestowal', as of a gift.

Too severe a training in regimented and punctilious bowel movements can lead to strange character anomalies in later life. The psychological association of faeces with property, and by extension, with money, has long been recognized, and is in fact almost universal. In the Germanic folklore figure called *Gelt-scheisserle*, 'excretor of gold coins', gold is identified with faeces. The lust for money is frequently connected with coprophilia, or 'dirt-love', which in turn links it with satanism. Gold, or money, becomes the 'excrement of hell'. 'Money', said Francis Bacon (d. 1626), 'is like muck', and, as the Scottish proverb has it, 'Where there's muck [faeces], there's luck [money].' The psychologist Sandor Ferenczi put it in even stronger terms: 'Money is nothing other than odourless, dehydrated filth, that has been made to shine.'

In psychoanalytic doctrine the anal-fixated person is petty-minded, obstinate, orderly, conscientious, preoccupied with trifling duties, and is obsessively concerned with personal possessions. He is also stingy. Being a miser he is constipated. He continues his childhood habit of holding on to his 'property' at all costs. Above all, the miser finds it difficult to love. For love involves giving. A man who cannot spend money cannot spend himself, that is, ejaculate. He holds on to his money and his semen, just as he earlier refused to part with his 'productions'.

Books

Bourke, J. G., *Scatologic Rites of All Nations*, Lowdermilk, Washington, DC, 1891.
Comfort, Alex, *The Anxiety Makers*, Nelson, London, 1967.
Dawson, B. E., *Orificial Surgery: Its Philosophy, Application and Technique*, Kansas City, 1925.
Freud, Sigmund, *Three Essays on the Theory of Sexuality*, Hogarth Press, London, 1953.
Huxley, Aldous, *The Devils of Loudun*, Chatto & Windus, London, 1952.
Pudney, John, *The Smallest Room*, London, 1954.

CONVULSIONS

Convulsions, or irregular and often violent contortions of the body, often accompany certain disorders of the nervous system such as epilepsy* and hysteria*, and also tetanus, advanced kidney degeneration and other disorders. In earlier days these spasmic twists and torsions were thought to be manifestations of heightened religious emotion, as in the case of ecstatic sects like the Tremblers (*c.* 1560) and the Convulsionaries (*c.* 1730).

Convulsions characterize certain xenophrenic* states, and the manifestations vary a great deal. They cease when unconsciousness or stupor supervene, and the victim may become cataleptic and lie as though dead, with a tetanus-like rigidity. The body becomes so inflexible that no amount of force can bend it, and helpers feel that if great force were applied it would snap like a dry stick.

Convulsions often attack those in the grip of mass hysteria, a phenomenon once common in convents. So-called demon possession is also sometimes marked by extraordinary convulsions. The victim falls to the ground, the rigid body is racked with spasms, the shoulder-blades and joints crack and snap, the bones seem to grate against one another. It seems as if some malevolent entity takes hold of the victim and alters the limbs and features into unrecognizable shapes. The body becomes distorted as though the self were making a tortured effort to get out of the fleshly element. To the victim it seems that people and things take on a strange unfamiliar aspect, become larger or smaller, assume grotesque shapes. Sometimes the afflicted cry out that they are being cut with knives, beaten with rods, scarred with red-hot pokers.

During the epidemic of 'diabolic' possession in Morzine near Lake Geneva in 1855 which afflicted more than two thousand people, girls and boys climbed trees and even walls with the agility of cats. The victims, adults and children, beat their heads against the wall or on the ground with all their might, with no ill-effect. Some like wild animals ran hither and thither in an aimless, erratic fashion, so that it was difficult to restrain them or know in which direction they were going.

Although most of such activity seems to be confused and unco-ordinated, it is often remarkably controlled, as in the case of those who perform dancing, gymnastic and eurhythmic movements of extreme complexity and grace. Their bodies acquire extraordinary elasticity. During another epidemic, in the convent of Louviers in 1642, one girl when caught by the arm turned her body over and over about eight times with remarkable ease and speed as if her arm were fixed to the shoulder by a spring. The force with which some victims are propelled is quite inexplicable. One girl seemed suddenly to be seized up and dragged through the room and thrown about from corner to corner.

While in the convulsive state, people seem to possess superhuman power, like the person who was described as having 'a giant's strength and a wild beast's ferocity'. Another witness writes:

A young possessed girl shot out her left arm and held my two hands in her single hand with a grip so firm it was as if it had been bound with stout cords. I made every effort to free myself but although I am of average strength failed to do so. She interfered with me in no other way, nor did she touch me with her right hand. Then as suddenly as she held me she let me go.

During an outbreak at a convent in Auxonne in 1662, one of the possessed girls delicately picked up a vase with her finger tips, raised it from its pedestal, turned it upside down and threw it on the ground as if it were made of papier-mâché. Actually it was of marble, 2 inches thick, 2 feet in diameter, and a little less than 1 foot deep.

An unnatural and tortured carriage of the head is characteristic of the possessed, the epileptic, frenzied, bacchanal, maenadic person. Greek writings describe dancers in Dionysiac ecstasy tossing their heads back and forth and flinging their hair to the skies, throats upturned and straining, the whole body jerking. Voodoo dancers throw back their head and then bring it forward till the chin touches the neck, and do this again and again, up and down, with such rapidity it seems the neck must break. Or the head is turned around to its fullest extent so that it appears the person is facing the other way. Says one chronicle, 'The neck was wrythen [twisted] so the face seemed to stand backward.'

The hands and feet are similarly affected. The arms twist about like snakes and tie themselves into knots. The hands are flexed back and forth in slow rhythmic movements, the fingers take on peculiar shapes reminiscent of the mystic hand gestures of Eastern yogis. The feet curve inwards with toes clenched. Or they may be stretched out with toes projecting in all directions. The ankle often seems to be disjointed while the foot twists back and forth and around and around.

The contortions that the body undergoes in certain hysterical states are quite incredible unless actually seen. For example, in what is called an *arc-en-cercle*, the person, usually a woman, starts from an upright position and arches over backwards till the head touches the ground and rests between the feet, and often proceeds to make movements in an exaggerated imitation of the coital act. This astonishing manoeuvre has been performed by people who in normal circumstances would be quite incapable of doing it. The position is held for a few minutes and then repeated, and this may be kept up for hours.

The facial appearance is no less extraordinary to the onlooker. The face may be suffused with hot flushes, or drained to a deathly white. The expression changes as if they were menaced by horrid spectres. There is a flood of tears or a menacing smile. The features are often so distorted as to be no longer recognizable, with grimacings and twitchings terrifying to behold. But strange to say, in some cases the face remains quite calm in spite of the other unbelievable contortions. The features remain unruffled, and the expression never alters, as if the victim is unaware of what is going on in the rest of her body.

The voice alters completely, probably because of the contraction of the larynx. Some of the sounds seem to emanate from the chest rather than the throat, and have a deep and frightening boom. Some scream as if in terror. The body is racked with uncontrollable sobs, agonized groaning and moaning, and shrill heart-piercing cries. Some talk in alien voices, in strange unknown tongues. There may be several incoherent sounds together; like a babble of many voices simultaneously. These alternate with hiccups, laughter, ribaldry and abuse, and sometimes a harsh whistling as if the breathing were obstructed (stridor). Another typical feature is what is known as theriomimicry, that is, the imitation of animal calls, so that they roar, bark, grunt, cluck, mew, hiss, neigh or moo. In 1556 during an outbreak at Xante in Spain, the nuns could not be restrained from bleating like sheep.

Respiration is often very rapid and panting, or troubled, asthmatic and difficult, with hissing intakes of breath, and sudden sounds as of strangulation. It may suddenly stop altogether, perhaps for as long as a minute. Both perspiration and breath have a curiously sulphuric smell. It is a clinical fact that the breath of hysterical epileptics has a very fetid odour. Jean Bodin (d. 1596), French jurist and demonologist, declared that possessed persons stank because the devil was within.

Sometimes the belly is 'huffed up', and often visibly swells, unnaturally distending the abdomen. In one instance the abdomen of a young possessed girl swelled up so much she looked as if she were eight months pregnant, and she remained thus for several hours. At other times the belly is suddenly puffed up and then as suddenly subsides and becomes flat again.

The eyes are sometimes closed, but more usually they are wide open, wild and staring and do not focus properly. But although the eyes are open, 'yet the soul sees not through'. The eyeballs roll alarmingly, as if they would jump from their sockets. Often nothing but the whites show, the pupils being turned up under the lids.

The mouth opens and shuts and the jaws move as though champing some hard substance. The teeth are gnashed and the mouth fills with a foamy saliva.

The mouth may open so wide it seems to be completely out of joint. Or the teeth and jaws suddenly snap to, with the force of a steel trap.

The tongue is 'bleared' and stretched out to a prodigious length, as far as the chin or the bridge of the nose, and sideways to the cheek. Or again, it may turn towards the roof of the mouth and back into the gullet as though the victim would swallow it; and it cannot be pulled back by those who try with their fingers to do so.

The neck often seems to get longer, and twists about so that the muscles stand out. Sometimes the throat swells out to such an extent it seems as if it would burst. In some cases there is a spasmodic contraction and relaxation of the throat as if the person were trying to swallow an obstruction. This is said to be caused by the closing down of the thyroid gland whose secretions are temporarily suspended.

The heart will either slow down considerably or accelerate far beyond the normal rate. This is reflected in the pulse. It has also been noticed that the blood turns very acid during convulsions and trance states, as also in certain other xenophrenic states. In fact, if the trance is prolonged there is a slight poisoning of the blood stream.

Books

Howton, R., *Divine Healing and Demon Possession*, London, 1909.

Nevius, J. L., *Demon Possession and Allied Themes*, New York, 1894.

Oesterreich, Traugott Konstantin, *Obsession and Possession by Spirits Both Good and Evil*, Kegan Paul, London, 1930.

Prince, R. (ed.), *Trance and Possession States,* Bucke Memorial Society, Montreal, 1966.

Tonquédec, R. P. de, *Les Maladies nerveuses et mentales et les manifestations diaboliques,* Paris, 1938.

ZilbOorg, G. and Henry, G. W., *A History of Medical Psychology,* Allen & Unwin, 1941.

CUPPING

A method of treatment in which a small cup-like vessel, a cupping-glass, is applied to the body, the air withdrawn from the vessel, and as a result of the vacuum so formed, the blood drawn to the surface of the skin. Sometimes the blood percolates through the skin surface, so that cupping occasionally serves as an alternative to bleeding*.

In many parts of the world, including Britain, Europe and America, expert cuppers still perform curative feats with cups of various sizes for different parts of the body. The most common way of withdrawing air from the cup, is first to shave the area to which the cup is to be applied, then burn a small piece of cotton dipped in alcohol in the cup and while it is still alight invert the cup over the spot. The flame consumes the air within the cup almost immediately, the skin is drawn upwards and the rim of the cup remains stuck to the body. Cupping is used to relieve headaches, aches and pains of various kinds, high blood pressure, abscesses and boils.

The method originated from primitive suction therapy, when the mouth was applied direct to the affected area and the blood drawn to the skin by sucking. Patients who are cupped are said to feel brighter in mind, lighter in body, and altogether rejuvenated.

Modern cupping devices have a tube fitted to the top of the cup (which is usually made of glass) with a small hand-operated suction pump to draw out the air and create the suction effect. In young girls, poorly developed breasts are said to be improved by this means. Similarly, special suction cups are made for men with poor development of the penis, but the after-effects of using such a device are generally believed to be disastrous. The blood vessels of the penis forcedly engorged by this means soon lose their normal elasticity and impotence almost invariably and rapidly follows.

Books

Brockbank, William, *Ancient Therapeutic Arts*, London, 1954.
Gordon, B. L., *Medicine Throughout Antiquity*, Philadelphia, 1949.
Law, D., *A Guide to Alternative Medicine*, Turnstone, London, 1974.

CYCLOTHYMIA

Cyclothymia (Gk. *thymos*, 'emotion'), also called manic-depression, circular psychosis, or periodic insanity, is latent in everyone, being part of the alternating cycle of exhilaration and dejection in the mood and behaviour of all normal individuals. But in most people the curve above and below the norm is not excessive, whereas in cyclothymia the upward swing of the manic or excitement phase, and the downward sweep into depression are both extreme and of considerably longer duration, and are accompanied by a loss of contact with reality sufficient to impair a person's efficiency in dealing with the practical problems of everyday life. Between phases there is usually complete normalcy lasting for varying periods.

The two extremes of emotional ups and downs are regarded as psychological opposites*, and may be either bipolar, as in cyclothymia, or unipolar, in which case they fall into the categories of mania* and depression*.

At the end of the last century the German psychiatrist Emil Kraepelin (d. 1926) in a study of manic-depressive psychosis gave primary importance to the changes of mood, and the tendency today is to classify it as an affective disorder. The diagnosis of cyclothymia is not easy, since the determining factors are not always clearly present or distinguishable, and the patient's condition is often diagnosed as schizophrenia.

The reasons for these periodical shifts of mood, whether in the normal individual or in the psychotic, are unknown, and are variously said to be chemical imbalance due to hormonal disturbance of the pituitary, adrenal or thyroid glands, or else external periodicities like seasonal changes or cosmobiological factors like lunar cycles, sunspots, or 'the stars'. Treatment is by psychiatry* or psychopharmacology.

Books

See under depression *and* mania

D

DEATH DIAGNOSTICS

The identification of symptoms by which the demise of a person can be determined beyond doubt. It is difficult, some indeed believe impossible, to say what death is, and at what stage or at which precise moment it occurs. Biologists tend to the view that we do not die all at once, but in bits and pieces. We know that certain organic functions continue even after what is ordinarily called death; for example, the hair and nails continue to grow for a time after a person is pronounced clinically dead.

There is reason to believe that the body continues to feel and the brain to function for some time after clinical death. Doctors experimenting at the Negovsky Resuscitation Laboratory in Moscow have stated that when for any reason the brain is suddenly cut off from its oxygen supply, it uses an emergency system that is effective for another five to six minutes. It would seem that sudden and violent death is not instantaneous, so that even when a man is shot through the heart, hanged or decapitated, he remains conscious for anything from three to fifteen minutes.

During the French Revolution some of the eye witnesses were convinced that the grimacing heads that fell into the basket at the foot of the guillotine, continued to think and feel for some time. One witness records that when the head of Charlotte Corday, assassin of Jean Paul Marat, was held up by the executioner and slapped, it showed unmistakable signs of indignation.

The opinion of the lay person regarding death is not of much use, and even medical opinion is not to be depended on entirely. In the past death was usually confirmed by the fact that the heart had stopped beating and respiration had ceased. Consequently many cases of catalepsy, suspended animation, trance, deep coma and other kinds of 'false death', were mistaken for death, and people buried prematurely. There is a case on record of a woman who was pronounced dead by six doctors applying the usual tests, and for whom a death certificate was issued. For some reason she was not buried for two weeks, and on the fourteenth day came back to life.

At the end of the last century Franz Hartmann, an Austrian physician, collected 700 recorded cases, in civilized countries alone, of people who were pronounced dead, laid out for four or five days, placed in coffins, and at some stage returned to life. Sometimes a knocking inside the coffin before interment has saved a person from premature burial. There are also records of people who were actually buried, but because of the unshakeable conviction of their relatives following a dream, voice or vision, the body was exhumed and found to be living, or showed terrible evidence of having been alive when buried.

The fear that one might be buried alive prompted many people to take precautions against it. The operatic composer Giacomo Meyerbeer (d. 1864) arranged to have bells tied to his extremities so that any movement on his part before or after he was placed in the coffin would call attention to the fact that he was still alive. Harriet Martineau (d. 1876), the writer, left her doctor ten pounds to amputate her head before burial. The novelist Wilkie Collins (d. 1889) always carried a letter with him, begging anyone finding him dead to send for a doctor to make sure. The novelist and journalist Edmund Yates (d. 1894) left instructions for his jugular vein to be severed before burial and left twenty guineas as a fee for the acting surgeon. The actress Ada Cavendish (d. 1895) did the same. Col. Edward P. Vollum of the US Army Medical Corps put forward a plan that anyone buried without an autopsy or without having been embalmed, should be interred with a bottle of chloroform within reach, so that if he revived he could end his life with a minimum of suffering. So great was the dread of premature burial that by the end of the last century, some 200 books were written on the subject, and numerous societies were formed to guard against the possibility.

Death in our own day, apart from being diagnosed by the usual outward signs, can be confirmed by precise scientific methods. The most obvious sign is the absence of any discernible activity in the body. All the reflexes are extinct. The pupils are fixed and dilated. This is associated with the total cessation of spontaneous breathing (breathing death), of heartbeat (heart death) and blood circulation. Ordinarily the brain undergoes irrecoverable brain damage if deprived of oxygenated blood for more than five minutes.

Today the definitive sign of death is considered to be the cessation of brain activity (brain death), which is determined by electroencephalograph (EEG) recordings of brain-waves, which must be completely flat, that is, the tracing must be a straight line (iso-electric line), for at least ten minutes. Here again it is to be noted that brain death may take place in bits and pieces. Thus, death of the cerebral cortex (cerebral or cortical death) is not necessarily true death. This must be confirmed by EEG tracings for all parts of the cortex, since one part of the cortex may be dead (as in stroke) while other parts are still functioning. It is possible that life is not extinct even in the case of cortical death, for the brain stem may continue to function. In other words, as far as present knowledge goes, death might be regarded as final only when there is both cortical and brain-stem death, that is, when there is total cessation of activity in all areas of the brain.

A matter for concern is that even today with a more precise definition of death, neither the family physician, nor, in most cases, the hospital doctor, feels it necessary to confirm death by EEG tracings, so that the possibility of premature burial remains as real as ever. Reports of people certified as dead, who revive in the morgue are not at all uncommon, even today.

Actually, we still cannot define death nor can we be certain that it has occurred. After a close critical examination of the data as it exists today, the biologist Lyall Watson concludes: 'Death has proved to be impossible to diagnose.'

A disquieting thought is the increasing use being made of the dead for salvaging organs and tissues to heal the living. The fact that all organs of the body do not die at once makes modern transplant surgery possible, but whether such partial death is true death or not is becoming a crucial problem that has to be solved.

Scientists now envisage the possibility of making much more extensive use of the newly dead (neomorts) for transplantation purposes. With present methods of intensive care and mechanical supportive aids, it is possible to preserve suitable corpses for one week, and it is hoped, as techniques of preservation improve, that bodies might continue a vegetable existence in a decerebrated condition for six months, and perhaps a year.

In future neomort banks, the bodily metabolism could be artificially maintained as in life. The organism would breathe, its heart would beat, it would absorb nourishment and it would excrete its waste. Transplant parts from the living dead like bone, bone marrow, blood, blood vessels, kidneys, heart, liver, skin, could be harvested for instant use whenever required. Moreover, as in life, the neomort would regenerate many of its tissues, including bone marrow, blood and skin.

Besides medical, legal and ethical issues, the question of death diagnostics assumes deeper occult dimensions. Unless we know more about the nature of the total human entity, including the human double, that is, the astral and etheric components of man, we can have no precise criterion of death.

In the occult view, death is defined as the severing of the astral cord, resulting in the permanent separation of the astral body, the seat of ego consciousness, from its physical container. The process of separation takes about three days, even after decapitation or cremation. During this time a kind of dim astral consciousness persists.

On the other hand the etheric body, which is the seat of the subego or vitalic consciousness, is more closely bound to the physical organism, and lingers till the vital impetus runs out. That is why some believe that physical death is final and irreversible only when putrefaction sets in. The human entity in its physical body conforms to an etheric blueprint, a bioplasmic counterpart which has a fixed vitalic potential. When this potential is exhausted, the blueprint begins its disintegration and life begins its dissolution. But when the potential is artificially maintained, the physical body is able to carry on its vegetative functions, and etheric death could be delayed. In this view an Egyptian mummy, however well preserved, is dead. The neomort might not be.

Books

Cooper, M. A., *The Uncertainty of the Signs of Death*, London, 1902.
Fletcher, M. R., *One Thousand Buried Alive by their Best Friends*, Boston, 1890.
Gannal, F., *Mort apparente et mort réelle,* Muzard, Paris, 1890.
Hadwen, W. R., *Premature Burial*, Sonnenschein, London, 1905.
Hartmann, Franz, *Premature Burial*, London, 1896.

DEGENERATION

Haweis, H. R., *Ashes to Ashes*, London, 1875.
Hibbert, C., *The Roots of Evil*, Penguin, Harmondsworth, 1966.
Oswald, John, *Suspended Animal Life*, London, 1901.
Tebb, W. and Vollum, E. P., *Premature Burial and How it May be Prevented*, 2nd edn, London, 1905.
Watson, Lyall, *The Romeo Error*, Hodder & Stoughton, London, 1974.

DEGENERATION

An earlier class of thinkers who studied the evolution of the human race was aware that human beings often reverted in their behaviour to more primitive types of the species. Such degeneration from the state already reached was usually gauged by the physical appearance of the individual in question, and an outward approximation to an animal type was regarded as betraying the presence of those animal characteristics in the individual. Thus there were leonine (lion-like), bovine (ox-like), leporine (hare-like), aquiline (eagle-like) or psittacine (parrot-like) men, with the characteristics of these creatures.

A physiognomist once read from the porcine (pig-like) features of the philosopher Socrates (d. 399 BC) that he was a brutal and sensuous man, inclined to drunkenness, and when his disciples objected to the incorrect reading, Socrates replied that the reading was correct, for such indeed was his natural disposition, although he had managed to overcome these tendencies.

Both Aristotle (d. 322 BC) and Galen (d. AD 201) spoke of the intimate relationship between physical peculiarities and quirks of character. The Neapolitan mathematician and philosopher Giambattista della Porta (d. 1615) attempted to show that man's nature was inextricably bound up with his body, and that crime was the consequence of various abnormal physical conditions. Henri Boguet (d. 1619) the French civil jurist declared that it was possible 'to conclude from the repulsiveness of a man's face that there was sufficient reason to expose him to torture to make him confess to a crime'. Some medieval laws went so far as to decree that when two persons were under suspicion for the same crime, the uglier or more deformed of the two was to be considered the guilty one.

Cesare Lombroso (d. 1909), whose main work was a study of degenerate human types, said: 'The atavism of the criminal who lacks every trace of shame or pity, may go back beyond the savage to the brutes themselves.' Sigmund Freud's picture of a civilized man's unconscious mind was not very different from Lombroso's picture of primitive man. But the classifying of human beings on animal analogies had been abandoned by the eighteenth century, and Lombroso in spite of the statement quoted above developed other criteria, and sought to detect incipient atavism and reversion to primitive strains from certain 'stigmata' or physical signs of decadence, by which degenerates could be distinguished.

He and his successors, notably Max Nordau (d. 1923), listed such features as long arms, flat feet, prehensile toes, heavy jaws, progenism (when the lower teeth normally close over the upper), defective backbone, projecting ears, ability to move the ears, poor hearing, abundant hair (degenerates are rarely bald), joined eyebrows, prominent eyebrow bones, high cheekbones, well developed canine teeth, large and uncouth nose, solitary lines on the palms, a squint or a curious fixed stare. There are besides certain general signs which sometimes indicate degeneracy in the young, such as tooth decay, prematurely grey hair, speech defects like stammering, left-handedness (even ambidexterity), weak eyes (spectacles betray an inherent genetic decadence), eye defects like nystagmus (the involuntary twitching of the eyelids), facial tics, deafness, lack of muscular co-ordination.

Benedict Augustin Morel (d. 1873), the psychiatrist, had a theory that almost all persons with chronic mental disturbances could be grouped under the heading of mental degenerates. This would include malingerers, or those who feign sickness, those who constantly criticize and complain, those who are boastful and exhibitionist, compulsive liars, the naturally destructive, those who have their bodies tattooed, males who titivate themselves, women who try to imitate men, sexual offenders, sexual perverts, homosexuals, moral delinquents and drug addicts.

More recent students of the subject, some of whose strictures have been very uncomplimentary, suggest that the increase in degenerative types in our day would seem to stem from the fact that young and impressionable people are ceaselessly exposed through news media, films and television to spectacles of crime and violence, and to sex and vice, which the weak-minded cannot witness without wanting to emulate. Their heroes are criminals and anarchists. Constant sensual stimulation has dulled the senses, which demand more and more stimulus. Hence the emphasis on vivid colour and above all loud music. This tolerance to loud music is sometimes cited as the chief mark of the modern degenerate. It makes a constant assault on his nerves and, without his knowing it, dulls his mental powers.

There is also the higher class of degenerate. Young men and women of this category win scholarships and fill the universities. The chief faculty of the higher degenerate is the excessive development of the speech centres in the cerebral cortex that gives them an extraordinary facility with words. But though remarkably articulate they seldom have anything original to say. They lay great emphasis on 'doing their own thing', but lack the stern individuality that is needed to live up to this doctrine. They easily form or join cults, follow all the latest fads, and are full of the arty jargon and peculiar cant of the group to which they belong. They pretend to broadmindedness, but are extremely bigoted, and cannot tolerate a viewpoint that is contrary to their own.

The type of career chosen by the higher degenerate is usually predictable. Many gravitate towards politics and as a rule belong to the left. Large numbers turn to the easy fields of sociology, which offers them wide scope for espousing or inaugurating some new doctrine of social sufferance for the moral shortcomings of the degenerate class to which they belong. Some turn to philosophy, usually materialistic, or contrarily, to Eastern religions or some current form of mysticism. Occultism is packed with their kind. The professions, such as the army, the church, business, law, medicine and science, are distasteful to them, and few of them are found in their ranks. Accordingly they despise most of these professions as making up the hated Establishment.

The lesser breed of the same class gravitate to what might euphemistically be called 'the arts', where the greater freedom from intellectual discipline and moral control provides them with a more suitable ambience for their type of talent. Many are protagonists and patrons of folk-rock musicals, pop art, pseudo-folk and pop music and the fringe theatre.

A number of degenerates reveal what is known as Tourette's syndrome (after Gilles de la Tourette who first described it) which is characterized by coprolalia, an uncontrollable compulsion to swearing and foul language. It is not a rare disease and is found among writers of pornography and those associated with the production of pornography. They are vociferous and at times violent advocates of obscenity in literature, art and life. Under the banner of freedom of expression they delight in what D. H. Lawrence calls 'doing dirt on sex'.

According to the psychologists who take this view, degeneracy implies above all a moral delinquency, and an attenuation of the instinct that respects the decencies of social behaviour. In this sense therefore, most degenerates can be called psychopathic*. They are morally deranged, suffer from personality disorders, and are in need of psychiatric attention. As such they make up the large and growing population of drug addicts, drop-outs, sexual perverts, layabouts, social misfits and petty habitual criminals.

Books

Carter, A. E., *The Idea of Decadence in French Literature*, University of Toronto Press, 1958.
Dallemagne, J., *Dégénérés et déséquilibrés*, Lambertin, Brussels, 1894.
Farez, Paul, *Stigmates de dégénérescence mentale et psychotherapie*, Paris, 1901.
Ferri, Enrico, *Criminal Sociology*, London, 1895.
Genil-Perrin, Georges, *Histoire des origines et de l'évolution de l'idée de dégénérescence en médecine mentale,* Leclerc, Paris, 1913.
Glueck, S., *Physique and Delinquency*, London, 1956.
Hibbert, C., *The Roots of Evil*, Penguin Books, Harmondsworth, 1966.
Lombroso, Cesare, *Crime: Its Causes and Remedies*, London, 1911.
Morel, Benedict Augustin, *Traité des dégénérescences physiques, intellectuelles et morales, de l'espèce humaine,* Paris, 1857.
Nordau, Max, *Degeneration*, London, 1895.
Rhodes, H. T. F., *Genius and the Criminal*, London, 1932.

DEPERSONALIZATION

The condition in which an individual loses his sense of relationship with his own personality and his sense of identity with the familiar self he knew. The world becomes unreal and he is a stranger to himself. He imagines that the face he sees in the mirror has changed, it seems to be the face of someone else; his voice is not his own, his thoughts are bizarre, his actions are automatic. He may feel he has no body, that he is not real, that he does not even exist, or is a shadow or ghost.

In some cases a tiny pinpoint of identity might remain, but only as a viewer, an outside observer. One might say that he has an I, but not a Me. He is conscious of a distant, aloof sense of selfness, but of non-involvement with the people around and the world in which they exist. Sensations, feelings and thoughts are present in the tenuous stream of his consciousness, but the over-all psychic experience is one of loneliness and isolation.

Depersonalization is to be distinguished from expersonation, which is the deliberate dispossession of the astral body of one person by that of another; in depersonalization the effect is usually that one is not oneself, and not so much that one has been ousted. It is also to be distinguished from 'possession', where an intrusive spirit entity takes over the personality; depersonalization does not involve the feeling of being taken over, but rather of being dissipated, dissolved and not 'present'.

This strange condition can spring from a number of causes. Mental disorders of various kinds, including schizophrenia* and serious memory disturbances, are frequently accompanied by symptoms of depersonalization. Mental patients are said to be estranged from themselves, or alienated, whence comes the now obsolete term, alienist, for a psychiatrist, one who restored the personality of a patient.

Persons with certain nervous diseases, like allochiry, where they lack self-perception of one half of the body, often suffer from a sense of partial or total depersonalization. Their limbs are not real limbs, or not their own limbs; their familiar surroundings become unreal; well-known faces assume a strange unreality and become unrecognizable.

It can occur in various circumstances that bring on xenophrenia*, including long periods of insomnolence or sensory deprivation. It can come as a result of epilepsy*, hysteria*, migraine, extreme torture or extreme pain, or great emotional stress. Psychedelic drugs can bring it on as well. Ecstasy and visionary experience may result in temporary depersonalization.

People who have met with sudden disaster or grief, or have received news affecting their security or their lives, frequently find themselves in a situation of unreality, as if the events were part of a phantasmagoria in which they had no part. Various conditions of angst*, melancholia* and fear*, are accompanied by depersonalization, partly as an attempt to escape from reality. Sometimes it springs from a pathological sense of guilt, or sin, that compels a withdrawal of identification with one's own body. Those who have been reprieved after having been at the point of execution or sudden death, have described the sense of unreality and personal 'absence' from the situation that comes over them. In terminal illness the immediate pre-mortem condition is one of depersonalization and loss of identity.

Psychologists observe that a periodical sense of isolation and alienation is becoming increasingly common today, even among otherwise perfectly normal people. A man sometimes becomes so perplexed with life's problems that the questions concerning the reality of the world and of his own existence assume a grave practical significance. He can only resolve his anxiety by believing, at least for a time, that the things that are taking place are not really happening to him.

This sense of unreality and non-participation in the events occurring all around has been experienced by many men of the highest genius, among them Leo Tolstoy (d. 1910), who was frequently overcome with a sense of great dread, which made him feel an alien, living in a hostile and uncaring world, isolated in the midst of things, out of touch with his family, his friends and himself.

Books

Dodds, E. R., *Pagan and Christian in an Age of Anxiety*, Cambridge University Press, 1965.

Hoch, P. and Zubin, J. (eds), *Anxiety*, Grune & Stratton, New York, 1950.

Kuhn, Helmut, *Encounter with Nothingness*, New York, 1951.

Meerloo, J. A., *Patterns of Panic*, New York, 1950.

Schilder, Paul, *The Image and Appearance of the Human Body*, John Wiley, New York, 1964.

Searl, M. N., 'A Note on Depersonalization', *International Journal of Psychoanalysis*, 12, 1932, 329.

Sypher, Wylie, *Loss of the Self in Modern Literature and Art*, Vintage Books, New York, 1964.

DEPRESSION

A common affliction, and there is no one who has not at some time or other, for no obvious reason, felt dejected, out of sorts, sad and despondent. In earlier medical practice it was treated as melancholia*. In psychological opinion today, depression has a more serious clinical significance, being one of the chief features of many modern neuroses, as well as a symptom of psychotic disorders.

In its bipolar form it figures as the downward phase of cyclothymia*, or manic-depressive insanity, but it is frequently a unipolar phenomenon, and is then treated as a separate malady. This kind of depression lasts longer than the situation warrants, and it is this persistence that characterizes true depression. It has been estimated that at any given moment about 8 million people in America and about 6 million in Britain and Europe are in need of professional help for depression.

The symptoms of depression are many and varied. The signs may progress from hypothymia (Gk. *hypo,* 'sub-', *thymos,* 'emotion'), or mild dejection, through more serious forms like involutional melancholia (sometimes associated with the menopause) to critical conditions leading to insanity and suicide.

An attack often starts with a feeling of fatigue and loss of energy. There is insomnia or difficulty in getting to sleep. When it does come sleep is light and the sufferer wakes up often during the night, or is up before the normal time, with a vague feeling of anxiety. The appetite is poor, the sexual drive low, there may be hypochondria and other symptoms of neurosis*. There is a lack of concentration, a loss of drive and will (abulia*), difficulty in making decisions, procrastination and a general sense of apathy and boredom.

The victim is hypersensitive to criticism and is easily hurt; he tends to cry without cause and become hysterical. Sometimes he has a feeling of being persecuted. At the same time he is also extremely self-critical, with bouts of self-accusation and self-reproach, and suffers a general lowering of personal morale. With the loss of self-esteem comes a sense of guilt and shame, a brooding over real or imagined failures, and a growing gloom. He feels hopeless, inferior, inadequate, rejected, ineffective, unworthy. Pessimism reaches black despair; he is full of fears and in a thoroughly demoralized and desperate condition.

By this time the victim has withdrawn from social contacts, is unresponsive to others and begins to have feelings of depersonalization, of not being himself, and yet of not knowing who he is. Not infrequently the overall mental and motor retardation degenerates into a state of stupor. Suicidal tendencies are ever present, although suicide is rare at the depth of depression, because of the lack of determination or will to do anything; but it is common during the recovery phase when the energies are on the upswing again.

The conjectural origins of depression may be *exogenous* or external, like financial loss; or *endogenous* or internal, like deficiency of noradrenalin in the brain. Most of the factors that produce stress* can bring on an attack. At the same time its true causes remain unknown. Whereas ordinary depression may arise from grief, loss of employment or similar cause, clinical depression has nothing to do with grief or loss, and in any case is out of all proportion to the apparent cause. Or it may be due to an imagined cause. It will afflict people who seem to have little or no reason to be depressed. According to psychoanalytic theory, depression is a self-imposed though unconscious punitive experience for the expiation of some deep-seated guilt.

Like the cause, the cure for depression is not known. The victim without realizing it may compensate by such things as overspending, overworking, oversleeping, overeating or sexual promiscuity. He may resort to stimulating drugs like alcohol or amphetamines that give him a momentary lift but actually only worsen the depression. Standard treatment includes psychosurgery, shock therapy, psychotherapy*, and above all, antidepressant drugs.

Books

Flach, Frederic F., *The Secret Strength of Depression*, Angus & Robertson, London, 1975.
Grinker, Roy *et al.*, *The Phenomena of Depression*, Hoeber, New York, 1961.
Hippius, H. and Selbach, H., *Das depressive Syndrom*, Munich, 1969.
Kendall, R. E., *The Classification of Depressive Illnesses*, London, 1968.
Kraepelin, Emil, *Manic-Depressive Insanity and Paranoia*, Livingstone, Edinburgh, 1921.
Ladee, G. H., *Hypochondriacal Syndromes*, Elsevier, Amsterdam, 1966.
Stack, John J., *Depressive States in Childhood and Adolescence*, Almquvist & Wiksell, Stockholm, 1971.
Watts, C. A. H., *Depression, the Blue Plague*, Priory Press, London, 1973.

DIAGNOSIS

The identification of disease from symptoms manifested by the patient, as revealed by external and internal examination, both at the bedside and in the laboratory. The patient's own statement, an understanding of his social background, home environment, hereditary influences and congenital predispositions, his past illnesses, making up his case history, and the likely aetiology* or cause of the disease, are among the other factors that help in diagnosis.

External diagnosis involves observing the skin (for flushes, pallor, spots, blotches), taking the temperature and determining the pulse rate. More detailed symptoms are sought in the analysis of blood, tissue, sputum, stool and especially the urine. Urinoscopy*, or diagnosis by examination of the urine, was a special branch of ancient and medieval medicine, and remains one of the chief diagnostic aids today. In addition, dozens of more unorthodox diagnostic methods exist, by which practitioners of fringe medicine reach their conclusions. Some include astrology, palmistry and other occult sciences, used mainly in psychodiagnostics*. In psychometry, the ailment is determined by a sensitive holding some personal possession of the patient, such as a handkerchief or ring, and by the 'vibrations' diagnosing the nature of the disease.

Certain sensitives specialize in aura diagnosis, by examination of the coloured radiations surrounding the patient, since a person's aura alters with the presence of disease. A still more advanced method is based on kirlian photography, which provides a picture of the life energy or bioflux field surrounding the body.

Others use radiesthesia or psionics, diagnosing by the oscillation, gyration, speed or direction of a rod or pendulum when brought into contact with the patient or a sample of his blood or saliva. In its more mechanized and sometimes electronic form radiesthesia is called radionics.

Related to radiesthesia is the black box, an electrically wired apparatus connected with a calibrated dial. A hair, or specimen of blood or saliva, taken from the patient, is placed in the box and the device turned on. Diagnosis is made from readings on the dial, and in some cases healing radiations, amplified in 'inverted phase', are transmitted through the same machine back to the patient. This form of treatment was pioneered by Dr Albert Abrams (d. 1924), professor of pathology at Stanford University.

Certain anomalies are to be noted about diagnosis. To begin with, many diseases have identical symptoms. Then some symptoms are false, and either do not reveal a disease or give a wrong and misleading clue. Again, hundreds of symptoms are psychosomatic*, which adds further complications.

Sometimes there is also found to be a difference between the symptoms listed by the clinician when the patient is alive, and those discovered by the pathologist at the post-mortem. The dynamic differs from the static. For example, when a man dies his arteries empty and the blood stagnates in the veins and capillaries, a fact that led physicians from the time of Hippocrates (d. 359 BC) to believe that the arteries transported the 'vital spirits'.

Similarly during severe illness the 'thymus gland shrinks considerably, so examination of the gland by earlier anatomists gave the incorrect impression that the thymus was smaller than it actually was. Examination of the thymus after sudden death (when the gland did not have time to shrink) showed the gland larger than normal, and death in such cases was often attributed to a mythical disease called *status lymphaticus*, or *status thymolymphaticus*.

Today the vast range of scientific aids and biotelemetric* devices makes diagnosis more accurate, detailed and certain. Laboratory machines can test 500 blood samples an hour, more accurately than technicians. The increasing refinement and speed of the process now involves feeding a computer with the results of a comprehensive clinical examination (itself mechanized) and accepting the computer's diagnosis.

On the other hand, the benefits of such mechanization are beginning to be treated with some caution. By intensive clinical scrutiny some kind of deficiency, abnormality or disease can most probably be discovered in almost every individual, no matter how healthy. Like the hundreds of bacterial species that inhabit our bodies, these 'diseases' do no damage and cause the individual no inconvenience. To bring insignificant disorders to light, and by the powerful drugs now at our disposal to eliminate them, when we still know so little about ourselves, might interfere with the delicate balance by which the body itself has adjusted to these idiosyncrasies, and stir up the dormant condition, perhaps causing an eruption of sickness of a more serious nature.

Books

Barr, James, *Abrams' Method of Diagnosis and Treatment*, Heinemann, London, 1925.

Butler, W. E., *How to Develop Psychometry,* Thorson, London, 1971.

Drown, Ruth, *The Science and Philosophy of the Drown Radio Therapy*, Artists' Press, Los Angeles, 1938.

Nichols, Beverley, *Powers That Be*, Jonathan Cape, London, 1966.

Payne, L. C., *An Introduction to Medical Automation*, Pitmans, London, 1966.

Reyner, J. H. *et al.*, *Psionic Medicine,* Routledge & Kegan Paul, London, 1974.

Tansley, David, *Radionics and the Subtle Anatomy of Man*, Health Science, Rustington, 1972.

DIET

Diet (Gk. *diaita*, 'mode of living') once referred to one's general way of life with regard to dress, behaviour and mental attitude, as a means of shaping one's destiny. Today the term is restricted to the food régime one follows, although the idea that it is connected with one's fate is often implicit in it. It is still believed that the nature of the food we eat influences our character, and that a man becomes what he eats.

The best food is said to be that which is grown or cultivated in one's own country; and for each season the fruits and vegetables of that season are the best. The true native eats the produce of his native soil and avoids alien and exotic foods, especially spices and condiments. The more a person partakes of foods from foreign climes, the more he is said to lose his native disposition and his natural wisdom.

Excessive eating is bad for body and mind. It leads to overweight, heart conditions and mental sluggishness. Seneca (d. AD 65) said: 'More people are killed through the stomach than by the sword.' Francis Bacon (d. 1626) recommended 'a sparse diet and almost a pathological'. Modern exponents invariably stress the value of periodical fasts as wonderfully rejuvenative. And indeed, the latest experiments with animals and men confirm the extraordinary benefits of fasting in the cure of many physical ailments, the restoration of health and vitality, vigorous hair growth, increased sexual power and a sense of wellbeing.

At the beginning of the present century the Russian pathologist Ilya Metchnikov (d. 1916) put forward the idea that man does not die or age naturally, but in fact poisons himself. Ill-health and senility are caused by autointoxication, resulting from continuous putrefaction in the large intestine. This process, he said, could be arrested by the lactic-acid bacillus contained in sour milk or yogurt. He pointed out that Bulgarian peasants lived so long because the chief article of their diet was cheese made from *koumiss*, or fermented mare's milk. Until his own death at the age of 71 the Metchnikov régime was very widely followed throughout Europe.

Today the most able defence of sensible diet comes from the naturopaths*, who recommend fresh fruit and vegetables, preferably compost-grown, without insecticides and artificial fertilizers, and unadulterated with chemical preservatives and colouring matter. Those who cannot tolerate a vegetable diet should in any case refrain from eating the meat of poultry and animals given sex hormones to fatten them or other additives to tenderize the flesh. Also recommended are wholewheat bread, butter, cheese, nuts and honey. What is called 'royal jelly', the substance produced in the bodies of the worker bees, and which is the sole nourishment of the queen bee, is also regarded as beneficial. The liquid intake should consist only of fresh fruit and vegetable juices, and other natural non-alcoholic beverages. Popular today is the macrobiotic, 'great life', diet based on Zen principles, consisting of simple foods like cereals, beans, seeds, whole oats and brown rice.

Experts on the subject find some strange anomalies in the whole modern concept of a balanced diet, and its insistence on minerals, vitamins and other supplements. They would like to know, for instance, how certain Papuan tribes of great physique, strength and stamina, have thrived for centuries on a diet that consisted almost exclusively of sweet potatoes. Or how many of the world's largest and strongest animals, including the elephant and rhinoceros, are purely herbivorous.

Altogether, the assimilation of food seems to have an occult aspect, of which little is known. We are familiar with the physiology of the digestive processes like salivation, chymification, chylification and the final absorption of the reduced food particles by the lymph vessels and the blood. This absorption is achieved through the villi, millions of very tiny hair-like projections that line the intestine like a coat of fur. Electron microscopy has shown that the villi are actually coarse structures, which themselves are bristling with microvilli, and these perhaps with still lesser and lesser villi reducing to vanishing point. It would seem that apart from the actual biochemical conversion by which meat and cabbage are transformed into blood and bone, the process of assimilation also involves the bioplasmic or etheric principle within the bodily apparatus.

The rosicrucians of medieval Europe, who inherited an earlier tradition, said that it was possible to live on a single meal taken every other day, if the body could be trained to absorb the 'essence' of the food, which is all that is needed for life and health. According to Paracelsus (d. 1541) the mouth is a stomach, and if one chews food sufficiently and then spits it out without swallowing, one can still be nourished.

For all we know our present emphasis on an all-round diet and on mega-vitamin therapy is misplaced, and we could thrive on a much more meagre diet than the one to which a prodigal society has habituated us, to our detriment.

Books

Belham, George, *The Virility Diet*, Corgi Books, London, 1967.
Carruthers, G. B., *Pocket Book of Diets*, Evans, London, 1955.
Davidson, Stanley *et al.*, *Human Nutrition and Dietetics,* Livingstone, London, 1959.
Hutchinson, M., *Food and Principles of Dietetics*, Edward Arnold, London, 1956.
Williams, Sue, *Nutrition and Diet Therapy*, Mosby, London, 1969.

DISEASE

According to the ancients, disease was a morbid condition of body, mind and spirit. From early times the concept of health, wholeness, healing and holiness were closely linked together. And so were illness and evil. A man's physical health and his spiritual state were believed to be interdependent. Sickness in primitive societies had an occult origin and occult consequences. It was attributed to malevolent spirits, or regarded as the work of sorcerers operating through the intermediary of demon entities. In some places the sick, though feared, were also regarded with awe, as being in contact with two worlds.

Students of pathology have always recognized an unknowable, almost occult, element in the cause and progress of disease. Even today, when the nature of illness is better understood, its incidence, severity and consequences are regarded to some extent as being 'in the lap of the gods', for they are never completely determinable. In the light of present-day research it is being increasingly realized that the true origin of disease may go much further than modern aetiology* suggests. Our relationship with the whole environment has to be taken into account.

We are not clear about the cause, and manner of spread, of many simple ailments. It is one of the perennial jibes against the medical profession that with all the resources of modern therapeutics, they have still not been able to cure the common cold. The cold is almost exclusively confined to human beings, and it has been found that while most viruses can be transmitted to experimental animals, no laboratory animals showed signs of suffering from the cold, nor could any be made to contract it. Human volunteers had to be used and continue to be used.

Damp, draughts, exposure and dozens of other so-called causes have in turn been tried, tested and disproved. Getting cold does not give one a cold, getting wet and sitting in a draught does not give a cold either. A person may be warm, comfortable, free from draughts and secure from exposure, and still

65

catch a cold. Colds are said to be 'caught' from others. Studies in air hygiene reveal that a sneeze, when expelled in the air, travels at supersonic speed, the droplets fragment and lose moisture and can remain suspended in the air for up to forty-five minutes. But it is now established that the theory of person-to-person spread is not always tenable.

The fact that the common cold often starts at a critical seasonal period, usually in winter, has suggested the possibility that it might itself be a means of building up immunity against more serious ills. Just as certain childhood infections seem to build up resistance in children, so it is thought that the common cold, with its short concentrated malaise, may represent an acquired ancestral immunization process against the more devastating winter diseases.

In the fatalistic view disease is a mode of destiny, and cannot be separated from the angst* and suffering that is the general lot of mankind. As such it has religious overtones. In popular Buddhism disease is a messenger from the gods to remind man of his mortal condition. Being a band in the spectrum of suffering, sickness can be a great teacher. Pain*, too, so often a part of sickness, contributes to the lessons that it has to teach. On a larger scale, as in an epidemic*, disease is a portent of divine wrath, whose lessons are learned at great cost to the whole community.

There are always those who see the significance of illness in its wider context against a philosophical setting. According to an old Pythagorean belief, the soul develops mantic, that is, psychic, powers, in advanced stages of disease, when the mind attains a state of ecstasy. In his *Timaeus*, Plato (d. 347 BC) says that true divinely inspired prophecy is only possible under certain conditions, 'as when the power of man's intelligence is fettered in sleep, or when it is distraught by disease, or by reason of some divine inspiration'. It would seem that sickness facilitates genuine paranormal perception, to which good health renders us obtuse.

Indeed, historians of pathology have suggested that there exists an alliance between illness and the intellectual faculties, supporting their thesis with the incidence of certain illnesses connected with genius*. Illness seems to favour the emergence of talent. Many of the world's greatest artists, writers, musicians and thinkers have suffered from chronic ill-health. Time and again, besides ordinary fevers*, we find evidence of a wide range of afflictions, tuberculosis, syphilis, cancer, epilepsy, migraine, melancholy, obsession and insanity, going hand in hand with outstanding gifts in the higher reaches of cultural activity. The toxins produced by infecting organisms seem to stimulate mental activity.

It has been suggested that in a perfectly healthy society we would have no geniuses, for the highest talents are created in the crucible of suffering. Immanuel Kant (d. 1804) said: 'In an Arcady all talent would be nipped in the bud.' The Superman of Friedrich Nietzsche (d. 1900), who was supposed to combine perfect physical and mental health with the highest genius, would be an impossible phenomenon, for such a combination cannot exist. Creative people have often found that they need a degree of discomfort in order to do their best work. Sigmund Freud (d. 1939) wrote: 'I have long known that I cannot be industrious when I am in good health.'

Some psychologists believe that physical disease has a therapeutic value in psychological complexes. According to Dr Felix Deutsch, it could be said that men and women would be most unhappy, or would tend to neuroses, 'if they could not fall sick from time to time'.

Books

Andrewes, Christopher, *In Pursuit of the Common Cold*, Heinemann, London, 1973.
Bett, W. R., *The Infirmities of Genius*, Christopher Johnson, London, 1952.
Cartwright, Frederick, *Disease and History*, Hart-Davis, London, 1972.
Crawfurd, Raymond, *Plague and Pestilence in Literature and Art*, Oxford, 1914.
Deutsch, Felix (ed.), *On the Mysterious Leap from the Mind to the Body*, International Universities Press, New York, 1959.
Henschen, Folke, *The History and Geography of Disease*, Delacorte Press, New York, 1966.
Lee, Roger, *Health and Disease: the Determining Factors*, Little, Brown, New York, 1920.
Pickering, George, *Creative Malady*, Allen & Unwin, London, 1974.
Scott, S. R., *Famous Illnesses in History*, Eyre & Spottiswoode, London, 1962.
Sigerist, Henry E., *Civilization and Disease*, University of Chicago Press, 1962.

DRUG THERAPY

Drug therapy, or chemotherapy, is the treatment of illness by natural or synthetic drugs. Associated subjects include: pharmaceutics, the art of preparing medicines; iatrochemistry, the study of the healing properties of drugs for diseases of body and mind; and pharmacogenics, which is concerned with the dangers of drugs because of their power to cause illness.

For over three thousand years the medical profession accepted the ancient principle of *vis medicatrix naturae*, 'the healing power of nature', and the physician as a rule prescribed medicines containing simple ingredients whose separate effects were known to him. The mixture or bolus, compounded by the apothecary, soothed the patient, and assisted the body in restoring the balance of its natural functions. The patient's own vital energies were brought to bear on his recovery. One of the best loved and most successful surgeons in the history of medicine, Ambroise Paré (d. 1590), used to say, 'I treat, God cures.'

Today there are hundreds of synthetic drugs that achieve miraculous cures. The success of short-stay, daytime and partial hospitalization, as compared with the long-stay hospitalization of the past, is mainly due to modern drugs. The doctor depends in 90 per cent of cases on drugs developed since 1950. But he does not know his drugs any more. Because of the increasing complexity of drug chemistry and the plethora of drugs being manufactured, the doctor is in difficulties in prescribing drugs. He discovers that the drugs he has been taught to use as a student soon go out of fashion.

As a rule the doctor does not know much about pharmacology, cannot keep abreast of new developments in drug treatment, knows progressively less and less about the chemical composition of the latest drugs, and usually confines his interest to their effects and side-effects. Once he has diagnosed a disease he has little more to do than prescribe one or more of the proprietary drugs manufactured by the pharmaceutical companies, which their catalogues and handbooks tell him are good for the disease in question. Doctors depend on drug companies to keep them up to date, and this is not without its drawbacks. A survey carried out in Canada some years ago on prescriptions for antibiotics showed that in over 62 per cent of cases the wrong drug had been prescribed.

But despite the danger signals, chemotherapy continues to hold sway over the whole field of modern medicine. Drugs are taken not only for physical and mental ills, but for various social reasons. They are used for the behaviour modification of unmanageable children and psychopaths; for increasing learning potential; for improving the memory. We have, or soon will have, truth pills, fertility pills, contraceptive pills, concentration pills, long-life pills and youth pills. For the obese there are fat-reducers; for the wrestler, muscle-builders. And, of course, there are the great standbys of the common man and woman: sedatives, sleeping pills, tranquillizers, mood-elevators, stimulants and pep-pills.

There are literally thousands of drugs on the market today, and so far no effective method of classifying them has been found. Classification by chemical composition is of academic interest and in any event cannot avoid considerable overlapping, so that the scheme becomes complex and unwieldy. One method, which is in accord with earlier practice, is to arrange them according to their effects on the various bodily organs and functions, so that we have laxatives, expectorants, emetics, antirheumatics, vesicants, analgesics, vermifuges, and in recent terminology, bronchodilators, cardiodepressants, vasoconstrictors, cataplexogenics, and so on.

The drugs that have an effect on brain and mind are more amenable to classification. The study of such drugs is called psychopharmacology, and the drugs themselves spoken of as psychotropics, or 'mind-altering' drugs, and also psycholeptics, 'mind-affecting' drugs. These drugs either stimulate or inhibit the activity of one or more of the neurohormones or enzymes released by the cells of the nervous system. In general, they have been grouped into four broad divisions: sedatives, tranquillizers, stimulants and hallucinogens.

Sedatives are said to be the class of drugs for those over fifty. They allay nervousness, anxiety, strain, excitement and usually promote sleep, and are therefore referred to as hypnotics. They include the bromides, calmatives and nervines.

Tranquillizers are said to be the drugs for those in their forties. They are called ataractics, giving 'peace of mind', or anxiolytics, 'releasing from anxiety'. The tranquillizers fall into three categories: the major tranquillizers, which are antipsychotic, 'contramadness', like chlorpromazine and reserpine; the antidepressants like the tricyclics (so called because of their three-ringed chemical structure), the MAOIs or MAO inhibitors (no longer in general use) and lithium used in the manic phase of cyclothymia* and schizophrenia*; the minor tranquillizers, which include meprobamate and diazepam.

The stimulants are the drugs for those in their thirties. They stimulate the control centres of the nervous system, induce wakefulness, alertness, excitement and improve mental performance. The stronger drugs of this class act as euphoriants, making a person taking them so witlessly optimistic that he is good for nothing. This class includes the amphetamines.

The hallucinogens create sensory and perceptual distortions, illusions and hallucinations, and are said to be the drugs for those on either side of 20. The drugs themselves are described as fantastics, producing fantasies of sight and sound; disinhibitors, removing the inhibitions that help to keep behaviour socially acceptable; confusants, causing mental confusion and perplexity; psycholytics, 'mind-loosening', and which in this sense form part of what is called psycholytic therapy; psychodysleptics, 'mind ill-seizing', because of their detrimental effects; chronoleptogenics, 'time weak-making', creating distortions of the time sense, so that it becomes difficult to distinguish hours and seconds, before and after, or cause and effect; psychotogenics, 'madness-creating', or psychotomimetics, 'madness-mimicking', because they produce for a time conditions similar to psychoses, especially schizophrenia; psychedelics, 'mind-revealing' or 'mind-expanding'; orgasmogenics, because they produce warm-flush pulsations in the lower abdominal region that are said to resemble sexual orgasm; these sensations lessen with addiction and may leave the addict impotent.

Because of the idiosyncratic reaction of different people to hallucinogenic drugs, it has proved virtually impossible to classify them in any acceptable scheme. Broadly they may be arranged under ten headings somewhat as follows: (1) *Cactus*: mescaline, peyote, teonanactl. (2) *Hemp*: cannabis, marihuana, hashish, dagga, bhang, ganja, kif. THC, or tetrahydro-cannabinol, is a purified extract of cannabis. (3) *Solanum*: belladonna, henbane, datura, stramonium, pituri. (4) *Banisterine*: yagé, caapi, harmine, ibogaine. (5) *Mushroom*: muscarine, psilocybin, fly agaric, bufontenin. (6) *Opium*: morphine, heroin, laudanum. (7) *Myristic*: nutmeg, epena, virola, parica. (8) *Convolvulus*: morning glory, ololiuqui. (9) *Coca*: cocaine, 'Charlie', 'C'. (10) *Synthetic*: LSD (lysergic acid diethylamide); DET (di-ethyl-tryptamine); DMT (di-methyl-tryptamine), milder than LSD; STP (di-methoxy-ethyl-amphetamine), its acronym said to be derived from the initials of 'scientifically treated petroleum', or 'serenity, tranquility, peace', which it is supposed to induce; it is also called DOM and is classed as a megahallucinogen.

The art of compounding medicines, known as pharmaceutics, was perhaps conterminous with civilization. In the Western world it is traced back to ancient Egypt, from whom the Greeks derived much of their knowledge. The art was a traditional one, confined to families who dealt in spices, fragrant oils (Gk. *myron*), perfumes, pomades, unguents, herbal drugs, medicines, poisons (Gk. *pharmakon*, from Egyptian *phar-maki*, 'drug-magic'), dyes and special wines of high spirituous content. The storehouse (Gk. *apothēkē*) where these commodities were kept was often under state supervision. From the Greek terms mentioned above come the words 'pharmacist', and 'apothecary'; as well as the Roman *myropola*, or 'perfumer'. From the Late Greek word for dried herbs (*xerion*) we have the word 'elixir', and also, by a circuitous route, the word 'drug'.

Few drugs today are compounded by a dispenser as in the past, since most are readymade and pre-packed, available for instant use by doctor or patient. Some preparations can be freely purchased across the counter, and others ('ethical drugs') can be given on prescription only.

A great controversy rages over the promotion and cost of drugs manufactured by the big drug companies. It is, of course, acknowledged that valuable advances have been made in modern chemotherapy as a result of their enterprise and endeavour. At the same time, investigations into the commercial side of the large pharmaceutical corporations have from time to time disclosed evidence of doubtful practice in some cases. Chief among these have been the following: the inflated and often misleading claims of their advertisements, and their tendency to play down the side-effects of their products; their dubious promotional methods, which must have an adverse effect on the medical profession; the exorbitant prices that are charged for drugs, enabling the companies to make profits of 300 to 5000 per cent; their unethical marketing and testing procedures. Drugs are sometimes marketed after insufficient clinical tests and with little concern for drug safety; or tests are carried out by manufacturers in countries where stringent standards are not insisted on; drugs that have passed their expiry date, or fail the required standards of efficacy or safety, are exported to the third world.

Closely connected with the subject of drug therapy is pharmacogenics, the study of 'drug-caused' diseases, which also embraces pharmacopathology, or the morbid changes brought about by drugs, and pharmacopsychopathology, or the abnormal mental effects produced by drugs.

An ancient axiom of the medical profession has been *primum non nocere*, 'above all, do no harm'. At times it is preferable to let the patient alone rather than give him medication. But today, because of pressure from patients and relatives, who insist on having drugs for trivial complaints, and because of their expectation of some tangible form of treatment, the doctor prescribes a drug. The problem arises from the fact that practically every modern drug is potent in more than one direction, and can therefore be harmful. Too much reliance on the very powerful synthetic remedies of today opens the way to many dangers, quite apart from the hazards of overdrugging, wrong medication, side-effects and addiction. No drug is totally harmless, non-toxic, non-addictive, free from side-effects. Its dangers are increased when other drugs are prescribed at the same time, because of the possibly mutual potentizing action of drugs and injections.

Western society, in particular, is overmedicated and is becoming increasingly drug-dependent. A growing tolerance to drugs makes them less effective in normal doses. The bacteria and viruses themselves are adjusting to the new pharmacology and building up resistance and immunity to it. Recent studies suggest that our triumph over infection* may well be premature and short-lived.

The natural resistance to the body is becoming weakened. Certain drugs actually undermine the body's natural defences, and lower the body's ability to fight disease, to heal wounds and to produce the biochemical agents that cause the blood to clot. Its basic immunological reactions are suppressed in order that transplant operations of all kinds might be carried out successfully. This is because foreign substances (and this includes the cells and tissues that are transplanted) tend to be rejected by the body receiving them, and the body has to be educated to accept them by the administration of drugs. The techniques of counteracting the natural process of rejection are known as immunosuppression. Such suppressive drugs also suppress the patient's ability to fight other kinds of infection.

Individual response to medication differs greatly. Some adverse effects arise from purely idiosyncratic traits in particular patients. Tolerance to drugs differs with the sexes; women of all ages and in all countries appear to be more sensitive to drugs than men, and more prone to react adversely. Genetic factors also play a part in the way people respond. There are apparently racial differences as well, and not only in drug response. Jews tend more than other races to Tay-Sachs disease, and Negroes to sickle-cell anaemia. The tolerance to opium is much lower in the white man than in the yellow; the tolerance to alcohol much lower in the black man than in the white.

Drug responses have been the subject of study for some time, and it is now admitted that notwithstanding the great benefits of modern chemotherapy, there has been at the same time, as Dr Wade says, 'an increase of adverse reactions to drugs of almost epidemic proportions'. Many drugs act as symptom-removers. A disease does not always vanish with medication. It often gives way to new and subtler complications. Every step forward in medicine increases the problem of healing, and we pay the price for new advances in manmade products. While old diseases are in retreat before the new drugs, these drugs themselves are sometimes responsible for what are virtually new diseases.

Many drugs have known short-term side-effects: headache, palpitations, sweating, flushing, rash, hypertension (high blood pressure), liver and kidney deterioration, deafness, dryness of the mouth, constipation, vomiting, diarrhoea, cardiovascular collapse and brain damage. But the long-term effects are still largely unknown. And they will only begin to be known after five, ten, even twenty years. Whatever they may be, whether physical, mental, chromosomal or etheric, they will leave their mark on future generations.

Sleeping pills, besides other side-effects, could cause REM-sleep starvation, which can lead to mental disturbance. Recent studies suggest a relationship between the growing dependence on sleeping pills and the progressive increase in mental illness. Barbiturates are responsible for thousands of deaths, resulting from the inadvertent drinking of alcohol at the same time. It has been suggested, on the analogy of tests carried out on rats, that a pregnant woman on barbiturates may give birth to a homosexual son. If she takes the masculinizing hormone progesterone (sometimes prescribed for women with a history of recurrent miscarriage), she may produce a clever but 'butch' daughter, as the drug causes virilization of the female foetus.

The effect of drugs taken by a pregnant woman on her unborn child forms the subject of a considerable and fast-growing literature. Like thalidomide, a number of other drugs 'cross the placenta' and can damage the foetus. Again, doctors confess that the effects of prolonged use of oral contraceptives are 'entirely unknown'. The pharmacological inhibition of a normal physiological function may, for all we know, have effects on body and mind still to be revealed.

The antibiotics have rightly been hailed as 'wonder-drugs' but their dangers are also considerable. The drugs used in organotherapy, including hormones, serums and steroids, also take their toll. The long-term effects of man's immunization programmes by means of vaccines, toxoids and antitoxins are beginning to give concern. Vaccine damage is now a growing problem because it can cause severe cerebral injury in children. Some drugs, such as those used in psychochemotherapy, pass the blood-brain barrier and have a direct and immediate effect on the nervous system, and we are still not clear how interference with the delicate balance of the neurohormones might influence the body at the level of the cells, chromosomes and nucleic acid molecules.

Voltaire defined medical treatment as the business of pouring drugs, of which doctors know little, to cure diseases of which they know less, into human beings of whom they know nothing. It was the opinion of the great English physician Sir William Gull (d. 1890) that 'medicines do most good when there is a tendency to recover without them'.

The critics of modern 'pharmapseudotherapy' aver that what Oliver Wendell Holmes (d. 1894) said of the drugs of his day, could with equal relevance be applied to some of the drugs used in our own time. 'I firmly believe,' wrote that famous anatomist, physiologist and physician, 'that if the whole materia medica could be sunk to the bottom of the sea, it would be all the better for mankind, and all the worse for the fishes.'

Books

Aaronson, B. and Osmond, H. (eds), *Psychedelics: the Uses and Implications of Hallucinogenic Drugs*, Hogarth Press, London, 1971.
Coleman, Vernon, *The Medicine Men*, Temple Smith, London, 1975.
Davies, Hywel, *Modern Medicine: A Doctor's Dissent*, Abelard, London, 1977.
Dunlop, D., *Medicines in Our Time*, Nuffield Trust, London, 1973.
Dunnell, K., *Medicine Takers, Prescribers, Hoarders*, Routledge & Kegan Paul, London, 1972.
Flach, F. and Regan, P., *Chemotherapy in Emotional Disorders*, McGraw Hill, New York, 1960.
Jones, Hardin and Jones, Helen, *Sensual Drugs*, Cambridge University Press, 1977.
Kefauver, Estes, *In a Few Hands*, Penguin, London, 1966.
Kline, N. S., *Modern Problems in Pharmacopsychiatry*, Karger, New York, 1969.
Meyler, L., *Side-Effects of Drugs*, William & Wilkins, New York, 1972.
Moser, Robert, *Diseases of Medical Progress: A Contemporary Analysis of Illness Produced by Drugs and Other Therapeutic Agents*, 2nd edn, Thomas, Springfield, Illinois, 1969.
Rhodes, Philip, *The Value of Medicine*, Allen & Unwin, London, 1977.
Talalay, Paul (ed.), *Drugs in Our Society*, Oxford University Press, London, 1964.
Wade, O. L., *Adverse Reactions to Drugs*, Heinemann, London, 1973.
Warburton, D. M., *Brain Behaviour and Drugs*, Wiley, London, 1976.

DYSGENICS

Dysgenics (Gk. *dys*, 'bad'; *genos*, 'race'), the study of factors responsible for the physical and intellectual decline of the human race, is complementary to the study of eugenics* or race improvement. It is established that there is a genetic component in mental and physical defects, and that many of them are transmissible to one's progeny, and dysgenics applies itself specifically to determining the agencies responsible for these defects and preventing the propagation of those who might carry them.

Scientific progress has undermined the law of natural selection that once ensured the survival only of the fittest. New preventive and remedial measures, advances in medicine, embryonics, genetics and intensive care have encouraged the perpetuation and propagation of all categories of people, including those with serious mental and physical handicaps, severe abnormalities, susceptibility to infectious diseases and transmissible genetic defects. This has resulted in the progressive multiplication of dysgenic qualities in the human race.

Intensive care includes all methods of caring for the desperately injured, hopelessly sick, the very aged and serious post-operative cases by extraordinary means, usually in a special hospital ward known as the 'intensive-care unit'. It involves the continuous observation and maintenance of a patient's vital functions during critical periods, until the emergency is over. Intensive therapy needs the services of highly trained staff, cardiac specialists, respiratory physiologists, anaesthetists, besides complicated and expensive equipment, usually computerized, electronic, automatic, with huge capital and running costs.

Many emergency resuscitation techniques, blood transfusions, potent drugs, heart machines, lung machines, kidney machines and other supportive techniques are brought into operation to maintain the life of a patient, and even revive a patient already dead. These methods in terminal and geriatric cases are so effective that life of a kind might be prolonged almost indefinitely. It is theoretically possible to extend without limit the physical functions of a dying person, like a piece of chicken tissue that is kept 'alive' for years in a laboratory.

Some people believe that such prolongation of a vegetable existence is morally indefensible. Socially it brings up the question of the utilization of necessarily limited resources. The economics of social concern will shortly place the doctor in a dilemma. The growing numbers of distressingly handicapped infants and adults, and hopelessly decrepit aged, will, they believe, eventually exhaust the available manpower and other medical resources. Problems of more and more accommodation, equipment, trained personnel, money, already raising their heads, will inevitably demand a drastic solution.

One of the first questions that confronts the advocate for race improvement and one that arouses bitter controversy, is the criterion of unfitness. This is bound up with the problem of determining at what stage it is desirable to let the chronically or incurably ill pass away. Two considerations are involved here, namely, the elimination of those who are beyond hope of cure, and the sterilization of the unfit to prevent them from perpetuating their defects.

The combined catalogue of eligible candidates selected by dysgenists for 'elimination' makes a formidable and frightening list: the insane, psychotic, feeble-minded, mentally defective, grossly subnormal; those in prolonged and irreversible coma; those with severe brain damage; those in the last stages of syphilis, leprosy, tuberculosis, chronic renal and heart disease, multiple sclerosis; those with high tetraplegia (paralysis of all four limbs resulting from damage to the spinal cord), or even paraplegia (paralysis of the lower body); epileptics; grossly deformed neonates (new born); all psychopaths with irremediable behaviour defects; the criminally insane. Also, incorrigible delinquents; repeated sex offenders; all criminals jailed for capital offences;

73

chronic alcoholics; incurable drug addicts; vagrants and tramps; the very senile.

The French-American doctor and Nobel prize winner, Alexis Carrel (d. 1944), writing of the vast sums spent on the maintenance of criminals and the insane, suggested that the ideal action would be to eliminate all such 'useless creatures' as soon as they proved dangerous. Philosophical theory and sentimental prejudice, he felt, were not entitled to a hearing in such a matter.

Linked with the question of dysgenics, is the problem of geneosis, or the diseases and abnormalities in the structure and constitution of the basic genetic material of an organism, leading to disablement or defect. Geneosis may result from natural process or artificial tampering, or be due to abnormalities in the gametes or sex cells (ovum or sperm), in the chromosomes, in the DNA molecules or in the genes.

The view has been expressed that humanitarian tolerance that permits the propagation of the unfit, is short-sighted, and while it may benefit the individual concerned, does great harm to the community and to the future of mankind. Similarly, allowing children born with severe dysgenic characteristics to live, imposes a lifetime's handicap on the child, places a heavy responsibility on the parents (which many seek to shirk) and is a strain on the limited resources of the state in terms of money, time, medical skill and nursing attention.

Nature has several ways of dealing with geneoses, and usually takes a hand in eliminating them, so that defects and abnormalities do not commonly recur. To begin with, genetic abnormalities in either partner will usually result in infertility and prevent conception. After conception special hormonal processes in the maternal body or in the fertilized egg come into operation and continue through every stage of pregnancy. If there is an abnormality such processes could trigger the expulsion of the developing entity out of the womb.

For a number of reasons many embryos still in the very early stages of development die in the woman's reproductive tract and are expelled. Because of the high percentage of genetic aberrations in the human being, thousands of women expel fertilized eggs in the very first phase of pregnancy, and this is hardly noticed by the mother. Between 12 and 15 per cent of all embryos die within a few days or weeks. The mother may have a missed period and the tiny creature will pass out in the form of a heavier than normal flow the month after. Between the second and sixth months about 10 to 15 per cent more will die as 'spontaneous miscarriages'. These are rejected by nature because of some fault. In Britain alone some 1,000 foetuses are spontaneously aborted every day. Miscarriages are a perfectly normal occurrence, and serve a useful eugenic function in eliminating the unfit.

Occasionally the defective foetus survives, but is then born before it is due. Premature babies do not stand a great chance of survival. The earlier the foetus leaves the womb, the less the chance of survival, and the greater the chance of mental and physical deficiency in later life. Even in cases of birth after the full nine-month period, defective or abnormal children do not normally survive more than a few hours or days. In brief, infertility, spontaneous miscarriage, premature birth, are among nature's ways of preventing the emergence or propagation of the unfit.

Today, this natural eliminative process has been subverted by genetic tampering, surgery, advances in remedial techniques and drug therapy, pre-natal and post-natal care. Parents, one or both of whom would normally be biologically infertile, are now helped to produce children. A previously barren woman can with the aid of fertility pills produce twins, triplets and further multiple births. Infant mortality has been reduced to a minimum. The vast majority of foetuses that are conceived, many of which in the normal course would have been aborted by nature as unfit, can now be maintained through all the stages of fertilized egg, blastocyst, embryo, foetus and brought successfully to full term. Almost all babies brought to full term, including the geneotic that would have succumbed to their defects, can now be nurtured through childhood, adolescence and maturity to preserve and propagate weak genes responsible for defects in mind and body.

A number of measures have been proposed to prevent what many see as a genetic disaster confronting mankind, some of which involve the curtailment of many human rights that are now accepted as basic. Among these measures are: test prospective parents for deleterious or incompatible genes; discourage, indeed prohibit, marriage between carriers of the same genetic defects or the same disease; sterilize the subnormal and genetically unfit; discourage any treatment, medication, surgery, interference (except to relieve pain) that assists the survival and transmission of heritable traits in the population; stop tampering with genetic processes that might damage the genes and chromosomes; allow the chronically sick and the senile with no hope of recovery to pass away in peace and quiet. It is being increasingly felt that natural selection should be allowed to operate in this area with its full ruthlessness, a viewpoint that is now being accepted with less reluctance in the face of the demositic catastrophe said to be facing mankind.

Demositis, 'population disease', covers the harmful social effects of highly accelerated population growth on a global dimension. Demographic or population studies show that the problem is now serious enough to be a matter of worldwide concern. Its implications can more readily be discerned from the following estimated figures of the world population:

in 1 AD	250 million
in 1600	500 million
in 1850	1,000 million
in 1900	1,500 million
in 1950	3,000 million
in 1976	4,000 million
in 2000	6,000 million
in 2200	400,000 million

Paradoxically, the greater the medical progress, the more crucial the problem becomes. The neo-Malthusians see nothing but catastrophe ahead, especially in the less developed countries. International agencies like the World Health Organization supply endless quantities of drugs to cure disease and stem epidemics, but provide little or nothing for feeding, clothing and housing the population after their deliverance.

The richer communities have their own problems. Students of the subject believe that Western countries are breeding down, and the general level of intelligence and other desirable qualities are on the decline. The more intelligent, cultured and 'fit', deliberately limit their families and are thus being bred out. The less intelligent, the unskilled, the degenerate, the unfit are multiplying unchecked, encouraged by a sentimental, 'humanitarian' approach to basic issues that is suicidally oriented. The proliferation of dysgenic elements in society is analogous, in the view of eugenists, to the rapid spread of cancer cells in a healthy body.

There has been an alarming increase in the incidence of transmissible mental and genetic disease. Recent figures suggest that 10 per cent of all admissions to hospitals in developed countries are for genetic diseases. In the United Kingdom alone, about 15,000 children are born every year suffering from severe genetic physical and mental disease and genetic predispositions. Babies with defects are increasing at 12 per cent compound each generation.

There is clear evidence that the rate of increase in the genetic defects of the general population will be beyond control unless the community or the medical profession take steps, in the words of Professor Darlington, 'to avoid the disastrous consequences of its own achievements'.

Books

Darlington, C. D., *Genetics and Man*, Allen & Unwin, London, 1964.
Emery, E. R. J., *Principles of Intensive Care*, English Universities Press, London, 1973.
Etzioni, Amitai, *Genetic Fix*, Macmillan, London, 1973.
Fishlock, David, *Man Modified*, Jonathan Cape, London, 1969.
Greep, Roy (ed.), *Human Fertility and Population Problems*, Schenkman, Cambridge, Massachusetts, 1963.
Hamilton, Michael (ed.), *The New Genetics and the Future of Man,* Eerdmans, Grand Rapids, Michigan, 1972.
Jones, Alun and Bodmer, Walter, *Our Future Inheritance: Choice or Chance?*, Oxford University Press, 1974.
Leach, Gerald, *The Biocrats*, Jonathan Cape, London, 1970.
McKusick, Victor, *Human Genetics*, Prentice-Hall, New Jersey, 1969.
Norton, Alan, *The New Dimensions of Medicine*, Hodder & Stoughton, London, 1969.
Penrose, L. S., *The New Biology of Mental Defect*, Sidgwick & Jackson, London, 1949.
Ramsey, Paul, *Fabricated Man: the Ethics of Genetic Control*, Yale University Press, 1970.
Thomson, Godfrey, *The Trend of National Intelligence*, Eugenics Society, London, 1946.
Vaux, K., *Who Shall Live?*, Fortress Press, Philadelphia, 1970.

E

ECCENTRICITY

Eccentricity literally signifies the state of being 'off centre', and the eccentric person, to use another mechanical analogy, has 'one screw loose'. Eccentricity implies a shifting of the personality out of the commonplace, so that an individual behaves in a manner that is out of conformity with accepted norms.

The true eccentric is often beset with phobias, obsessions and anxieties, and tends to be melancholic*. His quirks of character and conduct are quite inexplicable, often amounting to rank superstition, as in the case of people who never cultivate the friendship of anyone whose surname begins with a particular letter of the alphabet, or who ritually repeat some meaningless action.

The eccentric is odd, full of idiosyncrasies, impractical, non-conformist, and oblivious of the opinion of others. He often balances precariously on the borderline of insanity. Eccentricity is frequently regarded as one of the signs of great intellectual gifts (the absent-minded professor) and of genius*. The English philosopher John Stuart Mill (d. 1873) said, 'The amount of eccentricity in a society has generally been proportional to the amount of genius, mental vigour and moral courage it contained. That so few now dare to be eccentric marks the chief danger of the time.'

The following are a few instances of eccentricity among the great. John Milton (d. 1674) believed that cold hinders the free run of the imagination; he said that his muse was sterile in winter and therefore avoided writing poetry during the cold season. Jean-Jacques Rousseau (d. 1778) always turned his head to the full glare of the sun when pondering over new ideas, believing that its rays stimulated his brain. Samuel Johnson (d. 1784) was a confirmed hypochondriac, who felt he would get drunk if he ate an apple. He often felt madness approaching and would beg Mrs Hester Thrale to lock him in his room and place gyves upon his legs. When walking down the street he used to touch every lamp-post on the way; he knew exactly how many there were, and if he missed one he always returned and counted them over again, otherwise, he believed, he would fall ill.

Frederick II (d. 1786) of Prussia, surnamed the Great, was born of an iron-fisted dictator, and both were eccentric to the point of insanity. Vittorio Alfieri (d. 1803), the Italian poet, said: 'I have less perspicacity in the evening than in the morning, and have greater aptitude for creating in midwinter and in midsummer than in the intermediate seasons. With me writing depends on atmospheric and climatic conditions.' Friedrich von Schiller (d. 1805), the German poet and dramatist, found he worked best with his feet placed on ice for a time, and while inhaling the flavour of rotten apples. Giovanni Paisiello (d. 1816), an Italian musician who befriended and influenced Mozart, was able to compose only while he lay between six quilts in summer and nine in winter.

Ernst Wilhelm Hoffmann (d. 1822), the German novelist, musician and writer of tales, was so sensitive to atmospheric change that he drew up a meteorological scale from his moods and emotions during various weather changes, so that he might adapt his writing in accordance with it. Ludwig van Beethoven (d. 1827) was described as the housekeeper's nightmare, so untidy was he. He could never learn to dance, since he could not get his feet to keep time to music. He refused to change his suits and linen so that his friends had to take away his dirty clothes while he slept. He could not spell and never mastered the multiplication table. He was extremely absent-minded and morbidly suspicious.

Lady Hester Stanhope (d. 1839), niece of William Pitt, was a highly eccentric woman, who travelled to the East and lived among the tribes of Mount Lebanon, adopting Mohammedan garb, and preparing for the second advent of Christ. Frédéric Chopin (d. 1849) had a pathological fondness for silks and satins, and always wore gloves of a sickly pink colour. He never had thirteen to dinner and made no important decisions on Monday or Friday. Honoré de Balzac (d. 1850) used to get himself into a creative mood by drinking poisonous quantities of black coffee. In many other ways too he was eccentric in the extreme.

J. M. W. Turner (d. 1851), the English landscape painter, was also an eccentric, whose behaviour often verged on madness. Elizabeth Barrett Browning (d. 1861) felt that she wrote best when in a recumbent position. William Makepeace Thackeray (d. 1863) found his ideas flowed most freely in a congested club and while he held a quill in his hand. Charles Baudelaire (d. 1867) nursed many strange idiosyncrasies. He dyed his hair green and on one occasion went for a walk through a park leading a live lobster on a pale blue cord. Michael Faraday (d. 1867) felt that the body was most comfortable and received the best magnetic influences when it lay in an east—west direction. Charles Dickens (d. 1870) invariably slept with his head to the north (*see* magnetotherapy).

Alexandre Dumas (d. 1870) could write articles only on pink paper, poetry on yellow sheets, novels on blue. Ivan Turgeniev (d. 1883) got himself in a creative mood by keeping his feet in a bucket of water. Richard Wagner (d. 1883) worked in an overheated room perfumed with attar of roses, wearing a silk dressing-gown. He used to read his poems to his friends and ask for their frank opinion, but would fly into an insane rage if criticized. He could not bear to be contradicted.

Alfred Tennyson (d. 1892) felt the inspiration to write poetry more strongly during the spring and summer than in autumn and winter. Johannes Brahms (d. 1897) made a point of wearing shabby clothes even on important occasions and had a superstitious aversion to wearing socks. He loved children but was afraid of women and never married. Émile Zola (d. 1902), like Dr Johnson, used to count the gas jets in every street in Paris through which he walked, or even drove.

Books

See under genius

ELECTROTHERAPY

The use of static or dynamic electricity in the maintenance of health and the cure of disease. Among the experimenters with earlier and more primitive techniques were Carl Linnaeus (d. 1778), Swedish physician and founder of modern botany, Jean Paul Marat (d. 1793), French physician but better known as a revolutionary, and Benjamin Franklin (d. 1790). Later, electrodes were applied to the body and gentle currents of electricity allowed to flow through the system, and sometimes mild shocks given. A popular treatment consisted in wearing an 'electric belt', for neurasthenia, insomnia, muscular paralysis and other such ailments, but this was not found to have any long-term benefits.

In what is called diathermy, a modern method of physiotherapy, high-frequency electric current is used both for warming the deeper layers of tissue, and for alleviating inflammation, stiffness or pain in the joints and muscles, as also for the treatment of warts and tumours. Surgical diathermy can be used for simple 'bloodless' operations, since the diathermy blade cauterizes the tissues as it passes through the flesh leaving practically no bleeding. In electrolysis, electricity is applied to the skin to destroy glands at the roots of the hair, and thus remove superfluous hair. Variations of electro-therapy, usually in the form of radiation therapy, are ultrasonic, microwave, short-wave, X-ray, infrared, ultraviolet and actinotherapy.

Today biotelemetrical devices like the EEG, ECG and other electrical equipment, are standard aids in diagnosis*. In the 1930s electric shock treat-ment in the form of electroconvulsant therapy (abbreviated ECT) was intro-duced for severe forms of mental depression.

But besides the employment of such scientific apparatus, it is believed possible to bring to bear upon a patient the electricity freely available in nature. Electricity is regarded as one of the ultimates of the universe. It is present in everything, and the existence of opposite polarities makes its energy effective wherever it can be tapped. Experimental investigations carried out in the past decade confirm that trees, plants, animal and human subjects, are surrounded by a kind of envelope of electromagnetic energy. Professor Harold Burr, for over forty years a faculty member of the Yale Uni-versity School of Medicine, has said, 'So far as our present information goes, there is unequivocal evidence that wherever there is life there are electrical properties.'

Every living cell and blood corpuscle is electrical in character, and contains positive and negative electric charges; so do tissues, fibres, bones and limbs. The nerves, heart, brain, muscles and sex organs are complex networks of electrical 'wiring', which produce measurable bioelectrical discharges. Every ordinary physiological process, like eating, drinking, evacuation, sleeping, menstruation, ovulation, coition, orgasm, pregnancy; every energetic and healthy impulse; every malignancy and disease, has an electrical reaction. As Dr Leonard Ravitz, a Yale neurophysicist observed, 'Whatever else we may be, we are all electric machines.'

Lovers attract each other by the difference in their charges. It is more than a cliché that sexual activity is an exchange of electricity. According to Wilhelm Reich (d. 1957), 'Orgasm must be a phenomenon of electrical dis-charge.' Every emotion of love, hate, jealousy, rage and grief involves the mobilization of electrical energy.

The electrical potential in the individual undergoes a great increase at a certain age and during certain climacteric periods. Young people reaching puberty generate exceptionally strong currents of energy, and spontaneous electrical phenomena often take place in their presence. Objects become electrically charged, and electric shocks and currents are recorded when they touch things. Lulu Hurst (*c.* 1884), and other so-called 'electric girls', could send men sprawling by just touching them, and cause heavy furniture to move by a wave of the hand, according to contemporary reports.

Everyone has opposites within himself, which are electrical in nature. Different people have different potencies and charges, which either benefit or harm those with whom they come in contact. The application of bioelectric therapy is an extension of the old techniques of biomagnetism*.

One's personal bioelectric potential can be built up by breathing exercises, moderation in living habits and meditation. It is said that the wearing of synthetic fibres, and shoes made of plastic or having synthetic soles, draws out electricity from the system, depletes the etheric vitality and causes nervous disorders.

Books

Baines, A. E., *Studies in Electro-Physiology*, London, 1918.

Burr, Harold Saxton, *Blueprint for Immortality: the Electric Patterns of Life*, Neville Spearman, London, 1972.

Crile, George Washington, *The Phenomena of Life: a Radio-Electric Interpretation*, Norton, New York, 1936.

Frazer, M. A. B., *The Electrical Activity of the Nervous System*, Pitman, London, 1951.

Gibson, Walter, *The Georgia Magnet: Lulu Hurst*, St Louis, 1922.

Halacy, Daniel S., *Radiation, Magnetism and Living Things*, Holiday House, New York, 1966.

Lakhovsky, Georges, *The Secret of Life: Cosmic Rays and Radiations of Living Beings*, 2nd edn, True Health Publishing Co., London, 1951.

Lund, E. J., *Bioelectric Fields and Growth*, University of Texas Press, Austin, 1947.

Pines, Maya, *The Brain Changers: Scientists and the New Mind Control*, Allen Lane, London, 1974.

Ravitz, L. J., 'History, Measurement and Applicability of Periodic Changes in Electromagnetic Fields in Health and Disease', *Annals of the New York Academy of Science*, 98, 1962, 144.

Scott, Pauline, *Clayton's Electrotherapy and Actinotherapy*, Ballière, Tindall & Cassell, London, 1969.

EMBRYONICS

A new name for the study of all *ante-partum* (pre-birth) phases of the foetus, its genetics, biochemistry and physiology. Related studies include artificial generation*, molecular biology, geneosis and embryology.

But it is to be distinguished from embryology, which studies the development of the tissues and organs of the new entity from conception to birth. Broadly the embryological stages proceed as follows:

(1) Sperm deposited in the vagina travels up through the uterus and meets a ripened ovum or egg. (Normally one egg ripens every month during the process of ovulation.) The meeting takes place in the fallopian tube. This stage is called conception or fertilization.

(2) The fertilized egg moves down into the uterus and attaches itself to the wall of the uterus. This process of 'implantation' takes place within two or

three days of fertilization. A woman is said to be pregnant once this stage is reached. The coil, loop or IUD (intrauterine device) in birth-control does not prevent fertilization, but prevents the fertilized egg from attaching itself to the uterus, and effectively leads to abortion.

(3) Once implanted on the uterine wall, the fertilized egg, which is a single cell, divides and subdivides until in about one week there are about one hundred cells, forming a stage of development known as the blastocyst.

(4) From then on the cells multiply rapidly and the growing organism is referred to as the embryo. The organs begin the process of differentiating (organogenesis). After the third month of pregnancy, when the eyes, nose and limbs begin to form and the sex characteristics become recognizable, it is known as a foetus.

The susceptibility of the conceived and growing organism is an important part of the study of embryonics. Up to and including the stage of the blastocyst, that is, about ten days after fertilization, the embryo is apparently resistant to maltreatment. This is because the cells of which it is composed are not yet specialized, and any one of them can form any part of the whole individual. If a cell is destroyed at this stage, another cell grows to compensate for the loss.

It was once thought that, like the blastocyst, the embryo was immune to every influence, short of mechanical interference, gross poisons, and certain infections. But it is now known that after the organogenesis stage has begun the foetus is extremely susceptible to all kinds of agencies that can cause mutilation, mutation, deformity and death. It can be affected by X-rays, by nuclear radiation, by high concentrations of oxygen and by drugs. A number of genetic disorders in children can often be traced to damage during the embryonic stage: autism, mongolism, spasticism, cerebral palsy, aphasia.

The embryo is affected by many of the things that affect the mother: her diet, her dietary or vitamin (especially A and D) deficiencies, the hormone treatment she undergoes, and certain diseases, notably German measles. Serious infections such as smallpox frequently cause miscarriage. The mother's thoughts, her emotions, her way of life, all have a profound effect on the foetus. It is therefore of great importance that the child should be conceived and carried by the woman in a state of emotional contentment. The child should be wanted, and the mother should not have the burden of pregnancy if she rejects it emotionally.

There is also a great deal of mutual interchange, chemical and physiological, between mother and foetus. Although the blood of the mother does not flow into the foetus, which has its own circulatory system, some of the mother's hormonal secretions do pass through the placenta into the circulation of the foetus. The placenta is also permeable to certain drugs, which if taken by the mother can be toxic and damaging to the foetus.

A serious condition arises from what is known as the Rh factor (named from the rhesus monkey in which it was first discovered) in the blood of the human foetus. If the mother is Rh negative (does not have the factor in her blood), and the foetus is Rh positive, the factor can pass through the placenta and cause antibodies to build up in the mother, and these antibodies can then pass back into the foetus, causing erythroblastosis, which destroys the blood cells in the foetus. Such babies can develop jaundice (yellow babies), anaemia and feeble-mindedness. By natural rejection the mother should have a miscarriage, but to prevent this doctors carry out an exchange transfusion while the foetus is still in the womb.

Several drugs and chemicals also cross the placenta and can at times cause damage to the foetus. Pregnant women are being given drugs to alleviate the simple symptoms that have accompanied pregnancy from time immemorial, in order to save them from petty discomforts like nausea and morning sickness. Some doctors feel that while this is helpful in the short term, the long-term effects might not be so harmless.

Furthermore, there are the problems that arise from attempts to prevent spontaneous miscarriage which often occurs in the case of congenital defects. Modern drug therapy provides a means of stopping the natural emptying of the uterus, and the result is that the child is born with a defect.

It is now known that by interfering with the mother's metabolism, thalidomide, once given to women as a sedative, also produced congenital abnormalities, and at the same time prevented spontaneous abortion, allowing a defective foetus to reach full term. The babies were born with *phocomelia* (literally, 'seal extremities'), in which the long bones of the limbs are missing, and only rudimentary hands and feet are attached to the trunk. This tragedy occurred in the winter of 1961-2.

In animal experimentation drugs like penicillin, streptomycin, insulin, cortisone and even aspirin, have been shown to be teratogenic at this stage of development. Similarly LSD may lead to chromosomal breakage and is potentially a cause of congenital malformation.

Pregnant women addicted to heroin, morphine and related drugs may give birth prematurely; the children tend to suffer withdrawal symptoms after birth and to have higher perinatal mortality. They also become more prone to addiction when they grow up. Even mothers who smoke heavily can harm the unborn child.

Finally, the foetus is affected by its own hormones. It is a hormonal impetus from the foetus that triggers the onset of birth pains in the mother. This natural process is nowadays interfered with by drugs. The tendency in many hospitals is to induce labour artificially by injecting a pituitary hormone to stimulate the uterus or force the release of the amniotic fluid in order that the birth time should suit the hospital routine and not disturb the doctor and staff at an inconvenient time. Some authorities regard this as harmful. They believe that the natural course of cosmobiological as well as the hormonal processes that combine to determine the hour of birth are thereby disrupted, which will later lead to mental disturbances in the child.

Books

Hamilton, Michael (ed.), *The New Genetics and the Future of Man*, Eerdmans, Grand Rapids, Michigan, 1972.

Harrell, R. F. *et al.*, *The Effect of Mothers' Diets on the Intelligence of Offspring*, New York, 1955.

Jones, Alun and Bodmer, Walter, *Our Future Inheritance: Choice or Chance?*, Oxford University Press, 1974.

Liggins, G. C. *et al.*, *Foetal Autonomy*, CIBA Foundation, London, 1969.
Montague, A., *Prenatal Influences*, Springfield, Illinois, 1962.
Norton, Alan, *The New Dimensions of Medicine*, Hodder & Stoughton, London, 1969.
Penrose, L. S., *The Biology of Mental Defect*, Sidgwick & Jackson, London, 1949.
Rogers, M. E., *et al.*, *Prenatal and Paranatal Factors in the Development of Childhood Disorders*, Baltimore, 1957.
Wade, O. L., *Adverse Reactions to Drugs*, Heinemann, London, 1973.

EPIDEMICS

Epidemics and their aftermath have been a major factor in the shaping of history. Uncontrolled, they take a terrible toll of the population, paralyse agriculture and trade, bring armies to a halt, cause despair and demoralization, and change the direction of events. Epidemics, says Zinsser, 'have decided more campaigns that Caesar, Hannibal and Napoleon'. The chief diseases that have had these devastating effects on the course of civilization are typhus, typhoid, bubonic plague, cholera and dysentery.

Epidemic outbreaks have been recorded from earliest times. The Bible mentions several such calamities that beset the Israelites or their enemies. Among the earliest was a series of plagues, ending with the decimation of the Egyptian people (Exod. 12) that led to the freedom of the Israelites from Egyptian bondage. This was followed by the 'very great plague' (Num. 11:33) that in 1490 BC swept over the Hebrew tribes still lusting for the fleshpots of Egypt. Twenty years later another plague wiped out 14,700 Israelites (Num. 16:49) who rebelled against the leadership of Moses. In 1140 BC the Philistines who bore off the Ark after defeating the Hebrews were smitten with 'emerods', a word meaning 'swelling', variously interpreted to mean haemorrhoids, or a form of bubonic plague, or a venereal disease since it struck the 'secret parts' of the victims.

In about 700 BC the army of the Assyrian king Sennacherib besieging Hezekiah in Jerusalem was laid low by a plague, for as the Bible states (2 Kings 19:35), 'It came to pass that night that the angel of the Lord smote the camp of the Assyrians, and behold they were all dead corpses.' Herodotus places the event near Pelusium and adds that mice gnawed the bowstrings and shield-handles of the Assyrians, rendering them useless. The presence of mice would suggest bubonic plague.

According to Herodotus, Xerxes king of Persia, who in 480 BC marched against Greece with an army of 800,000 men, was forced to abandon his campaign and return home when a devastating epidemic reduced his forces to less than 500,000 men. The Greek historian Thucydides tells how a great plague brought from Ethiopia and Egypt ravaged Athens in 430 BC and killed over 50,000 people, including the Athenian statesman Pericles. The direct consequence of this disaster was that the Lacedaemonians for long retained their advantage over the Athenians in the internecine Peloponnesian war.

Diodorus Siculus describes an epidemic that attacked the Carthaginian armies besieging Syracuse in 414 BC, and again in 396 BC, compelling them to raise the siege. This was probably a decisive factor in the course of world history, for if the Carthaginians had established a base in Sicily, then in the Punic Wars between Rome and Carthage a century and a half later, Hannibal could easily have displaced Rome as the dominant power in the Mediterranean.

Many devastating plagues struck Rome as well. Livy, the Roman historian, describes an outbreak that afflicted the city in 462 BC, resulting in the loss of thousands of lives. While the Senate ordered prayers and supplications to the gods for relief, priests performed expiatory rites and offered sacrifices, and men, women and children filled the shrines and begged remission of the divine displeasure. In 433 BC another terrible plague visited Rome and lasted for a full year. Intermittently, epidemics of equal severity struck the city, first in 399 BC; again in 364 BC, 347 BC, 330 BC and 293 BC; during the Punic War in 212 BC; and again in 208 BC, 183 BC and 176 BC. Each visitation was a full-scale calamity that decided the outcome of critical battles, changed policies and altered historic decisions.

Tacitus tells of an epidemic of 'extraordinarily destructive virulence' that spread unchecked over Rome and the cities of Italy in AD 54, causing untold suffering. Ten years later the emperor Nero looking for a scapegoat for the miseries of his people blamed the Christians not only for the plague and its consequences, but also for the burning of Rome.

The plague of Galen, physician to Marcus Aurelius Antoninus, so named because he described it, broke out in AD 164, when the army of Verus campaigning to the east against Parthia, looted a temple. It spread rapidly among the soldiers, swept like a whirlwind through the Roman empire, veered upward towards the tribes of the north and did untold damage to several Germanic warrior peoples, including the Marcomanni. In AD 250 there occurred the great epidemic of Cyprian, named after St Cyprian who related the events associated with it. As many times before, it started in Ethiopia, spread swiftly 'from Egypt to Scotland', playing havoc with the Roman armies *en route*, and providing the opportunity for the barbarians to start harassing their outposts. The fall of the western Roman empire is largely attributed to the recurrent waves of disease that paralysed the military strategy and administration of the Roman governors and so played a major role in the downfall of Rome.

Between the fifth and sixth centuries there was a widespread *Völkerwanderung*, a great 'wandering of peoples'. The Huns erupting from China stormed westwards towards the Caspian and Black seas in the direction of Constantinople, which at the time was ill-prepared to meet them. But because of an epidemic of an unknown nature they were forced to change their course and were joined by the Alans. Together the Huns and Alans converged on the Goths who were driven back into Roman territory. The repercussions of these mass encounters led to a large-scale movement of other barbarian tribes, the Avars, Ostrogoths, Visigoths, Suebi, Burgundi, Vandals, Lombards and others, who swarmed in their hordes over Western Europe invading Italy, Gaul, Spain, Britain and North Africa. The Vandals held the Roman provinces of Numidia (Algeria) and Mauretania (Morocco) until a plague almost wiped them out, thus in turn making them an easy prey to the Muhammadans.

The Byzantine empire was in like manner rendered ineffective by epidemics and she too fell victim to the incursions of the barbarian tribes. Plague after plague racked Constantinople and her provincial cities and towns. The plague of Justinian, brought from Ethiopia in AD 540, lasted for fifty years and so shattered the imperial economy that it became one of the chief contributory causes of the decline of Byzantium.

The history of the Crusades continues the sad chronicle of crippling epidemics which determined many a victory or defeat. In Europe itself the story of the struggle for existence of the newly emerging nations is repeatedly marked by disease. Petty princes won unexpected kingdoms because an epidemic had reduced the army of their more ambitious neighbours, and great provinces fell to usurping rivals because a disease had rendered the populace too weak and helpless to resist. The English soldiers before the battle of Crécy in 1346 were called 'the bare-bottomed army' by the French, because they were riddled with dysentery.

In the middle of the fourteenth century Europe was visited by one of the greatest epidemics in recorded history. Originating in India, a virulent type of bubonic plague travelled swiftly across Persia and Turkey, and then spread a swathe of destruction over the Western world. This was the notorious Black Death of 1348-52. A pall seemed to settle over the continent, and people were persuaded that the end of the world was at hand. The dead could not be buried fast enough, and Pope Clement VI (d. 1352) was obliged to consecrate the Rhône so that the corpses could be dumped straight into the river. It is estimated that this terrible pestilence took the lives of 42 million people in Europe, or one-third of the total population. In less virulent form it recurred at regular intervals in 1361, 1371, 1382 and so on through the fifteenth and sixteenth centuries.

The Black Death gave rise to many strange societies, both secular (whose members spent their days in reckless merrymaking) and religious (largely devoted to caring for the sick and burying the dead). Also curious dances (the danse macabre, and St Vitus's dance later applied to a nervous disorder), sects (the Flagellants, Beggar Societies, the Eleutherians), several strange characters, the most notable being the semi-legendary Pied Piper of Hamelin, and a curious literature both gay and morbid. The memory of the Black Death remained deeply etched in the psyche of Europe for centuries.

Another kind of epidemic, the English 'sweating sickness', an unidentified inflammatory fever, broke out in 1485 and spread rapidly through the kingdom, brought agriculture and trade to a halt, forced the universities to close down, and caused the virtual paralysis of the country's social, academic and commercial life.

The first syphilis* epidemic, imported from the New World in 1495, infiltrated into every corner of the continent of Europe and by the seventeenth century brought the infection to most of the royal houses.

In 1520 smallpox came to Mexico from Cuba along with the Negro slaves brought over by the Spaniards. The Aztecs were not used to the new disease, and before the end of the century a succession of epidemics killed over 18 million out of the total population of 25 million people. It caused considerably more devastation than the Spanish conquerors.

Back in Europe the epoch-making struggle between Francis I of France

(d. 1547) and Charles V was terminated when an epidemic killed over half the French army in a single month. Says Zinsser, 'Charles V was crowned ruler of the Roman Empire by the power of Typhus Fever.' The struggles between the Italian cities, the wars between France and Italy, the English Civil War, were all frequently resolved by epidemics. The Thirty Years' War in all its phases was dominated by disease. The Great Plague of London of 1665 described by Daniel Defoe and Samuel Pepys was only a minor episode in a lengthy chronicle of calamities that ravaged Europe throughout this period.

In 1792 the French Revolution might have been ended had not the armies of Prussia and Austria, which were moving against the revolutionaries and could easily have crushed them, been halted by an outbreak of dysentery, thus giving the French time to consolidate their position. In Napoleon's career the impact of epidemics that laid low his army time and again decided the fate of more than one important battle. In his Russian campaign his task army numbered 265,000 men; only 90,000 reached Moscow, the greater number killed not by snow but by typhus, months before they reached the capital.

The American Civil War tells the same story of the determining influence of disease on the outcome of war. In the Federal armies alone almost 45,000 men were killed in battle, and almost 50,000 died of wounds, but 185,000 died of sickness. After the First World War an influenza* epidemic carried off more people in a few months than had been killed on both sides in four years of fighting.

The European colonizers were able to establish vast empires overseas largely because malaria, plague and other epidemics had made the native populations lethargic, inefficient and backward. In Africa diseases of various kinds such as those carried by the tsetse fly did much damage to their live-stock, and made them still more vulnerable.

The study of epidemic diseases clearly shows that they constitute one of the most mysterious 'chance' factors in history. Their onset is unpredictable, their effects beyond calculation. Because of their terrible nature, they were regarded almost universally as a visitation of God. Accounts of ancient and medieval epidemics and pestilences show that people were stricken with a sense of extreme terror, saw portents in the sky and phantom shapes in streets and houses, and all kinds of superstitious notions as to the cause and remedy were rife. Even today there is a theory that the outbreak of epidemics might be linked with natural phenomena having cosmobiological effects, like volcanic eruptions, earthquakes, abnormal weather conditions, eclipses, comets, sunspots and cosmic rays.

Notwithstanding the establishment of the microbe* origin of disease, we can no more say what actually triggers an outburst of virulent germ activity than we can explain the sudden periodical breeding explosion among certain animals like the lemming. The microbes that cause most diseases* are present everywhere, yet they do not cause epidemics. Some medical authorities feel that there will always remain an unknown factor in epidemiology, and our ignorance of the true nature of infection* suggests that there may yet be some unpleasant surprises in store for us.

Books

Cartwright, Frederick, *Disease and History*, Hart-Davis, London, 1972.

Colnat, A., *Les Epidémies de l'histoire*, Paris, 1937.

Crawfurd, Raymond, *Plague and Pestilence in Literature and Art*, Clarendon Press, Oxford, 1914.

Creighton, Charles, *A History of Epidemics in Britain*, Cambridge University Press, 1891.

Gill, M., *The Genesis of Epidemics and the Natural History of Disease*, Ballière, Tindall & Cox, London, 1928.

Greenwood, M., *Epidemics and Crowd Diseases*, Macmillan, New York, 1935.

Hecker, J. F. K., *The Epidemics of the Middle Ages*, Sydenham Society, London, 1844.

Longmate, N., *King Cholera*, Hamish Hamilton, London, 1966.

McNeil, William, *Plagues and People*, Basil Blackwell, Oxford, 1977.

Morris, R. J., *Cholera*, Croom Helm, London, 1977.

Nohl, Johannes, *The Black Death*, Allen & Unwin, London, 1960.

Prinzing, F., *Epidemics Resulting From Wars*, Oxford, 1916.

Scott, H. H., *Some Notable Epidemics*, Edward Arnold, London, 1934.

Shrewsbury, J. F. D., *The Plague of the Philistines*, Gollancz, London, 1964.

Smith, Geddes, *Plague on Us*, Commonwealth Fund, New York, 1941.

Zinsser, Hans, *Rats, Lice and History*, New York, 1967.

EPILEPSY

A generic term applied to a group of diseases of the central nervous system usually marked by such symptoms as convulsions and the sudden impairment or complete loss of consciousness. In Greek mythology Hercules was a sufferer from epilepsy, which came to be known as the disease of Hercules. Till Hippocrates (d. 359 BC) decreed otherwise, it was regarded by the Greeks as the 'sacred disease', an affliction sent by the gods. The Romans too regarded it as supernatural, and called it *morbus sacer*, 'sacred illness', or else *morbus demoniacus*, 'devil's disease'. When a member of the comitia, the Roman people's assembly, was attacked with epilepsy while the assembly was in session, it was taken as a sign of divine displeasure, and the comitia was dissolved. It was therefore also known as the *morbus comitialis*, 'comitial disease'. At one time people referred to it as the 'filthy disease', probably because general muscular impairment accompanies seizure; the patient can sweat profusely, and may become temporarily incontinent, involuntarily discharging urine and faeces.

The symptoms of epilepsy vary to some extent, but in general it proceeds on the following lines. In certain forms a strange premonitory warning is received which gives the patient time to find a place of seclusion and safety. The ancients said that an epileptic who felt an attack coming on rushed home or to a deserted place, and covered his head, either from shame of the disease or dread of the deity. Sometimes, indeed, there is an inexplicable sense of terror.

The premonitory sensations are spoken of as the epileptic 'aura' (Lat. 'breeze'), which often feels like a gust of wind playing on some part of the body and moving up towards the head. The victim feels that an external power is rapidly taking possession of him. This may be accompanied by a peculiar sense of the immanent revelation of some great mystery. Hence the common notion that the spirit or breath of God was infusing the individual. However, such epileptic auras are not always present.

Sometimes the victim feels as if he had received a blow in the epigastrium, and there is tension and constriction in the stomach. Other symptoms include palpitations, dizziness and interior noises, a ringing in the ears, dimness of eyesight, spots before the eyes, a sensation of cobwebs covering the face and approaching confusion. The patient is conscious of his surroundings, but only vaguely, as if in a trance or dream. In this dreamy state patients sometimes have the experience of being transported elsewhere to places that seem strangely familiar (*déjà vu*), or of seeing panoramic scenes of childhood or hearing voices of people who are not present. At times the victim suffers an epileptic furor or delirium; he becomes violent, rushes about, vociferates loudly. Some have even been known to commit murder at such times. Aretaeus (*c.* AD 80), a physician of Cappadocia, compared the behaviour of an epileptic during an attack to that of an ox whose throat had been cut.

Hippocratic writings used the name 'great disease' for epilepsy. This, translated literally into Latin, was *morbus maior*, which in turn became the medieval French *grand mal*, today a standard designation for the great epileptic attack accompanied by convulsions. This is to be distinguished from *petit mal*, which is a momentary blackout for a few seconds, without convulsions. The patient may just suddenly cry out and fall down unconscious.

Convulsions* are characteristic of the more serious form of the disease. There are violent contortions and writhings of the whole frame, jerkings of the head and limbs with the legs kicking in all directions. Males have an erection of the penis and sometimes a discharge of semen. To summarize some of the other concomitants: the arms are twisted, the hands cramped, the whole face swollen, red and distorted, the veins on the neck stand out. The cheeks tremble, the eyes roll about, the pupils are dilated, the mouth dry, the teeth clenched and gnashing, or the tongue protruding and often bitten, the lips pursed or retracted into a grimacing smile. Strange sounds issue from the mouth, which begins to fill with foam. So shocking is the sight that a sensitive onlooker is liable to succumb to a mild attack himself.

In a very literal sense epilepsy is a brain storm. It was in fact so described by medieval writers who compared it to a tempest: here too were the premonitory warning signals, the dark and tumultuous clouds, the thunder and lightning and the devastating effects of the onslaught. After the seizure comes the calm, and the victim is usually quite unaware of what happened during the attack.

A number of factors thought to predispose one to epilepsy: heredity, constitution, age, sex and the seasons. The moon, which according to the ancient theory had the same cold temperament as the brain, is liable to inflict headache and epilepsy. Hippocrates said that epilepsy befalls phlegmatics and never cholerics. Melancholics*, too, tend to epilepsy. Catarrh is a predisposing factor since the phlegm and other fluxes in the head become tainted, and these cerebral excrements lead to oppilation or 'blocking' of the ventricles of the brain and thus cause epilepsy. Anything directly affecting the brain can bring on a fit: foetal disease, birth injury, infectious disease, cerebral injury, brain tumour. Furthermore, certain kinds of violent disruptive sounds have a disturbing effect on some people and what is known as musicogenic epilepsy can be precipitated by certain kinds of music.

Medical experts regard epilepsy as a syndrome, a group of symptoms rather than a specific disease. Physicians speak of the epilepsies, in the plural rather than in the singular. The focus of the various types can often be fairly well defined in a specific brain region. In physiological terms electrical energy piles up until it reaches a point where it discharges. But an epileptic discharge is always potential in the central nervous system, and with sufficient stimulation, whether electrical, chemical, mechanical or emotional, any person can have a fit, for everyone is a latent epileptic.

It is commonly recognized that certain disturbances associated with adolescence include not only schizophrenia* (originally called dementia praecox, 'insanity of youth'), and the type of schizophrenia still known as hebephrenia (from another word meaning 'youth'), but epilepsy itself, which occurs most frequently in the early period of life. On the other hand, it has been remarked that epilepsy and schizophrenia are 'opposite' diseases, and those who suffer from the one never suffer from the other. Medieval writers sometimes contrasted hysteria* which affected males with hysteria which affected females.

Medical terms with the suffix '-lepsy' (Gk. *lēpsis*, 'seizure'), such as epilepsy, catalepsy, narcolepsy, and analepsy; and the suffix '-plexy' (Gk. *plēssein*, 'to strike'), such as cataplexy and apoplexy, retain evidence of their supposed epileptic origin.

Two kinds of epilepsy were once distinguished, namely *idiopathic*, which started in the brain owing to an obstruction of the ventricles and which extended downwards; and *analeptic*, arising from vapours generated in a lower organ such as the epigastrium and ascended to the brain. In women analepsy was thought to originate in the womb and erupt in hysteria. For centuries it was believed that hysteria was an 'opposite' variety of epilepsy.

Various forms of paroxysm, convulsive seizure, syncope (a sudden fainting fit arising from anaemia of the brain), coma, clonus (muscular spasms such as myoclonus), tetany (painful muscular cramps) and ataxia (lack of muscular co-ordination) are characterized by symptoms that have a strong family resemblance to epilepsy.

Many simple ailments and everyday phenomena have likewise been ascribed an epileptic origin. The ancient Greeks said that those whom they regarded as the 'ancients' in their day, called vertigo a 'little epilepsy', and indeed giddiness has at times been given an almost supernatural significance.

The Stoics compared anger to epilepsy, pointing out that the trembling of the limbs, the dilated eyes, the contorted face and the heavy breathing were symptoms identical with the falling sickness. Plutarch (d. AD 120) advised the person who felt his rage rising to flee and hide himself until he regained his composure, just as the person who felt an epileptic attack coming on ran off and hid to save himself embarrassment.

Jean Baptiste van Helmont (d. 1644) believed that asthmatic attacks were related to epilepsy, and referred to asthma as 'the falling sickness of the lungs'.

Cesare Lombroso (d. 1909) commented that 'many cases of headache (migraine*) or simple loss of memory are now recognized as forms of epilepsy'.

John Hughlings Jackson (d. 1911), one of the greatest authorities on nervous diseases, said that even 'a sneeze is a sort of healthy epilepsy'.

It would seem that from the cradle to the grave our normal lives are punctuated at intervals by epileptic attacks. Every night just before falling asleep we experience a light myoclonic jerk. Aristotle (d. 322 BC) went further; he said: 'Sleep is similar to epilepsy and in some way sleep is epilepsy.' Hippocrates said, 'Coitus is a light epileptic attack', and indeed the convulsive spasms of orgasm have often been compared to the disease. If therefore conception is rooted in 'epilepsy', so is birth. The growing foetus in the womb suffers periodical seizures. A month or so before birth the child begins to get more regular convulsive seizures which increase as the time of birth approaches. Labour pains preceding birth are thought to be triggered by the more violent epileptic paroxysms of the infant half-suffocated in the womb. And finally, the throes that precede death may represent the terminal convulsions of an epileptic seizure marking the surrender of life.

Among the cures prescribed for epilepsy in earlier times were: blood-drinking, especially human blood, swallowing the powdered skin of a lizard, drinking a posset made with the rennet of a seal, and similar outlandish medicaments. A mixture of vinegar and honey was highly recommended. Fever, particularly if it could be induced in a patient, was believed to banish epilepsy; it is said that this was tried in an attempt to cure Louis XI (d. 1483) of France of this ailment. Grated bits of human skull mixed with food and eaten was another common remedy; even great and fashionable physicians like Robert Boyle (d. 1691) advocated this. Crocodile dung was prescribed by Alexandrian physicians (c. 220 BC), and the dung of various other animals continued to be prescribed till the seventeenth century in Europe. Trepanning, cauterization, scarification, setonization, fumigation, massage, emetics and purgatives were of course recommended as well. Castration was one of the more drastic remedies. According to Hector Boece (d. 1536) it was customary among the Scots to castrate men with hereditary diseases, including epilepsy.

Among the things to be avoided were: sexual intercourse; baths; crossing the hands and feet at any time, whether standing, sitting or lying down; black garments. Also to be avoided were onions, garlic, seafish, quail and, especially, the meat of goats, which animal is 'most seized with epilepsy', and whose flesh is impregnated with the quality that can communicate it.

Among the saints associated with epilepsy and whose intercession was sought in the Middle Ages were St Lupus, St John, St Valentine and St Vitus. Because the three wise men 'fell down' (Mt. 2:11), their names, Gaspar, Melchior and Balthasar were invoked in various supplicatory chants.

In its extreme form epilepsy has long been associated with delusional fantasies, and also with religiosity and mystical experience. The early Greeks, as already stated, regarded it as sacred. They believed that the epileptic during his seizure was a mouthpiece of the gods, and treated him with great respect. Epilepsy sometimes has a resemblance to possession, mediumship and multiple personality. Its symptoms may include speaking in tongues, or in a strange voice, and experiences of *déjà vu*. The phenomena associated with the Convulsionaries, Pentecostalists, Flagellants and other ecstatic sects, as well as with those afflicted with the dancing mania, the jerkers at revival meetings, with various convulsive outbreaks in schools, convents and women's wards, and similar historical instances of individual and mass hysteria*, bear distinctly epileptic features.

It has been observed that the highest faculties of the mind have a strange connection with epilepsy. Aristotle, in fact, related epilepsy to genius. Other early writers too have noted the close relationship between the sudden impact of inspiration that descends on poets, sibyls, prophets and diviners, and the sudden seizure of the epileptic. Modern psychiatrists have also pointed out the resemblance; Lombroso, for instance, spoke of the epileptoid nature of genius.

The following is a chronological list of a few famous people who were epileptics. Hercules, the Greek mythological hero after whom epilepsy was also called the Herculean disease; King Saul (fl. 1095 BC), mentioned in the Bible; Cambyses (d. 522 BC), the Persian king who invaded Egypt and killed himself in an epileptic frenzy; Socrates (d. 399 BC), Greek philosopher and teacher of Plato; Alexander the Great (d. 323 BC); Callimachus (d. 240 BC), head of the Alexandrian library; Julius Caesar (d. 44 BC); Caligula (d. AD 41), Roman emperor; St Paul (d. AD 67), apostle of the gentiles; Muhammad (d. AD 632), prophet of Arabia; Duns Scotus (d. 1308), one of the greatest of the medieval schoolmen; Francesco Petrarch (d. 1374), Italian lyric poet; Charles V (d. 1558), in his day the most powerful ruler in Europe; Benvenuto Cellini (d. 1571), goldsmith and sculptor; St Teresa of Avila (d. 1582); Torquato Tasso (d. 1595), Italian poet; William Shakespeare (d. 1616), who probably died of an epileptic seizure; Cardinal Richelieu (d. 1642); Molière (d. 1673), French dramatist; Henri de Turenne (d. 1675), French general; Jacques Bossuet (d. 1704), churchman and orator; Peter the Great (d. 1725), ruler of Russia; Jonathan Swift (d. 1745), author of *Guilliver's Travels;* George Frederick Handel (d. 1759) and Wolfgang Amadeus Mozart (d. 1791), famous musicians; Warren Hastings (d. 1818), greatest of Indian administrators; Napoleon Bonaparte (d. 1821); Lord Byron (d. 1824), who had several attacks before he died; Nicolo Paganini (d. 1840), who was both epileptic and consumptive; Felix Mendelssohn (d. 1847), composer; the Duke of Wellington (d. 1852), who suffered with fits throughout his career; Alfred de Musset (d. 1857), dramatist, novelist and poet; Charles Baudelaire (d. 1867), French poet; Hector Berlioz (d. 1869), whose death was preceded by epileptic fits; the brothers Jules (d. 1870) and Edmond (d. 1896) de Goncourt, French novelists; Gustave Flaubert (d. 1880), French novelist; Fyodor Dostoevsky (d. 1881), Russian novelist; Modest Mussorgsky (d. 1881), Russian composer; Vincent van Gogh (d. 1890), Dutch post-Impressionist painter; St Teresa of Lisieux (d. 1897); Algernon Charles Swinburne (d. 1909), English poet.

Books

Ajmone-Marsan, C. and Ralston, B. L., *The Epileptic Seizure*, Thomas, Springfield, Illinois, 1957.

Alström, Carl Henry, *A Study of Epilepsy in Its Clinical, Social and Genetic Aspects*, Munksgaard, Copenhagen, 1950.

Barrow, R. L. and Fabing, H. D., *Epilepsy and the Law*, Hoeber-Harper, New York, 1956.

Gastaut, Henri, *The Epilepsies*, Thomas, Springfield, Illinois, 1954.

Gowers, W. R., *Epilepsy and Other Chronic Convulsive Diseases*, London, 1881.

Green, J. R. and Steelman, H. F. (eds), *Epileptic Seizures*, Williams & Wilkins, Baltimore, 1956.

Janz, Dieter, *Die Epilepsien*, Thieme, Stuttgart, 1969.

Lennox, W. G., *Science and Seizures*, Harper, New York, 1941.

Murphy, Edward L., 'The Saints of Epilepsy', *Medical History*, 3, 1959, 303–11.

Penfield, Wilder and Jasper, Herbert, *Epilepsy and the Functional Anatomy of the Human Brain*, Little, Brown, Boston, 1954.

Reynolds, J. R., *Epilepsy: Its Symptoms, Treatment and Relation to Other Chronic Convulsive Diseases*, London, 1861.

Rolleston, J. D., 'The Folk-lore of Epilepsy', *Medical Press and Circular*, 209, 1943, 154–7.

Sieveking, Edward, *On Epilepsy and Epileptiform Seizures*, London, 1858.

Temkin, O., *The Falling Sickness*, 2nd rev. edn. Johns Hopkins Press, Baltimore, 1971.

Turner, William Aldren, *Epilepsy: a Study of the Idiopathic Disease*, Macmillan, New York, 1907.

Unverricht, Heinrich, *Die Myoklonie*, Leipzig, 1891.

EROTOMANIA

An overactive eroticism manifesting in excessive and persistent sex desire. As there is no fixed norm of sexual activity, the precise definition of what can be regarded as excessive is not determinable. Erotomania may arise as a result of unsatisfied sexual urges, a lack of response from the partner, lack of self-confidence or a feeling of insecurity. It may also be symptomatic of mental illness so that the patient constantly seeks but seldom achieves satisfaction. It is to be distinguished from the normal tides of desire found in all animals, including human beings.

In men, erotomania is known as satyriasis, named after the ancient Greek satyrs, who with phallus erect were always chasing and ravishing the fleeing woodland nymphs. Where the penis is in a state of constant or prolonged erection or semi-erection, we have what is known as priapism, which is usually unrelated to sexual desire and is a physiological disorder. It often appears in epilepsy*, tuberculosis*, inflammation of the kidneys, acute prostatic infection and spinal injury.

Men who cannot find satisfaction with one woman, but change their partners frequently, acquiring the reputation of a Don Juan, Casanova or Lothario, are very often trying to convince themselves of their own masculinity. Some men seek the company of prostitutes because of a pathological need to indulge their pornomania (Gk. *pornē*, 'prostitute'), for it is only in one or other of the forms of aberration that prostitutes provide that they achieve sexual fulfilment. True satyriasis does not seek reassurance of manhood nor perverse sex.

Erotomania is more prevalent among women, as seen in nymphomania, where satisfaction may be sought in perverse ways as in lesbianism, although it is usually obtained from males, and specifically termed andromania (Gk.

andros, 'man'). As a rule the inordinate desire for sexual stimulation and intercourse arises from her inability to achieve complete orgasm in the way she wants, but there may be hormonal reasons. 'Nymphomania,' writes Richard Burton (d. 1890), 'is always attributed by Easterners to worms in the vagina.'

A very distressing kind of nymphomania is what was once known as *furor uterinus*, 'excitement of the womb', believed to be a furor* inspired by Aphrodite and Eros. This is a severe nervous disorder often arising from enforced celibacy and once common in convents. In this condition sexual desire is constantly present, highly salacious images come to the mind, the subject raves in erotic frenzy and the genitals undergo uncontrollable spasms that crave sexual satisfaction.

There is a striking similarity between the language used by female saints and ecstatics during their experience of the *unio mystica*, the 'mystical union' of the soul with God, when they are in the highest stages of religious rapture, and the language of erotic frenzy. Indeed they themselves speak of the *incendium amoris*, 'fire of love', a burning sensation that consumes the heart and melts the limbs, terminating in a 'liquefaction of the soul with God'. Some psychologists attribute all so-called spiritual states of this nature entirely to erotomania (*see* medical materialism).

A more distinctive manifestation of erotomania is found in sexual deviation, particularly homosexuality, in which a person finds normal modes of sexual satisfaction inadequate. The causes of such deviation have been variously sought. In some cases it is thought to be due to the drugs taken by the mother during pregnancy. Others believe it arises from continuous exposure to sexual situations and sexual stimulation from an early age, which results in a blunting of the sexual centres and leads to experimentation into more intensive areas to obtain sexual satisfaction.

Some regard sexual perversion as a sign of emotional immaturity and a regression to the infantile; an unwillingness to accept the responsibilities of growing up; a refusal to make lasting attachments with the opposite sex; a rejection of family life. It is a form of protest against society. Again, the decline of religious and moral standards, the anathema placed by modern psychology against creating feelings of guilt and shame, and the consequent lack of parental and social disapproval, leads to a growing tolerance of perversion. Some would treat sexual perversion as an etherosis*, an illness of the second body.

Others again would point out that besides being a pathological manifestation in the individual, erotomania as an inflammation of the libido is actually a commonplace symptom of a deeper sociopsychosis* infecting the whole of Western civilization, as seen in the cryptopornography or incipient pornography of public advertising, the mass media and entertainment. Modern man is obsessed with sex. He receives in one way or another, thanks to psychological and sociological progress, constant reminders of sex every hour of the day, every day of the year. Sex is all-pervasive, and there are few features of life and activity that are not saturated with sexual overtones. We are, some believe, becoming sex-mad.

Books

Bienville, T., *Nymphomania: a Dissertation Concerning the Furor Uterinus*, London, 1875.

Burton, Sir Richard, *Love, War and Fancy*, Kimber, London, 1964.

Ellis, Albert and Sagarin, Edward, *Nymphomania*, London, 1968.

Hirschfeld, Magnus, *Sexual Anomalies and Perversions*, Francis Aldor, London, 1944.

Laurent, E. and Nagour, F., *Magica Sexualis*, Falstaff Press, New York, 1934.

Lilar, Suzanne, *Aspects of Love*, Thames & Hudson, London, 1965.

Longworth, T. C., *The Devil a Monk Would Be*, Herbert Joseph, London, 1936.

Masters, R. E. L., *The Hidden World of Erotica: an Objective Re-Examination of Perverse Sex Practices in Different Cultures*, Lyrebird Press, 1973.

Taylor, G. Rattray, *Sex in History*, Thames & Hudson, London, 1959.

Wellesley, Gordon, *Sex and the Occult*, Souvenir Press, London, 1973.

ETHEROSIS

A disorder of the 'second body' of man, forms the subject of etheric pathology. In occultism the second body is asomatic or non-material and is made up of the astral and etheric systems. The astral body is associated with the pathemic or emotional side of the individual, and his higher intellectual faculties. The etheric body co-ordinates the vitalic processes in the human organism, and is subject to certain diseases connected both with the somatic or physical system, and the astral or emotional system. The etheric body carries the bioplasmic current of life-energy, controls the animal, procreative and survival instincts, is the seat of the five senses, of brain consciousness, sensual passion, the sexual drive, pleasure and pain. It interacts with the physical body in the areas of the plexuses, and the pineal and perhaps other endocrine glands. Expressions like 'second sight', the 'third eye', the 'fourth dimension', the 'sixth sense', and many paraesthetic* phenomena relate to the sphere where the etheric body operates.

Like the physical body, the etheric body is prone to various pathological conditions. In the occult view many diseases, physical and mental, are etheric in origin, so that an awareness of the second body is basic to an understanding of many aspects of health and healing. The etheric blueprint determines the vitalic potential of the individual. Senility is the decline, and death the disintegration, of the etheric blueprint. Disease like cancer*, migraine*, epilepsy* and certain psychosomatic* allergies, could perhaps be better understood when considered as the malfunctioning of the etheric system within the physical, or a faulty co-ordination between the two.

Asthma could perhaps be included in the latter category. It is a fit of laborious breathing, in particular difficulty in breathing out, and a prolonged attack can be very distressing to the onlooker. It is associated with the most diverse factors, including the weather, diet and occupation. As there are types of people who are prone to migraine and tuberculosis, so there are types who get asthma. They are usually introspective, nervous and anxious. The condition is aggravated by emotional shock, or emotional factors such as an unhappy home situation. Indeed, some regard asthma as almost entirely psychosomatic and an unconscious appeal for sympathy.

In some cases asthma may be due to an allergy, which is the hypersensitivity of an individual to a certain substance, known as an allergen, which is normally quite harmless and to which others remain immune, but to which he over-reacts with an abnormal response. The effect of an allergy is entirely personal and its ultimate cause remains a mystery. The physiological reason for allergies is the release of a substance called histamine, ordinarily locked up in the body cells, which results in histamine poisoning of the system. Physicians use antihistamines to allay allergic manifestations.

People can be allergic to all kinds of things. A baby can be allergic to its own mother's milk. Some people are allergic to special colours, like a particular shade of red. The presence of summer pollen in the air will give violent hay fever to the sensitive. Persons can be allergic to drugs and injections, the administration of which can produce anaphylaxis, a kind of serum-sickness. Curiously, the body can be allergic to its own tissues and to substances manufactured by itself, the condition being known by the inappropriate term, autoimmunity ('autoallergy' has been suggested as more accurate). Auto-immune diseases include goitre, pernicious anaemia, haemolytic anaemia, nephritis and rheumatoid arthritis.

Allergies can cause phobic reactions as well, and many irrational physiological responses are associated with morbid fears. Some curious allergies and allergic phobias have been recorded of historical personalities. Julius Caesar (d. 44 BC), it is said, could not bear to see a fowl, and was unable to hear a cock crowing without a shudder. The Italian poet Ludovico Ariosto (d. 1533) broke into a rash whenever he had a bath. Desiderius Erasmus (d. 1536) got fever whenever he ate fish. Jerome Cardan (d. 1576), mathematician and physician, could not suffer eggs. Henry III (d. 1589) of France could not bear to remain in a chamber with a cat and would collapse in a faint if one touched him. Tycho Brahe (d. 1601), the great astronomer, felt his knees give way whenever he saw a hare or a fox. Joseph Scaliger (d. 1609), the great scholar, trembled at the sight of ordinary cress. Maria dei Medici (d. 1642), though she loved flowers, could not bear to see a rose, and felt faint if she saw even a painted rose.

Severe emotional reaction to a situation or a person is also a form of allergy and can give rise to many strange symptoms affecting respiration, the heart, the skin and viscera. As a rule these are not amenable to antihistamine treatment. Psychotherapy is sometimes recommended in cases of chronic allergy where a psychosomatic origin is suspected.

The phobias, obsessions* and peculiar psychological quirks that seem to be linked with some allergic attacks have raised puzzling questions as to their actual source. Some psychologists have suggested that there are deeper subconscious reasons for certain allergies which may go back to the individual's early history or even an ancestral experience, the memory of which is inherited and lies latent in the bodily cells. It is a legacy bequeathed to the second body.

Mental illness in most of its manifestations, such as psychosis, cyclothymia*, some kinds of monomania*, neurosis* and hysteria*, could be explained as temporary or permanent disorders within the second body. Similarly certain xenophrenic* and so-called occult states are said to be due to a displacement of the second body. Catalepsy*, cataplexy*, epilepsy and sus-pended animation represent the separation of the physical and etheric (or astral) systems. Nightmares are believed to arise from a torsion of the astral cord during sleep, producing hallucinations and terrifying dreams. Possession*, multiple personality*, expersonation and psychic vampirism* represent the involvement or entanglement of alien forces with one's etheric double.

All so-called nature spirits and elementals are life-forms of the etheric dimension. Ghosts, wraiths and other apparitions (where they are not astral projections of living people), are usually earth-bound entities who have not been able to shed their etheric vehicle in the normal way after death. The emanations of the etheric body constitute the ectoplasm of spiritualistic séances; and physical mediumship and séance-room phenomena such as apports and materializations occur through the intermediary of the etheric element.

Several types of psychopathology* could be regarded as inflammatory conditions of the etheric system. In their gross form these frequently mani-fest in abnormal preoccupation with some bodily substance. The patient constantly thinks and talks about it, and has a strong urge to touch and even eat it. This may be faeces, as in coprophagy, or dung-eating; or urine, as in urodipsia, a yearning to drink urine; or blood, as in haemolagnia, a lust for blood; or semen, as in spermepotation; or forbidden flesh, as in cannibalism, or necrophagy, eating dead bodies.

The major pathological symptoms, however, are associated with sex, and usually lead to erotomania* and deviations of various kinds, ranging from pornography to sex murder. Thus, trans-sexualism, in which the victim feels that he is of the sex opposite to that which he manifests in his outward sexual appearance; and transvestism, the uncontrollable desire to wear clothes appropriate to the opposite sex, are probable indications that through some genetic quirk the physical counterpart differs in gender from its etheric blue-print.

In the occult view most forms of sexual deviation stem from etheric disorders, including homosexuality or sexual interest in one's own sex; bestia-lity or sexual congress with animals; necrophilia or sexual intercourse with corpses; and algolagnia including sadism and masochism. An unusual manifes-tation of etheric sexuality is found in what is called *congressus subtilis* or intercourse with a succubus or incubus, which is said to be practised by black magicians. All the more sinister forms of occultism seek power from debased etheric sources, including satanism, demonolatry, witchcraft, sorcery, necro-mancy, voodoo, wanga and obeah.

Rare and extreme examples of etherosis or ethero-pathology could lie behind the deep-rooted beliefs we find enshrined in folklore throughout the world. These centre around the zombie, the vampire and the werewolf. In Haitian belief the zombie is said to be a fresh corpse that has been reanimated by the *bokor* or sorcerer so that it behaves as if alive. Occultists have sug-gested that this would imply the empowering of the etheric counterpart of a dead person before its separation from the physical (*see* death diagnostics). The vampire, on the other hand, is popularly regarded as the reanimated body of a dead person who periodically rises from the tomb and seeks nourishment by sucking the blood of the living. This tradition may again be based on the apparition of an earthbound entity, or possibly the materialized etheric double of a left-hand adept who is able to replenish his etheric energy by drawing nourishment from the etheric bodies of others while they sleep.

Again, certain obscure pathologies might create in the victim the belief that he is an animal. This could account for the common folk-tradition of therianthropy, where the form of a man allegedly changes into that of a wild beast, so that he becomes a were-animal. It is also known as shape-shifting, and in Europe usually takes the form of lycanthropy, in which the person becomes a werewolf. The Norse sagas speak of the *berserker*, a class of savage fighters who wore bear skins, growled like bears and sexually mated with the wild animals that crossed their path.

Several theories have been put forward to explain therianthropy. Thus, in a rare disease called lupinomania (or *folie louvière*) the victim has a sensation of extreme dryness in the mouth and suffers inordinate thirst, which may drive him to savage others and drink their blood. A related form of paranoic insanity called zoanthropy gives the victim the delusion of being an animal, and where opportunity offers expresses itself in cannibalism, sadism, erotomania, sodomy, bestiality, and haemothymia or pathological excitement at the sight of blood. In the condition known as lycorexia, probably the result of glandular disturbance, the person believes he is a wolf; he howls like a wolf, feels wolfish hunger and thirst for blood.

In addition, certain drugs like the alkaloids found in the roots of the gelsemium give one the sensation of the skin being covered with thick hair. There are, of course, a number of recorded cases of wolf-children who were reared by wild animals to become feral men. Therianthropy has also been explained in terms of an atavism, or reversion to an earlier evolutionary phase of development.

The aetiology* of etherosis includes many of the causes that give rise to other ordinary physical and mental diseases. Diagnosis* requires a special intuitive faculty and psychic sensitivity. Radiesthesia and auroscopy may be useful in detecting the condition of the bioplasmic aura. Treatment is difficult. Some drugs have a disastrous effect on the second body, causing inadvertent dissociation and thus aggravating an already discordant state. Exorcism*, religious therapy*, prayer and related psychotherapies seem to be the most effective.

Books

Copper, Basil, *The Vampire in Legend, Fact and Art*, Robert Hale, London, 1973.

Eisler, Robert, *Man Into Wolf: an Anthropological Interpretation of Sadism, Masochism and Lycanthropy*, Routledge & Kegan Paul, London, 1951.

Farson, D. and Hall, A., *Vampires, Zombies, Monsters, Monster Men and Mythic Beasts*, Aldus Books, London, 1975.

Fortune, Dion, *Psychic Self Defence*, Aquarian Press, London, 1952.

Graham-Bonnalie, M., *Allergies: Asthma, Hay Fever, Dermatitis, Migraine and Others*, David & Charles, London, 1970.

Kemp, Robert, *Understanding Bronchitis and Asthma*, Tavistock Publications, London, 1963.

Reyner, J. H., *Psionic Medicine*, Routledge & Kegan Paul, London, 1974.
Sinistrari, L. M., *Demonality, or Incubi and Succubi*, ed. by Montague Summers, Fortune Press, London, 1927.
Walker, Benjamin, *Beyond the Body: The Human Double and the Astral Planes*, Routledge & Kegan Paul, London, 1974.
Walker, Benjamin, *Encyclopedia of Esoteric Man*, Routledge & Kegan Paul, London, Stein & Day, New York, 1977.

ETHICS AND HEALING

Ethics and healing have always been linked together. From earliest times all forms of therapy were associated with an ultrarational element, be it magic, superstition or religion. The earliest physicians were usually members of a priestly class, and even when the separation occurred the practice of healing was circumscribed within the bounds set by religion. Hippocrates (d. 359 BC) expressed the view that the profession of healing could not endure without a sound moral philosophy.

Medical science has brought enormous benefits to society, and doctors form a very special class in the social cadre. The general tendency has usually been to exempt them from any imputation of negligence, incompetence or wrong-doing for what happens in the course of their professional practice. But there has been strong evidence in recent times to suggest that a steady erosion is taking place in the high standards we have come to expect from them, and many people feel that we need clearer moral imperatives to control the decline. The ethics underlying therapeutic practice is full of grey and twilight areas, where it is not always easy to determine whether what is being done is right or wrong, and the solution to these problems has been the monopoly of the medical profession.

In common law it is recognized that certain types of conduct, though not criminal, are immoral. For example, lying, drunkenness, promiscuity, adultery, homosexuality. Human nature being what it is, such activities are bound to exist, and are tolerated, but they cannot pass the test of the highest moral code. That is why all religions condemn these misdemeanours on principle.

People are sometimes led to believe that what is possible is permissible; that because something can be done there is no objection to doing it. Thus, as soon as a scientist is capable of carrying out an experiment, it is perfectly justifiable to go ahead with it. But others hold that the cost-benefit equation in all matters should not overlook the moral issues likely to be involved. The pursuit and increase of knowledge as such is not the over-riding mission of medical science, and not everything is permissible in the name of progress.

In medicine the need for a reassessment is especially relevant because of the growing moral cynicism of the scientist, his rejection of sentiment, his impatience with 'value'-judgments concerning right and wrong, his belief that what is 'natural' (by which he means 'possible') cannot be unethical, forgetting that murder, the Nazi concentration camp and brainwashing are all 'natural'.

There is hardly any aspect of modern medicine that has not raised religious, moral, ethical, legal or social issues of the highest order, and it is impossible to avoid a consideration of these issues when such matters are debated. A few topics of current interest might be considered here.

For instance, problems arise in the modern medical practice of transplantation (also spoken of as biological engineering, or spare-part surgery), in which various cells, tissues, organs and parts are taken from one body and used on another body. To be of any use transplantable organs must be extracted and transplanted within a certain time limit of the donor's death. The question of 'death diagnostics'* has to be solved here, without which the possibility would be created of an organ, such as a kidney, being removed from the body of a donor who is not yet dead. The public rightly fear the prospect of overzealous doctors (dubbed 'transplant vultures') waiting anxiously over a dying patient in order to excise an organ to save another patient's life. Cases are also on record of doctors removing certain expendable organs, such as a kidney, from a patient undergoing surgery for some other reason.

Advances in the techniques of transplantation have opened up the possibility of brain transplants. At present these pose certain difficulties, chief among them being those concerned with connecting the 'wiring' of the nerve channels, and with nerve restoration, since tissues of the central nervous system do not regenerate. Scientists also envision the day when they will be able to transplant the entire head of one man on to the trunk of another man. Such brain and head transplants would create a number of intriguing legal and moral problems. With what, for example, is the identity of the individual to be linked: is it with the body and all its physical organs, or with the brain and all its acquired experience? Who is the donor, the one who donates the body, or the one who donates the head?

Again, the practice of intensive therapy borders on the region of ethics, besides raising disquieting demositic and dysgenic* problems. Some people question whether it is incumbent on the doctor to prolong a person's life at all costs and despite a 'vegetable' prognosis. In this view, to keep the physical body ticking over by mechanical and chemical aids when all else has failed, is socially unjustifiable and morally indefensible. There are staunch advocates, even among the moralists who maintain that when a patient is faced with the prospect of permanent and irreversible coma, to take but one example, the doctor should turn off the respirator, the stimulator and other sustaining artifices, and allow the patient to breathe his last. Their position was summed up by the precept of the poet Arthur Hugh Clough (d. 1861), 'Thou shalt not kill; yet need'st not strive, officiously to keep alive.'

A related area of concern is that of geriatrics (Gk. *gēras*, 'old age'; *iatreia*, 'healing'), the study and treatment of the diseases of old age. No one as yet understands the reasons for senility. Robert Prehoda refers to a recent monograph on gerontology that lists 120 different explanations of senescence. In the occult view the gradual disintegration of the body's etheric blueprint after the expiry of its vitalic potential, results in the irrevocable decline of the physical apparatus. After a set span of years, the bioplasmic supply peters out. Little can be done to arrest the decay. 'My diseases are asthma and dropsy,' said Dr Samuel Johnson (d. 1784), 'and, what is less curable, seventy-five.'

99

Pneumonia, once cynically described as 'the old man's friend', because it carried him off at a reasonable time of life and saved him from the indignities of doddering imbecility, has now been conquered with the aid of sulphonamides and antibiotics. Today the majority of the sick are the elderly. Two-thirds of all deaths are associated with geriatric diseases. More people die in old age than in all the younger age brackets. According to the experts, before long the number of people who will survive into advanced age will become the major problem of industrial civilization.

Those who presume to take the realistic view believe that as the struggle for survival becomes fiercer in the progressive demositis that will prevail in the world, the senile will inevitably figure high in the category of expendables. The community's dwindling resources will not be squandered on those who have lived their lives, when they will be more urgently needed for those who still have their lives to live.

Recently there has been a renewal of interest in the subject of euthanasia. Those who oppose it state that a man should be allowed to die naturally and with dignity. Those in favour point out that needless medical interference prevents precisely this. The final moments of many dying persons today do not resemble the death scenes of the idealized past, with the aged patriarch propped up in a clean bed and uttering a few memorable last words, and then gently giving up the ghost, to the grief of all concerned. Today's death scene is much more likely to be that of a sedated, comatose, subhuman wreck, with catheters and tubes sticking out from all his bodily orifices, who even his loved ones fervently wish would pass on to his eternal rest. This, they maintain, does not prolong life; it prolongs death.

Most advocates of euthanasia are clear that the termination of life is not for the patient with a good prognosis, or for anyone, however old or sick, who is cheerful, alert and active. But in certain circumstances, as when there is no reasonable prospect of recovery from illness (whether mental or physical) which if prolonged would in the immediate future cause severe or protracted pain and distress and render him incapable of rational existence, the patient should not be kept alive by artificial means. All further treatment should be withheld, although he should, if necessary, be given drugs to keep him free from pain, so that he can die in comfort.

Though accused of espousing an immoral cause, euthanists maintain that while it is the duty of the state to care for its aged citizens, it is not so clear that it should instantly press into service all the resources of intensive care in order to ensure the survival at any price of the decrepit and near moronic who totter aimlessly in geriatric wards, each time they are on the brink of natural death. The real immorality, they insist, does not lie in allowing them to go to their rest in peace and quiet, but in providing them with the means of attaining this kind of obscene perenniality.

A few of the other major problems of medical ethics might be itemized in the form of a simple questionnaire. In view of the demositic threat to mankind, should fertility pills be given to women? Is the sterilization of normal persons morally acceptable as a method of birth control? Is abortion a form of infanticide? While every individual has rights, does not the pregnant woman have special responsibilities with regard to the rights of her unborn infant? Do we need to take steps to eliminate the unfit by positive eugenic* methods, or can we allow dysgenic traits in the population to multiply unchecked? Should time, money and resources be spent in trying to keep alive a defective embryo that would normally be rejected by the womb? Why are geneotic babies, born with severe abnormalities, allowed to survive? Is it time that we reduced the area where intensive care should be allowed to operate? Should any form of experimentation on human beings be permitted? Should we put an end to animal vivisection? Should the transplantation of organs, in particular brain transplants, be allowed? Are test-tube babies and other forms of artificial generation morally acceptable modes of reproduction? Are genetic engineering and molecular biology morally justifiable? How do we prevent the spread of VD without moral sanctions or social disapproval of promiscuity and permissiveness? Should the manufacture, sale and use of drugs, and the determination of their safety be left entirely to the pharmaceutical industry?

Books

Clark-Kennedy, A. E., *Man, Medicine and Morality*, Faber & Faber, London, 1969.
Cohen, Lord, *Morals and Medicine*, BBC Publications, London, 1970.
Downing, A. B. (ed.), *Euthanasia and the Right to Death*, Peter Owen, London, 1969.
Fletcher, J., *Morals and Medicine*, Gollancz, London, 1955.
Harrington, Alan, *The Immortalist*, Panther Books, London, 1973.
Illich, Ivan, *Medical Nemesis*, Calder & Boyars, London, 1975.
Longmore, Donald, *Spare-Part Surgery*, Aldus, London, 1968.
McFadden, C. J., *Medical Ethics*, Burns & Oates, London, 1961.
Marshall, John, *Medicine and Morals*, Burns & Oates, London, 1960.
Prehoda, Robert, *Extended Youth: the Promise of Gerontology*, Putnam, New York, 1968.
Schmeck, Harold, *The Semi-Artificial Man*, Harrap, London, 1966.
Torrey, E. F. (ed.), *Ethical Issues in Medicine*, New York, 1968.
Trowell, Hugh, *The Unfinished Debate on Euthanasia*, SCM Press, London, 1973.
Vaux, K. (ed.), *Who Shall Live?*, Fortress Press, Philadelphia, 1970.

EUGENICS

Eugenics (Gk. *eugenēs*, 'well-born'), the scientific improvement of the race through marriage between individuals of the best stock, has formed part of the racial ideals of communities old and new. The nobility in many countries is perpetuated on the principle of eugenics or good breeding, by marrying into the right families.

In its modern form eugenics owes its revival to Sir Francis Galton (d. 1911) who defined it as 'the study of agencies under social control which impair or improve the racial qualities of future generations'. He wrote a book entitled *Kantsaywhere*, which he submitted to a publisher a few weeks before he died; it was refused, and Galton told his niece to destroy the manuscript. But some parts were preserved. It envisioned a kind of Utopia, in which he described how a eugenically selected community should be organized. Prospective parents had to sit for an examination and their joint results determined the number of children they could have.

Eugenics implies race improvement as a means of helping the evolution of humanity. All factors that hinder such improvement form the subject of dysgenics*. Eugenics is considered in two ways, positive and negative.

Positive eugenics deals with planning for quality, in which social selection replaces personal and natural selection. Early marriages between healthy partners with desirable hereditary characteristics should be encouraged, to accelerate the increase in the number of their children in order to preserve, perpetuate and improve the stock. If necessary, it could include the artificial insemination of mentally and physically healthy women with the sperm of suitable donors of high genetic quality. Selective breeding could be still further ensured through controlled mutations (*see* molecular biology).

Negative eugenics concerns itself with the elimination of the unfit, that is, those who are genetically unsuitable; including their sterilization, so that they cease to propagate. This will ensure that serious mental and physical defects will not be transmitted to future generations. And it will prevent the social burden, responsibility, expense and manpower that would otherwise be needed to care for their progeny. There should be suitable legislation to ensure that this is done. Eugenists feel that we can carry too far the absurd UN declaration of human rights according to which every married couple has the basic right to have a child and 'found a family'.

Several objections have been raised to the principles of eugenics. Its too zealous application could hold serious risks of abuse, which have been vividly illustrated in the racist ideology of the Nazis, who had their own criteria of what was genetically suitable. Even if we do not accept a racial basis for eugenics, we are confronted with the problem of determining who is fit and who is not. The human genetic mechanism is extremely complex, and we still do not understand more than a few of its workings. Normal and perfectly healthy parents, no less than those who are ostensibly unfit, can carry defective transmissible genes.

But eugenists point out that carriers of transmissible disease of high 'penetrance' (where a disease easily manifests itself) can be separated from those who carry diseases of low penetrance (which seldom reveal themselves). Again, whatever obscure ingredients make up the best human stock, we do know the obvious physical and mental qualities that are desirable, and we could start from there. The best are those who are judged to be best by common sense and general consensus.

Books

Blacker, C. P., *Eugenics: Galton and After*, Duckworth, London, 1952.
Cook, Robert, *Human Fertility*, London, 1951.
Fisher, R. A., *The Genetical Theory of Natural Selection*, Clarendon Press, Oxford, 1930.
Ramsey, Paul, *Fabricated Man: the Ethics of Genetic Control*, Yale University Press, 1970.

EXORCISM

The rite by which demons, earth-bound spirits, and elementals, which are believed sometimes to possess people or animals, or to haunt objects and places, are formally banished. A possessed person exorcized in this way is thereby freed from his psychic uncleanliness, sin, disease, mental malady or other evil caused by the presence of the invading demon.

Belief in possession by spirits and in the power of exorcism is common to all religions. In one form or another the rite was performed in all ages and in all countries, in primitive societies, and early civilizations, and continues to be performed today. Priests specializing in exorcism are found everywhere in the Middle East, central Asia, India and the Far East. The Japanese Buddhist sect of the Nichiren has made exorcism its particular task, and their temple at Nalayama near Tokyo is devoted to this end.

In Hebrew legend Solomon had command over demons, and was able to capture, imprison or exorcize them by magical arts. In Greek tradition the orator Aeschines (d. 314 BC) and the philosopher Epicurus (d. 270 BC) were both the sons of female exorcists, and were both reproached, the first by Demosthenes, and the second by the Stoics, for tolerating and in fact assisting their mothers in practising the art.

In the New Testament it is written that Christ travelled all over Galilee preaching and driving out demons. He told his disciples that those who believed would cast out devils in his name (Mk. 16:17). The early church, therefore, upheld its faith in the efficacy of exorcism. The Council of Antioch (AD 341) mentions a minor order of exorcists, and a century later the Council of Carthage (AD 430) describes their ordination. Priests of the Church of Rome were given power by the bishop, of laying hands upon the *energumen* ('the one possessed') and driving out the spirits.

There were several early church manuals on exorcism, all of which were later codified in the *Rituale Romanum*, under orders of Pope Paul V in 1619. St Benedict of Nursia (d. 543), founder of the Benedictine Order and of Western monasticism, is the patron saint of exorcism. According to tradition he was confronted by extraordinary manifestations of evil spirits who obstructed the building of his monastery on the crest of Monte Cassino, where satanism had previously been practised. Medals of St Benedict are given to those possessed by spirits.

Today the Roman Catholic Church only rarely permits the full ceremony of solemn exorcism, and then only after stringent investigation and under strict supervision. There have been far too many ignominious failures. The exorcist usually works with another helper, and the ritual is always preceded by prayers and preparatory observances, including a 24-hour fast. The rite itself consists of readings from the Bible, the invocation of the name of the Most High God, the Lord Jesus Christ and the Most Holy Trinity, the use of the crucifix and the sign of the cross, the laying on of hands, the sprinkling of holy water and anointing with holy oil, along with continuous adjuration and solemn command to the spirit to depart.

The spirit speaks through the victim, whose appearance and voice alter hideously during possession*; he often gets into a fury, cries aloud and abuses the exorcist. Sometimes the spirit, when ordered, reveals his name, and this is said to make matters easier for the exorcist. Many exorcisms take on a dramatic quality with a lively dialogue taking place between priest and spirit. It has been pointed out that the sessions between exorcist and possessed strongly resemble those between psychiatrist and schizophrenic*.

It appears that the possessing spirit always has knowledge of the exorcist's character and career. A spirit exorcized by Christ declared, 'I know thee, who thou art, thou Holy One of God.' And the oracular spirit possessing the woman of Philippi identified Paul and Silas as 'servants of the most high God' (Acts 16:17). The demon is thus in a position to reveal the private secrets of the exorcizing priest, not infrequently to his and the church's embarrassment. The exorcist is therefore usually a newly ordained priest who presumably has no sins on his conscience (Leslie, 1964, p. 17).

At the beginning of the seventeenth century the Church of England, suspicious of the 'egregious popish impostures and cozenage', prohibited exorcism, except by very special sanction. But recently a number of priests have performed the rite when called upon to do so, usually to clear haunted houses.

Because the rite of exorcism is believed to be beset with danger, it is performed in all religions by specially trained exorcists, be they medicine men, shamans or priests. Not the least of the dangers is that the exorcist, being in the vicinity of the demon, arousing his anger by his commands, threats and adjurations, might himself become possessed. An eighteenth-century French manual on exorcism states that 'nearly all exorcists are exposed to infection and most are tainted by their ministrations as a result of which they are vexed by demons and suffer persecution from them in the form of bodily aches and pains, general malaise, dizziness, vomiting, hallucinations, and impure thoughts'. A great deal of nervous and physical energy is expended during an exorcism. It has even been said that 'the more successful the exorcism, the sooner the exorcist dies' (Strachan, 1972, p. 36).

Books

Kraft, H., *Historie vom Exorcismo*, Hamburg, 1750.
Leslie, Shane, *Ghost Book*, Four Square, London, 1964.
Omand, Rev. D., *Experiences of a Present-Day Exorcist*, Kimber, London, 1970.
Pearce-Higgins, John, *Life, Death and Psychical Research*, Rider, London, 1975.
Petitpierre, Dom Robert, *Exorcising Devils*, Robert Hale, London, 1976.
Richards, John, *But Deliver Us From Evil*, Darton, Longman, Todd, London, 1974.
Strachan, Françoise, *Casting Out Devils*, Aquarian Press, London, 1972.
Woolley, R. M., *Exorcism and the Healing of the Sick*, London, 1932.

EXPERIMENTAL MEDICINE

A comparatively recent development of medical practice, includes experiments to test new drugs or try out new techniques; experiments to determine the outcome of certain processes, as in artificial generation*, molecular biology* and transplantation; and vivisection or experiments on living animals.

Animal experiments, usually on dogs, cats, guinea pigs and other small animals, began to be systematically carried out from the beginning of the present century, some of them quite extraordinary. In 1908 an American physiologist, Charles Claude Guthrie transplanted the head of a dog onto the body of another dog. The operation lasted one hour. On awaking from anaesthesia both heads appeared to be quite normal. The animal lived for one day. In 1950 the Soviet surgeon Vladimir Demichov of Moscow transplanted the head, neck and forepaws of one dog on to the neck of another larger dog. The transplanted head could smell, see, eat and bark. The larger dog tried to shake off the load from its neck, but the little dog bit its ear. This two-headed animal lived for 29 days.

Since the 1960s scientists in the USA and Japan have 'kept alive' the brains of monkeys and cats for days, even months. Japanese methods of vivisection are particularly callous, and it is said that Japanese researchers make an annual pilgrimage to a shrine to offer homage to the souls of animals they have 'sacrificed'.

The often paltry conclusions arrived at after a long series of ghastly experiments would, in the opinion of many people, hardly justify the time and labour spent on them, nor warrant the agony suffered by the victim. Many of the experiments are scientifically valueless, and their objective trivial. For instance, hundreds of experiments involving the blistering or blinding of animals by applying caustic chemicals to their eyes, nasal passages, and sensitive mucus membranes, are done in order to test cosmetics. In any event, say the critics, it is not clear whether the results of animal tests have much direct relevance to human beings.

Although researchers point out that their experiments are strictly controlled under a stringent licensing system and supervised by a state inspectorate, the opposition point out that these controls have been enforced after fierce public outcry and in the teeth of strong opposition and resistance from scientific and commercial interests.

Some, especially earlier, animal experiments were conducted with such cruelty and callousness that doubt has been cast on the mental health of the experimenters themselves. Even today animals continue to be cut up, castrated, mutilated, blinded, starved, frozen and drowned. They are given electric shocks, stupefying drugs and poisons, dosed with X-rays and injected with germs to give them painful and protracted diseases.

Experimentation on human beings has not been far behind in ruthlessness and brutality. It reached its nadir in Hitler's Germany, when the state authorized research experimentation on non-Aryans. The Nuremberg trials revealed the full horror of the experiments carried out on living prisoners by top-ranking Nazi doctors, leaders of German science and medicine, and hundreds of devoted ancillarists, to test biological responses to drugs and diseases, and to various adverse stress conditions, and in general to observe the limits of human endurance.

The Nuremberg Code (1947), the Helsinki Declaration (1964) and other post-war standards of practice were set out to prevent similar occurrences in future. But there is ample evidence that unnecessary, painful and dangerous research on men, women and children still goes on, besides hundreds of almost routine experiments to test new drugs. The eminent surgeon Sir William Ogilvie spoke of experimental medicine as 'something new and sinister'. Since the Second World War, doctors in many advanced countries have carried out experiments both privately and in hospitals, without the knowledge or consent of the patients or their relatives or guardians. The subjects of these experiments have included pregnant women, infants, the mentally subnormal, the insane, the very poor, the elderly, the very sick and the dying. The extent of medical malpractice in this area as revealed in fully documented books and periodicals recently published, has been described as shocking, reprehensible and immoral.

Such work is sometimes performed without proper medical or legal control, in order to avoid the interposition of disturbing factors that such controls would create. To allow observations to be made in a 'pure' state, controls are reduced and risks thereby increased, leaving the ignorant patient exposed to possibly serious complications. When consent of the patient is required by law, ways of evading it are easily found. The nature and purpose of the experiment and the dangers involved are not always explained, and salient facts necessary for forming the basis of informed consent may be withheld for fear that it might be refused. Often the patient is given the impression that there is no alternative to the treatment proposed by the doctor.

There is always a minority of professional men to whom patients are primarily resources, placed at their disposal; or experimental objects, furnishing raw material for a pet project. They are more interested in advancing medical research than in the welfare of the patient entrusted to their care.

It is known that surgeons sometimes interfere and tamper with or take sample tissues from healthy organs when operating on an adjacent diseased organ.

Experiments may be carried out, more or less as an extension of surgery, that may have nothing to do with the organ operated on. Operations are performed that are not related to the disease from which the person is suffering.

Some doctors experiment merely to prove or confirm a theory. Some indeed feel, when the patient is conveniently there and ready to hand, that they are entitled to have a go and test the result of their theory. Experiments are carried out to perfect a technique, to establish a principle already known in theory, and to 'get the hand in', that is, for practice.

Most experiments are performed because it is believed they will be advantageous to science, although it is now generally admitted that the value of medical research is far from commensurate with the vast number of experiments officially or unofficially carried out. Much of current research, with all its lavish expenditure of time, money and talent, produces little of value. Not infrequently, say the critics, the conclusions drawn are ludicrous, based almost exclusively on the mechanics of experimental procedure, and seldom touching on the underlying problems involved. It would, they claim, occur to the researcher to recommend for a weeping woman who has lost her child, the surgical removal of her tear glands.

Experimental medicine is said to provide occupational therapy* for aspiring doctors. It is less arduous than bedside medicine, and considerably more rewarding in terms of personal advancement. Many of those who presume to do experimental work 'for the good of society', look on it as a short-cut to promotion and obtaining grants. Writing for scientific journals is the shortest way to success in the academic world.

Critics also point out that doctors resent what seems to them like unwarranted public meddling in their private preserve. Often where there is public debate and news comment on the exposure of some scandal, the medical profession closes ranks and the doctors concerned receive considerable support from official quarters. It would seem that humanitarian considerations do not loom large in the mind of the dedicated researcher.

Books

Beecher, H. K., *Experimentation on Man*, Thomas, Springfield, Illinois, 1959.
Bernard, Claude, *Introduction to the Study of Experimental Medicine*, Abelard-Schuman, New York, 1962 edn.
Freund, Paul (ed.), *Experimentation with Human Subjects*, Allen & Unwin, London, 1972.
Goldman, Louis, *When Doctors Disagree*, Hamish Hamilton, London, 1973.
Hutchings, M. and Carver, M., *Man's Dominion: Our Violation of the Animal World*, Hart-Davis, London, 1970.
Jackson, D. M., *Moral Responsibility in Clinical Research*, London, 1958.
Ladimer, I. and Newman, R. W. (eds), *Clinical Investigations in Medicine: Legal, Ethical and Moral Aspects*, Boston University Press, 1963.
Pappworth, M. H., *Human Guinea Pigs: Experimentation on Man*, Routledge & Kegan Paul, London, 1970.
Smith, Colin, *Alternatives to Vivisection*, National Antivivisection Society, London, 1969.
Vyvyan, John, *The Dark Face of Science*, Michael Joseph, London, 1971.

FEAR

Fear arises as the natural response of an organism to a real or imagined threat, when danger is sensed or pain anticipated. It is expressed in instinctive animal reaction, prompting fight or flight. It may include vocalization, retreat, escape, concealment or, occasionally, a motionless and mute reaction, as when animals play possum and feign death.

Fear is an inbuilt reflex against danger in the struggle for survival, for the animal without fear will not run to save itself. In human beings fear largely arises from the threat of pain, poverty, illness, change, the loss of love, accidents and the other hazards of daily life.

Fear is a safeguard, but at the same time it is one of the most destructive of all emotions. According to the old saying: where the plague kills one, fear of the plague kills ten. Physiologically, bodily changes result from the arousal of the autonomic nervous system. Adrenalin is passed into the blood stream;

FEVER

the pulse rate is increased; sugar is released from the liver into the blood; the hair rises (horripilation); the pupils become dilated. There is a feeling of tenseness as if the body were held in a vice.

Because it can cause these instant chemical changes, fear is one of the principal psychosomatic* agents, contributing to cardiac, respiratory and alimentary diseases, and one of the chief factors in stress*. It both precipitates and prolongs physical and mental illness, and interferes with the action of drugs used in treatment. Man cannot avoid fear. In spite of increasing security, he still finds things to become disturbed and fearful about, and this manifests in the vague pervasive disquiet that characterizes human existence.

In a spiritual sense fear is dangerous because it creates the very situation one wishes to avoid. As the afflicted Job laments: 'The thing which I greatly feared is come upon me' (Job 3:25). The Chinese sages of old believed that when a man fears something, his very breath (ch'i) attracts the spirit related to his fears, and thus gives it an actual reality.

Related to fear are a number of other kindred emotions. Anxiety* is fear from an unknown source, and is usually prolonged. Angst* might be called an existential fear, with deeper religious implications. A phobia is an obsessive and persistent fear of a single object or situation, as is found in various kinds of monomania*. Pavor (Lat. 'fright') is a feeling of unreasoning terror, found more frequently in children than in adults, and at night rather than in the day. Panic is a sudden seizure of blind fear, usually of short duration, during which a person, either alone or in a group, completely loses control of his behaviour. It is named after the Greek god Pan, who was believed to inspire men with such emotions.

Books

Hall, Stanley, *Study of Fear*, London, 1925.
Kierkegaard, S., *Fear and Trembling*, Doubleday, New York, 1954.
Marks, Isaac, *Fears and Phobias*, Heinemann, London, 1969.
Meerloo, J. A., *Patterns of Panic*, New York, 1950.
Schultz, D. P., *Panic Behavior,* Random House, New York, 1964.

FEVER

The physical condition of the body when the temperature rises above the normal 98·4°F. At any one time there are slight variations of temperature in different parts of the body surface and external apertures: skin, armpit, mouth and anus. Various internal organs are also believed to have different temperatures. So far no one understands the principle of homeostasis, by which a constant internal environment is maintained in the bodily processes of living things, such as the heart rate, blood sugar level, body temperature, and so on. It remains a mystery.

Fever is usually accompanied by a flushed skin, a more rapid pulse, changes in breathing, a sense of heat and cold, restlessness and malaise. When fever is very high, coma supervenes. Both temperature and the pulse rate normally rise in different physical situations; they fluctuate at different times during the waking hours, and are slightly different during sleep. They are higher in the late afternoon and evening and lower at night during sleep. The temperature may also go up or fall in highly emotional situations such as anger, terror, frustration and deep annoyance.

Fever usually accompanies infections, but there are many fevers of obscure origin that cannot be explained in these terms. Fever is not a disease but a sign. It is a symptomatic reaction of defence. Many germs die when the body temperature is raised. It is also the body's method of providing immunity and resistance. A feverish cold may be no more than a building up of antibodies against winter ills.

The old name for fever, especially for malaria, was ague, when fever was usually accompanied by acute chills and shivering. According to an old superstition, ague was outside the physician's reach; it could only be cured by some wise woman's nostrum. For example, put a spider in a raisin and swallow it. Or take pills of compressed cobwebs before meals. Fright was another cure, based on the principle that the shaking of the fright would overcome the shaking of the ague. One old Anglo-Saxon remedy reads: 'For a fever take the right-foot shank of a black dead hound, hang it on the arm; it shaketh off the fever.' A medieval cure was: reduce a toad to powder by baking it dry, then put it into a bag and place it under the armpit.

But in many instances fever was believed to be an effective remedy for various diseases, both physical and mental. The ancients regarded it as a specific therapeutic agent against various forms of mental disorder. The venom of moon-madness, for example, was desiccated by febrile heat. Internal cankers withered and noxious vapours were dispersed. Similarly sores brought on by overindulgence in erotic encounters were healed by fever. Even modern physicians until the beginning of the present century, believed that venereal diseases including syphilis* could be cured and medication helped if the patient had fever.

Fever was regarded as a specific for epilepsy*. An old Greek legend relates that when Teucer the Cyzican was asked by the god Asclepius whether he would like to be cured of his epilepsy in exchange for a lesser evil, he agreed, whereupon the god gave him quartan fever. Hippocrates (d. 359 BC) pointed out: 'People with quartan fever do not get epilepsy. If during an epileptic attack quartan fever supervenes the victim is released from epilepsy.'

The treatment of disease by artificially induced fever is known as pyretotherapy (Gk, pyretos, 'fever'), but the problem here lies in the extreme difficulty of producing artificial fever, and of maintaining it, without actually giving the patient a disease. There is an extremely powerful built-in thermostatic regulator for stabilizing the normal temperature of the body that resists external influences. That these difficulties were already recognized in ancient times is evidenced in the remark by Rufus of Ephesus (fl. AD 90), who said that any physician able to cure by wilfully provoking fever ought indeed to be classed with the gods, for alas, humans did not possess such power.

A favourite method used in early times to provoke a short-term fever was to place an onion under the armpit and stand in the sun. A temporary rise in temperature was also induced by making the patient sit in a sweatbox, a small heating chamber called a hypertherm, to induce perspiration. Several strange methods were tried in the Middle Ages. The famous Catalonian physician Arnold of Villanova (d. 1312) suggested that in order to bring on fever for the treatment of epilepsy and other diseases, leeches should be applied over the spleen, followed by a poultice of pigeon's dung mixed with raven's eggs. This would draw the morbid matter from the afflicted part and generate a fever, thus effecting a cure.

Franz Anton Mesmer (d. 1815), the pioneer hypnotherapist, could increase and decrease fever in subjects by suggestion; sometimes his mere presence was enough to raise or lower the temperature of a patient. A Belgian physician, Albert Selade (c. 1840), who had under his care two chronic epileptics, towards the end of winter exposed them half-clad to intense cold for one hour daily, then put them into a warm bed till they perspired profusely. They were both cured, one permanently, and the other, who had a relapse after two years, was eventually cured in the same manner.

The ancient Greek philosopher Parmenides (d. 480 BC) said, 'Give me the power to produce fever and I'll cure all disease.' The Viennese psychologist Julius Wagner-Jauregg (d. 1940) inspired by Parmenides and, noticing the effect of fever on the mental condition of psychotic patients, originated a treatment for paresis (partial paralysis) by inoculating a person with live malaria parasites to induce fever and thus halt further deterioration. Attempts were also made to treat GPI (general paralysis of the insane, a late manifestation of syphilis and epilepsy by the same means. These are forms of inductance therapy, which is the curing of one disease by inducing another. Yet another method of inducing hyperthermia or high fever, is the intravenous injection of dead typhoid bacteria. The opposite of pyretotherapy is cryotherapy, or treatment by freezing an afflicted limb or organ (see thermosomatics).

The fact that fever has been successfully used as a therapeutic aid in mental diseases, has suggested to some researchers that there perhaps exists a correlation between fever and a heightening of the intellectual faculties. The relationship between feverish sicknesses of various kinds, and a high degree of creativity in literature and the arts is adduced in support of this theory. William James (d. 1910), the great psychologist, said: 'For aught we know to the contrary, 103° or 104° Fahrenheit might be a more favourable temperature for truths to germinate and sprout in, than the more ordinary blood heat of 97 or 98 degrees.'

Books

Bett, W. R., *The Infirmities of Genius*, Christopher Johnson, London, 1952.

Cannon, Walter B., *The Wisdom of the Body*, rev. edn, Kegan Paul, Trench, Trubner, London, 1939.

Cockayne, T. O., *Leechdoms, Wortcunning and Starcraft of Early England*, vol. I, Holland Press, London, reissued 1961.

DuBois, E. F., *Fever and the Regulation of Body Temperature*, Springfield, Illinois, 1948.

James, William, *The Varieties of Religious Experience*, Longmans, Green, New York, 1902.

Lakhovsky, Georges, *The Secret of Life*, 2nd edn, True Health Publishing Co., London, 1951.

Terry, Gladys, *Fever and Psychoses. A Study of the Literature and Current Opinion on the Effects of Fever on Certain Psychoses and Epilepsy*, Hoeber, New York, 1939.

FLORITHERAPY

Floritherapy, or healing by exposure to the influence of flowers, is a branch of phytotherapy*, or healing by plants and trees in general. Again, inhaling the aroma of flowers is part of the healing system of pneumopathy*, based on the principle that people can be affected by the fragrant atmosphere surrounding flowers. Floritherapy combines the benefits of chromotherapy* (colours) and aromatherapy* (scents).

Floritherapy was once widely practised in certain countries, and achieved a high degree of sophistication in the Far East. It figured in the mythology of the ancient Greeks, who attributed the beneficent virtues of medicinal herbs and flowers to the deities. The Romans believed that the perfume of flowers was strong enough to subdue the intoxicating effects of wine, and during their sybaritic feasts crowned their heads with floral wreaths, or adorned themselves with flowers.

In medieval Europe in time of epidemics, garlands of thyme and rosemary were worn about the neck, both as a disinfectant and a cure. The nursery rhyme, 'Ring a ring o' roses', still recalls this remedy.

Flowers send forth a constant radiance that heals and calms, and they in turn respond to love and care. The great American Negro agricultural chemist, George Washington Carver (d. 1943), used to say, 'All flowers talk to me, and I reply.' In recent years one of the chief exponents of floritherapy was Edward Bach (d. 1936), a Welsh physician who gave up his practice to concentrate on the curative virtues of flowers. He regarded them as 'the quintessence of nature', and worked out a system by which he was able to find the corresponding relationship between flowers and human moods. He extracted flower essences by steeping fresh petals in spring water and exposing them to the sun; the impregnated water was then used in various ways.

Though many manufactured perfumes have a floral base, flowers themselves represent a pure, unmixed fragrance that has wonderful natural potency. A knowledge of their properties enables the expert to choose particular flowers, or posies and bouquets of mixed flowers, for particular purposes. It is claimed that there is practically no disease that cannot be cured by flowers, and no mood that cannot be evoked by them.

The perfume of flowers is said to have an extremely powerful effect on the psyche, and helps to counteract the ill-effects not only of other smells, but of the auras emanating from evil presences. But a thorough understanding of these effects is very essential. Some flowers, especially the more exotic, cloying varieties can harm the psyche.

Flowers containing as they do the plant's reproductive organs, represent some of the transcendent qualities of the plant. Growing even in the most unpromising soil, they blossom in every colour under the sun, and give forth perfumes of all kinds that scent the air for miles around. Their beauty, fragrance and colour, have great psychotherapeutic value and are a source of delight and comfort at all times. In the sickroom they are a valuable supplement to other healing methods, providing a soothing ambience for the recovery of the patient.

Depending on its colour and perfume, and the species to which it belongs, each flower has its own distinctive effect, some good and some bad, exerting its influence either singly or in combination with other species. These floral attributes are usually based on the ancient doctrines of signature, sympathy and correspondence. Some therapies take account of seasonal variations, since it is considered injurious to make use of flowers that are out of season, or incompatible with the country where they are used, as in the case of exotic flowers.

A brief list of the more common varieties and the mental state with which they are associated is given below:

Agrimony, lessens anxiety
Amaryllis, creates pride
Anemone, provokes small worries
Antirrhinum (snapdragon), makes one short-tempered
Azalea, induces fickleness
Begonia, creates incompatibility
Camomile, inspires devotion
Carnation (red), turns the mind to worldly concerns
Centaury, gives feelings of independence
Chrysanthemum, promotes mysticism
Clematis, inspires courage
Convolvulus, makes one flirtatious
Cornflower, tends to staidness and sobriety
Crocus, tends to superficiality
Daffodil (or Narcissus), makes one deceitful
Dahlia, inspires exoticism
Daisy, provokes outspokenness
Dandelion, incites to jealousy
Delphinium, gives superior airs
Gentian, dissipates depression
Gladiolus, makes for stability
Hollyhock, helps resolution
Hyacinth, arouses suspicion
Impatiens, removes irritability

Iris, creates indifference
Jonquil, incites to obstinacy
Larkspur, makes for petty annoyances
Lavender, inspires tender love
Lilac, engenders trouble
Magnolia, arouses combativeness
Marigold, creates jealousy
Mimulus, arouses nervous fears
Nasturtium, is good for conjugal love
Pansy, makes for flightiness
Peony, creates feelings of shame
Petunia, arouses anger
Phlox, arouses a sense of oppression
Poppy, makes for carelessness
Primrose, makes for inconstancy
Rose (red), arouses poetic feelings
Rosemary, demands exclusive love
Sunflower, aids falseness
Sweetpea, inspires conservative attitudes
Tulip, provokes admiration
Valerian, induces tenacity
Verbena (or Vervain), arouses artistic feelings
Violet, gives feelings of placidity and modesty
Zinnia, makes one cautious

Books

Adams, G. and Whicher, O., *The Living Plant and the Science of Physical and Ethereal Spaces*, Goethean Science Foundation, Clent, Worcs., 1949.
Anonymous, *Fishes, Flowers and Fire as Elements and Deities in the Phallic Faiths and Worship of the Ancient Religions*, London, 1890.

Bach, Edward, *Heal Thyself*, Fowler, London, 1931.
Crow, W. B., *The Occult Properties of Herbs*, Aquarian Press, London, 1969.
Dowden, Anne, *The Secret Life of Flowers*, Odyssey Press, New York, 1964.
Friend, H. I., *Flowers and Flower Lore*, George Allen, London, 1884.
Grigson, G., *The Englishman's Flora*, London, 1955.
Guilcher, J. M., *La Vie cachée des fleurs*, Flammarion, Paris, 1951.
Jinarajadasa, C., *Flowers and Gardens: a Dream Structure*, Theosophical Publishing House, Adyar, Madras, 1913.
Skinner, C. M., *Myths and Legends of Flowers*, London, 1925.

FUROR

A state of wild emotion during which a person's mind is enveloped in a blinding flame that overwhelms normal consciousness, and raises him to a pitch of such intense excitement that he loses all control over himself. A man in the grip of such an overpowering passion is deaf to reason, lost to all sense of shame and responsibility, and acts blindly in pursuance of his monomania* as long as the fury lasts. The Greeks believed that in the human being the midriff (*phrēn*) was the seat of the passions, and that if the feelings engendered in that organ were malignant or violent they infected the spirit with ill-humours. This gave rise to the idea of *phrensy* (frenzy), a xenophrenic* state like temporary insanity that possesses a person as if he is in the grip of a demon.

Plato (d. 347 BC) discusses the fevered condition of the mind when consumed by various passions. Cicero (d. 43 BC) refers to the 'convulsions of the soul', and during the Middle Ages these convulsions of the agonized, tormented and inflamed psyche were analysed, classified and elaborated upon. On the basis of Plato's theory the Renaissance scholar Marsilio Ficino (d. 1499) developed the theory of the four furors (prophetic, religious, poetic, erotic), and his commentators added two more as follows:

(1) Religious furor (*furor divini*) covered all forms of theomania* and religious fanaticism. Its patron deity was Dionysus.

(2) Prophetic furor (*furor fatidicus*) afflicted those persons through whom the gods desired to make their wishes known, and usually culminated in vaticination, or oracular prophecy. Its patron was Apollo.

(3) Poetic furor (*furor poeticus*) culminated in poetical or musical expression. Its patrons were the Muses.

(4) Erotic furor (*furor amatorius*), or erotomania*, afflicted the copulatory organs and culminated. in intercourse and orgasm. It was inspired by Aphrodite and Eros.

(5) Melancholic* furor (*furor melancholicus*) brought deep depression, feelings of angst* and grief, and darkened the soul, sometimes terminating in insanity. It was inspired by Saturn.

(6) Martial furor (*furor bellicosus*), the fury of the warrior, inspired by the god Mars. A good example is the Nordic *berserker,* whose frenzied rage in the battlefield spread terror in the enemy ranks.

Books

See under xenophrenia

G

GENIUS

The unique inborn faculty that makes a man outstanding among his fellows. He infuses things with his creative imagination, takes a fresh look at the world around him, and presents it with a new significance, highlighting what has been unknown or hidden, and thus bringing to society and the world new values and insights. He is an innovator and regenerator.

Genius has little relationship to cleverness or a high IQ. Many great geniuses have been like somnambulists, notoriously lacking in those qualities that make for success in practical affairs. Nor does there seem to be any connection between genius in one art and talent in another art related to it. Robert Burns (d. 1796), whose melodious lyrics have made immortal songs, had a 'remarkably dull' musical ear, and could hardly distinguish one note from another.

The genius pays a high price for his endowment of exceptional gifts; he is invariably racked with disabilities of some kind, physical, mental or spiritual. Often he has struggled against bodily deformity. Geniuses have been deaf like Pierre de Ronsard (d. 1585), Jonathan Swift (d. 1745), Beaumarchais (d. 1799), Ludwig van Beethoven (d. 1827) and Goya (d. 1828); blind, like Homer (d. 800 BC) and John Milton (d. 1674); squint-eyed, like Albrecht Dürer (d. 1528) and Francesco Guercino (d. 1666); ugly, like Comte de Mirabeau (d. 1791); deformed, like Alexander Pope (d. 1744), Henri Toulouse-Lautrec (d. 1901), or Lord Byron (d. 1824), whose club foot was a source of great humiliation to him; stutterers like Demosthenes (d. 322 BC) and Camille Desmoulins (d. 1794).

Geniuses have been impotent or lacking in sexual drive, like Isaac Newton (d. 1727), Immanuel Kant (d. 1804), Arthur Schopenhauer (d. 1860) and Thomas Carlyle (d. 1881). The marriage of Edgar Allan Poe (d. 1849) was never consummated, and he may have been impotent. So too might have been John Ruskin (d. 1900), whose marriage was annulled. Many have been notorious womanizers, like François Villon (d. 1463), Robert Burns (d. 1796), Lord Byron (who had a harem in Venice), Hector Berlioz (d. 1869), and Richard Wagner (d. 1883); or homosexuals, whose names, like those of womanizers, crowd the catalogues of geniuses.

Often they have been obsessed with a maddening perfectionism. Frédéric

Chopin (d. 1849) deleted, re-wrote, struck out, corrected, transposed, until he was desperate and would feel completely worn out and depressed. Gustave Flaubert (d. 1880) would struggle for hours over a single phrase. On one occasion he struck out and re-wrote the word *mais* eleven times before finally allowing it to stand in a sonnet he was writing.

The powerful imaginative faculty of great writers forces them to empathize with their creations. The characters of Honoré de Balzac (d. 1850) were as vivid to him as people in the flesh, so that he often spoke of them as friends. Charles Dickens (d. 1870) could hear his characters talk aloud as people would in ordinary conversation. While writing the dramatic poisoning sequence in *Madame Bovary*, Gustave Flaubert swore that he felt the taste of arsenic in his mouth.

Imaginative, impressionable, passionate, morbid, the genius is almost invariably a moody individual, beset with angst* and phobia, and dogged by phases of deep mental depression*. Edgar Allan Poe, himself a tormented genius, wrote: 'The question is still unsettled whether all that is glorious and profound does not spring from the disease of thought; from moods of mind exalted at the expense of the general intellect.'

Neither physical health nor peace of mind is among the privileges of genius. If we remove from the list of the world's great names in all fields the chronically sick, the consumptive, the syphilitic; and those afflicted with epilepsy, melancholy and chronic migraine; the drunkard, the eccentric, the idiosyncratic, and the mentally unbalanced, the best of them are gone.

In madness the unconscious breaks through into consciousness, and often reveals states of consciousness experienced in dreams. A more primitive, simple and natural level of awareness is reached, akin to the free and fresh perspective of the child or the savage. 'The man of genius,' said Goethe, 'experiences a repetition of adolescence, whereas other people are only youthful once.'

Insanity is sometimes linked with a very high degree of mental and even spiritual development. In many ancient communities madness was regarded as sacred, putting the victims into an inaccessible supranormal plane, nearer that of divinity. The insane were treated with a frightened reverence. They were the holy ones, friends of the deities, in communion with spirits. Their words, however nonsensical, were listened to and pondered over for hidden meanings and messages. The Turks used to say that it is not always possible to distinguish a *deli* (lunatic) from a *veli* (saint). Like the madman and the lover, the genius is 'possessed'.

Most geniuses are cyclothymes*, alternating between wild enthusiasm and euphoria, when they are optimistic, active and aggressive; and deep depression, when they are shut in with their own morbid thoughts, retiring from the world to produce their masterpieces in solitude (*see* melancholy). Some are schizophrenics, believing themselves without peer, or morbidly suspicious. And all of them are neurotics in greater or lesser degree.

Socrates (d. 399 BC) said, 'Our greatest blessings come to us through madness.' According to the Greeks of his day the insane were touched by the divine hand. Those who affronted the gods, those who were favoured by the gods, those whom the gods inspired, went mad. The philosopher Democritus

(d. 361 BC) said that all sane poets are excluded from Helicon, the mountain sacred to the Muses, since there is a close connection between the inspired state and the state of the mentally unbalanced. Aristotle (d. 322 BC) commented on how often great men displayed morbid conditions of mind. Seneca (d. AD 65) declared, 'There never has been a great talent without a touch of madness.'

'How near is genius to madness', cried Denis Diderot (d. 1784). 'Genius is nearer to madness than to the average intellect', wrote Arthur Schopenhauer. Alphonse de Lamartine (d. 1869) spoke of 'that malady which one calls genius', and Marcel Proust (d. 1922) remarked, 'Everything great in the world comes from neurotics.' Ernest Jones (d. 1958), psychologist and biographer of Freud, said, 'Neurotics are the torchbearers of civilization.' In the opinion of Harold Nicolson (d. 1968), literary critic and diplomat, 'All creative writers are hypochondriacs.'

Below is a brief catalogue of some famous personages who were either themselves insane, or suffered from profound neurosis, hypochondria, melancholia*, manic-depression, schizophrenia* or other psychosis; or, in earlier parlance, 'came of tainted stock'. (The list can be further supplemented by reference to articles on eccentricity, epilepsy, melancholy, tuberculosis and syphilis.)

Michelangleo (d. 1564) was severely psychopathic and showed signs of schizophrenia. Torquato Tasso (d. 1595), Italian poet, composed his poetry during paroxysms of near-insanity, and was eventually confined for seven years because of it. Tycho Brahe (d. 1601), the astronomer, became imbecile in his declining years. Francis Bacon (d. 1626) was the son of a woman who was insane for some years before her death. Johann Kepler (d. 1630), the astronomer, came of deranged and psychopathic stock. Salvator Rosa (d. 1673), Italian painter, sank into imbecility towards the end of his life. John Bunyan (d. 1688) went insane in the medical sense of the term, for three or four years of his life. Nathaniel Lee (d. 1692), English dramatist, was subject to spells of insanity, and died drunk in the snow.

Isaac Newton (d. 1727) was profoundly neurotic and suffered bouts of melancholy and temporary 'alienation of mind'. Richard Savage (d. 1743), English poet, came of insane stock, and himself behaved like a madman. Jonathan Swift, the 'mad parson', was often on the verge of insanity. George Frederick Handel (d. 1759), a paralytic, once came so near to total mental breakdown that he had to spend a year in retirement. William Pitt (d. 1778), the Earl of Chatham, known as the Elder Pitt, was insane for over a year and died of an apoplectic seizure. Jean-Jacques Rousseau (d. 1778) was mentally disturbed, with persistent mania of persecution and phobias concerning his health and sanity, and it is doubtful if he was wholly sane during the last fifteen years of his life. Wolfgang Amadeus Mozart (d. 1791) broke down mentally and physically at the age of 30, and died of 'inflammation' of the brain. Comte de Mirabeau, the French writer and statesman, was a 'supreme degenerate', who looked and behaved like a lunatic. Maximilien Robespierre (d. 1794), one of the most bloodthirsty leaders of the French Revolution, had schizoid tendencies.

William Cowper (d. 1800), English poet, spent eighteen months in a lunatic asylum, while Immanuel Kant, Germany's greatest philospher, became imbecile in his declining years. Heinrich von Kleist (d. 1811), German dramatist and poet, suffered from schizophrenia, and shot himself. Percy Bysshe Shelley (d. 1822), a profound hypochondriac, was nicknamed 'mad Shelley' because of his eccentric conduct and strange ideas. John Kemble (d. 1823), famous actor, and his equally famous sister, Mrs Sarah Siddons (d. 1831), were both considered 'half mad'. William Blake (d. 1827) was 'cracked', but, said Edith Sitwell, 'that was where the light came through'.

G. W. F. Hegel (d. 1831), German philosopher, had a sister who went insane, and himself was eccentric in the extreme. Johann Wolfgang von Goethe (d. 1832) also had a sister, who was severely deranged mentally. Edmund Kean (d. 1833), the famous actor, died insane. Charles Lamb (d. 1834), whose temperament Thomas Carlyle described as 'not genius but diluted insanity', was not quite free from the family taint of madness. He had a mental breakdown at puberty which necessitated his temporary restraint. His sister Mary, in a fit of insanity, stabbed their mother to death.

Robert Southey (d. 1843) married a woman who went insane, and himself died in a condition of imbecility. Felix Mendelssohn (d. 1847) came of stock where deformities, blindness, apoplexy, paralysis and epilepsy were present in unbroken succession. François Chateaubriand (d. 1848), French writer and politician, belonged to a family in which insanity was present. He himself displayed strange idiosyncrasies of behaviour. Gaetano Donizetti (d. 1848), Italian composer, spent the latter years of his life in an asylum. Edgar Allan Poe, although never placed under restraint, was said to have been undoubtedly insane.

William Wordsworth (d. 1850), although not himself unbalanced, came of tainted stock, and his sister Dorothy (d. 1855) in her later years lost her mind. The mother of J. M. W. Turner (d. 1851) died in a private asylum. The English architect Augustus Pugin (d. 1852) died insane. Johann Hölderlin (d. 1853), German poet, had periodic bouts of insanity over a period of nearly forty years. Gérard de Nerval (d. 1855), French writer, long intermittently insane, ultimately hanged himself. Robert Schumann (d. 1856), composer, died in a lunatic asylum. Auguste Comte (d. 1857), founder of Positivism, was confined to an asylum for a year.

Arthur Schopenhauer, the prophet of pessimism, had markedly schizoid traits. Elizabeth Barrett Browning (d. 1861) was a neurotic, while Walter Savage Landor (d. 1864), English poet and writer, was a quarrelsome eccentric, described as having 'an insane temperament'. Charles Baudelaire (d. 1867) was a syphilitic and drug addict, which led to his eventual derangement, of which he apparently had intimations. In 1862 he wrote in his diary, 'Today I had an ominous warning. I suddenly felt the wings of insanity brush my mind.' Edward Bulwer Lytton (d. 1873), English novelist, was subject to ungovernable fits of tempestuous rage amounting to insane mania. Edwin Landseer (d. 1873), English painter, was hopelessly insane during the last four years of his life.

Gustave Flaubert, French novelist, suffered from brain disease, a euphemism for insanity. Fyodor Dostoevsky (d. 1881) used to suffer from epileptic fits and bouts of insanity. Charles Darwin (d. 1882), a hypochondriac, suffered most of his life from a deep psychoneurosis. Victor Hugo (d. 1885) came from a family in which insanity was positively known to exist. Richard Dadd (d. 1887), English painter, in a fit of insanity stabbed his father to death and spent over forty years in institutions. Vincent van Gogh (d. 1890), Dutch post-Impressionist painter, went insane and shot himself. Herman Melville (d. 1891), author of *Moby Dick*, came of tormented stock; his brother Gansevoort died insane in London. Alfred Tennyson (d. 1892) was a hypochondriac most of his life. Guy de Maupassant (d. 1893) went insane a year before his death.

Friedrich Nietzsche (d. 1900) died insane; so did John Ruskin, English writer; and so also did Hugo Wolf (d. 1903), Austrian song composer. Florence Nightingale (d. 1910) was driven by a blazing obsession to carry on her extraordinary work. She was neurotic and compulsive. Mary Baker Eddy (d. 1910), founder of Christian Science, was a suspicious and neurotic hypochondriac. August Strindberg (d. 1912), Swedish playwright, was subject to mad fits. Marcel Proust, French writer, was neurotic from an early age. Sigmund Freud (d. 1939) did his most important work when suffering from a psychoneurosis. Vaslav Nijinsky (d. 1950), dancer of semi-legendary fame, suffered a nervous breakdown in 1916 and ended his days with a mind benighted by insanity.

Books

Bett, W. R., *The Infirmities of Genius*, Christopher Johnson, London, 1952.
Clissold, Augustus, *The Prophetic Spirit in Genius and Madness*, London, 1870.
Cox, C. M., *Genetic Studies of Genius*, Harrap, London, 1926.
Ellis, Havelock, *Study of British Genius*, Hurst & Blackett, London, 1904.
Galton, Francis, *Hereditary Genius*, Macmillan, London, 1869.
Hyslop, T. B., *The Great Abnormals*, London, 1925.
Jacobson, A. C., *Genius: Some Revaluations*, Adelphi, London, 1926.
Kemble, J., *Idols and Invalids*, Methuen, London, 1935.
Kretschmer, Ernst, *The Psychology of Men of Genius*, Kegan Paul, London, 1931.
Lombroso, Cesare, *The Man of Genius*, Walter Scott, London, 1891.
Marks, J., *Genius and Disaster*, John Hamilton, London, 1928.
Nisbet, J. F., *The Insanity of Genius*, Ward & Downey, London, 1891.
Pickering, George, *Creative Malady*, Allen & Unwin, London, 1974.
Révész, G., *Talent und Genie*, Berne, 1952.
Terman, Lewis M., *Genetic Studies of Genius*, London, 1936.

GEOTHERAPY

Geotherapy (Gk. *gē*, 'earth'), healing by physical contact with the earth, is based on the principle that the earth, being the womb of nature from which all life emerges and by which all living things are nourished, has inexhaustible reserves of vital power to invigorate and heal. Its magnetism attracts beneficent influences from sun, moon, planets and constellations, which it stores for the use of all creatures. Each kind of zone, affected by cosmobiological forces, has its particular potencies: desert, jungle, mountain, steppe, each has its specific therapeutic virtues.

In itself, the earth has refreshing and rejuvenating properties. Francis Bacon (d. 1626) in his *Sylva Sylvarum* held that the smell of earth, especially fresh earth newly turned up with the spade was a great tonic, and inhaling its vapours would preserve life. He said, 'I knew a man that lived long, who had a clean clod of earth brought to him every morning as he sat in bed, and he would hold his head over it a good pretty while.' Following a plough as it turned up the earth was excellent for invigorating the spirits and improving the appetite. Pouring malmsey or Greek wine into a hole dug in new earth and inhaling, was also recommended. Bacon said that women would do themselves much good by weeding. Spring was the best time for all these matters, before the earth had spent its energy and its 'sweet breath' in the task of growing plants and vegetables for summer.

The notion of the strength-giving power of the earth is common to all parts of the world. Legend relates that Hercules on his way to perform one of his labours came upon the giant Antaeus, son of Neptune and Ge (water and land). During the ensuing wrestling bout he discovered that the giant seemed to gain more strength each time he touched the earth (his mother), whereupon he lifted Antaeus off the ground and strangled him in the air. The close rapport between *homo* (man) and *humus* (soil) was recognized from ancient times, and there are rural communities to this day where rites of homage are performed in honour of Mother Earth.

Occultists refer to the invisible geomagnetic energy as *telluric* force (from Latin, *tellus*, 'earth'). They believe that a man can recharge his energies by walking barefoot on natural soil, grass or sand. In the eighteenth century, James Graham (d. 1794) a 'magnetizer', recommended earth-baths, which he used to demonstrate with his female companion; they would be buried side by side with only their heads protruding. This total bodily contact with the earth, he claimed, enabled the pores to draw in all the nourishing elements from the soil.

In many ancient and primitive communities, women knelt at childbirth and gave birth upon the ground. Among the early Germans, Scandinavians, Romans and Japanese, babies were placed on the ground immediately after birth so that the magic power of the soil might pass into the child's body, and only after this rite were they washed and dressed.

As with the new-born child, so with the ailing. In accordance with the laws of geotherapy, the sick are placed on the ground to receive the vitalizing currents from the land. Mud-baths and clay compresses are prescribed for aches and pains. In some countries those who are dying are similarly placed on the bare earth, so that the ancestral spirits who are thought to dwell underground might receive them. The desire still expressed by civilized people to be buried in their own country is an echo of this instinctive urge to return to one's native soil in the bosom of the earth. The symbolism of burial is that while the soul returns to its Maker, the body made of clay is restored to earth.

The land is alive and breathes and needs nourishment. Belief in the earth as an organism is strong in eastern and southern Asia. The Baiga tribe of central India never tilled their fields for fear of ripping the breast of Mother Earth with the ploughshare. Primitive people in certain parts of the world regard the building of long stretches of metalled road and large concrete earthworks such as dams and embankments in their territory, as tending to stifle the breathing of the earth. The areas where such constructions have been made are regarded as unwholesome.

Certain prehistoric cults of ancient Greece connected with the sacred oak and the double-headed axe, and later associated with Zeus and Ge, were headed by priests known as *khamai-eunai*, 'ground-sleepers', who slept direct on the naked soil in order to energize themselves with the emanations from the earth. Popularly they were called *anipto-podes*, having 'unwashed feet', because they never washed their feet so that the soil of the sacred enclosure in which they served the goddess might not be dissipated. The semi-mythical poet, prophet and healer, Melampus, 'blackfoot', was the most famous of their fraternity.

Pilgrims returning from visits to sacred places often refrain from washing their feet so that the dust of the hallowed soil might cling to them as long as possible; during this period they also refrain from sexual intercourse. Many modern occultists discourage the wearing of rubber shoes and certain other articles of clothing because they act as insulators and cut off the vital radiations from the earth.

The place of one's birth or the land where one's ancestors originated is regarded as specially holy and sacrosanct, for its soil has a special affinity and therefore special virtues for the person concerned. There is an almost universal feeling of kinship with one's native soil. Love for one's country and patriotism in general are intimately bound up with this mystical link with the soil. A Bolivian tribe, when they feel the need to renew their vitality, return to the place supposed to have been the cradle of their ancestors. Jews, wherever they dwell, feel a strong urge to visit the land of the patriarchs, to traverse the regions trodden by their forefathers.

The topological features and the nature of the land in each locality determine the physical appearance and character of the people who dwell in it. The nutriments in the soil, its mineral content, its acidity and other chemical components, porosity, gas-content, fertility, the micro-organisms within and the vegetation upon it are strong factors in determining the diseases with which the inhabitants might be afflicted. To a large extent an organism, whether human or animal, is the biochemical product of the environment in which it lives. The presence or lack of certain elements can result in metabolic disorders and predispose one to anaemia, tuberculosis, goitre, thrombosis, diabetes and cancer*. The total environment, landscape, climatic conditions, even the water-level work their influence on the mind and spirit of the people, on their outlook, and ultimately on their religion, art, philosophy and culture.

The idea, first expressed by Hippocrates (d. 359 BC) and Polybius (d. 123 BC), the Greek historian, was further developed by modern writers like Henri Taine (d. 1893), French historian, and Friedrich Rätzel (d. 1904), German ethnographer and originator of the concept of *Lebensraum*, 'living space', and geopolitics. It was found, for instance, that the skull and pelvic measurements of all immigrants to America become 'indianized' by the second generation, and the American, be he Nordic, Mediterranean or Negro in origin, can be recognized as a type. Animals removed from their native country and pure-bred in another country lose some of their original characteristics and acquire those belonging to the fauna of the new homeland. As Carl Gustav Jung said, 'The soil of every country holds some such mystery.'

Books

Derrey, F., *The Earth is Alive*, Arlington Books, London, 1968.
Dieterich, Albrecht, *Mutter Erde, ein Versuch über Volksreligion*, 2nd edn, Leipzig, 1913.
Durrell, Lawrence, *Spirit of Place*, London, 1969.
Jung, C. G., *Civilization in Transition*, London, 1964.
Stringer, E. T., *The Secret of the Gods: an Outline of Tellurianism*, Neville Spearman, London, 1974.
Voisin, André, *Soil, Grass and Cancer*, Crosby Lockwood, London, 1959.

GROUP THERAPY

Psychotherapy involving any form of group activity under the guidance of a therapist. Groups can, of course, be studied in many situations: the family, school, college, club, workshop, hospital, asylum, jail, army unit, business, factory. As such this becomes the province of social, political, industrial, occupational or educational psychology. In one sense group therapy can also be applied to any method designed to improve the larger social background, and in this sense is known as social, milieu or situation therapy. Broadly, it studies the social setting in which people become and remain sick because of the stressful environment in which they find themselves (*see* sociopsychosis).

The chances of the useful application of group therapy in institutionalized or larger community situations are poor. To be effective from the therapeutic standpoint, the presence of a not too obtrusive specialist observer is important, but he can most usefully make observations only within a manageable group system. As commonly understood a group is defined as a small collection of between 3 and 12 persons (which includes the observer) who come together spontaneously or otherwise for purposes both diagnostic and therapeutic. Individuals are observed as they interact, verbally and non-verbally, with others in the group, and remedial treatment if necessary is suggested accordingly.

There is a dynamic interaction (group dynamics) among the members of a group, and inevitably a holistic and synergistic concept arises that can only be maintained by democratic participation, co-operation, sharing responsibility, and by accepting the need for discipline, faith, loyalty, respect for others, comradeship and other intangibles that do not form part of the goal, but make for coherence and group morale and strength, and are implicit in successful goal achievement. Psychologists are once again beginning to realize that these qualities, so long maligned, must be reinstated since they are essential not only for the social good, but for one's personal wellbeing too.

The origins of group therapy are somewhat obscure, but it seems to have started with the T-groups (training groups) of the late 1930s, consisting of educational courses for army officers, and later, business executives, who came together for brisk sessions of mutual evaluation and the exchange of ideas. It received fresh impetus under the brand of Gestalt psychology introduced by the Austrian-born American psychoanalyst, Frederick ('Fritz') Perls (d. 1970), which attempts to integrate or make 'whole', the individual who has been subjected to the fragmentation influences of modern life. A further boost came in 1962 with the Esalen movement (named after an Amerindian tribe) at Big Sur in California, founded by Michael Murphy.

Literally scores of group therapies have been evolved during the last two decades, ranging from the orthodox specialist studies associated with psychodrama*, music therapy* and art therapy*, to wilder forms which encouraged uninhibited personal, emotional and sexual expression. Some of the better-known variants of group therapy may be briefly listed.

In couple therapy two or more couples talk out their problems in the presence of a leader. Families come together for family therapy, when issues are often found to be rooted in the family head, who may be too liberal or too despotic, restrictive or permissive, patriarchal or matriarchal. In co-operative group therapy, two untrained people help each other, with a regular therapist in attendance. Any form of group therapy which lasts for up to 36 hours at a time is spoken of as marathon group therapy. In network therapy several families or groups may talk out their problems together.

In the group called Synanon, various asocial individuals, from drug addicts to petty thieves, meet others who have been through the same mill but are now reformed, and talk it out with them, with no holds barred. In contract therapy people come together by tacit or implicit contract for a specific purpose and often for a fixed period of time. Among the more individualist therapies are transactional analysis, founded by Eric Berne; client-centred therapy developed by Carl Rogers; and reality therapy, developed by William Glasser.

There are many therapies of extreme unorthodoxy, the most curious being that known by the generic name of encounter therapy. Some forms of this treatment have assumed the nature of a cult, where methods of 'turning on' were tried out. It became linked with the subculture of the beatniks and hippies. Inevitably some encounter groups received Zen, yoga, sufi and subud admixtures, with their quota of gurus, swamis, roshis (Zen adepts) and other masters, teaching meditative methods with personal Sanskrit phonemes, or giving training in Eastern sex techniques, archery and the sitar. Many intellectuals and fringe psychologists have gravitated towards it.

Encounter 'workshops' have evolved as a direct reaction against established psychiatric treatment, and the formal, rigid and doctrinaire approach of the professional consultants. The atmosphere is informal, the practitioner (leader, facilitator, guide or trainer) sympathetic and friendly. While one needs a medical degree to practise as a psychiatrist, anyone can lead an encounter group, be he minister, social worker, teacher or general friend of the neighbourhood.

The actual techniques of encounter groups vary considerably, and range all the way from passive meditation to energetic group activity. In what is called movement meditation, the members of the group just sit around, or stand, until first one, and then the others begin to swing or sway rhythmically, or make continuous sounds of humming, hissing, shh-ing, oh-ing, ah-ing, om-ing, and so on. In dyadic eye-fixation, two people, preferably of opposite sex, sit and gaze into each other's eyes, for ten minutes to an hour at a time, without saying a word. Often participants go off into a trance and some even claim to attain 'Allah consciousness' by this means.

It is important that all those who participate in encounter therapies should act with spontaneity and talk with complete frankness, to get rid of the deep-seated and suffocating inhibitions that choke normal intercourse. In truth-labs, people sit around, confess their likes, hates, their secret desires, their sins, and receive sympathy, reprimand, forgiveness. Often they undergo a kind of religious conversion, and groups in fact speak of grace and redemption.

Sometimes one member occupies the 'hot seat', a position in the centre of a circle of sitters, and talks freely about himself. He confesses his bad habits and defects of character, and this painful self-examination may lead to heated confrontation with the others. It is important that he should disclose any 'pathogenic' secrets, such as masturbation or deviant sexuality, or anything that has caused hidden feelings of guilt, shame or a sense of failure. He is offered 'feedbacks', that is, given the reactions of the group, who make comments about him, which are often hostile and humiliating. Sometimes they badger him to make him lose his temper, or even reduce him to tears, in order to effect a catharsis.

Many groups have their own jargon, much of it incorporating the older clichés. Everything is a game. People are beautiful. Everyone must do his own thing. Other slogans are connected with the concepts of: communicating, commitment, relating, involvement, belonging, being accepted, maturing.

Encounter therapy encourages people to sound off and let off steam. Such 'fight-training' is said to be highly beneficial. Vilification and abusive attack are permitted, even encouraged, and these may be directed against anyone: one's own mother, spouse, friend, child, boss or society in general, who for all one cares can all 'drop dead', another once-common cultic cliché. Often the person hysterically screams out his hatred, rage and resentment at the top of his voice until he is all 'screeched out'.

A still further stage, the hate-in, involves direct action, when the person not only verbalizes his feelings, but acts them out. A pillow or mattress is provided as a substitute for the object of his hate, and at the height of his bitter railing he will assault, pull, slap, throttle, and kick the imaginary enemy. This psychomotor therapy gets rid of any latent hang-ups, resentments and tensions, clears the mind and enlivens the body.

All encounter groups are basically body-oriented. The essence of much of the treatment lies in touching, to provide sensory awareness, body awareness and sensitivity training. Civilized society, they point out, frowns on physical contact, even to the extent of discouraging the mother from fondling her baby, and this embargo results in tactile deprivation that makes touching all the more necessary.

Sensory awareness is developed in many ways. Couples stand back to back, eyes closed, and have 'back talk' by rubbing up and down and sideways. Or a person covers himself or herself with a sheet and makes silent contact with others similarly covered with sheets. Groups of two or more persons, preferably blindfolded, touch one another's face, hair, shoulders, hands, legs. Electricity is exchanged and the psyche recharged.

Sessions may take in larger numbers during what is called a group-grope, sometimes in the nude and with no restrictions on sexual intercourse. In nude marathons such sessions can last for hours. Or bathers get naked into a pool together and soap one another's bodies, and afterwards massage one another with oil.

Like the orthodox methods they have censured, the extreme wing of the encounter groups have their own cynical critics, who attack their methods, suspect their motives, and doubt the validity of their philosophy. Ostensibly a 'therapy for normals', it is mostly the lonely, the sex-starved, the neurotic, the sex-deviant, who is attracted to their ranks, and is none the better for all the workouts. They have many features of various 'underground' groups of unwholesome intent. But there are other, more specific objections as well.

The leader of these groups is as much a victim of his therapy as his followers. He lacks professional standards. He is the blind leading the blind; a phoney fostering a false dependence in his victim. For all his democratic pretensions, he tends to assume messianic qualities, and with a smattering of psychiatric *patois* makes dogmatic pronouncements about his particular brand of therapy. Often he is more like the conductor of a satanic sabbat or a witch coven than a therapist.

Opponents of the system state that to encourage weak-minded people to give vent to their rage or hatred is not sound psychology. And as for pounding a pillow to take it out of your mother, wife, husband or child, it is ethically indefensible. To encourage even the expression that someone might 'drop dead' is hardly in consonance with the aim of encounter groups to spread sweetness and light.

Indulgence in anger or tantrums can never lead to a serene disposition or ease tension. It only helps to make resentments expand and multiply. It is a commonplace observation that those who are traditionally known to display their temper with impunity, the sergeant-major, the autocratic father, the bully, grow more, and not less irascible and arrogant. In a notable treatise entitled *On the Passions of the Soul*, the Greek physician Galen (d. AD 201) taught that the first step in the mastery of one's passions was to abstain from any crude and emotional outburst of passion.

Again, physical contact while desirable between mother and child, and permissible between lovers and intimate relations, is not to be encouraged between strangers without considerable reserve. There is a deep-seated natural instinct in the whole animal kingdom that opposes bodily contact or even contiguity, except in very special circumstances. Only the psychologically ignorant, it is argued, can believe that indiscriminate and promiscuous touching is natural and desirable.

Touching, starting with contact of hands and hair, provides an excuse for holding, hugging, fondling and greater sexual intimacy. What purports to begin as sensitivity-training in interpersonal growth, ends in undisguised sensuality. This is clearly evidenced in those love-ins where male or female partners are provided, and nakedness and sexual intercourse frankly encouraged. The final tenet of this doctrine states bluntly that sex facilitates 'interpersonal honesty', and is the best way of getting to know someone. Critics point out that sex-ins are not love-ins. And these love-ins, so called, like hate-ins, are fantasies that do more harm than good.

It is further pointed out that confessions are best made privately to those who are trained to receive them and give advice. Public self-disclosure to a group of other neurotics produces no benefit. It encourages a distortion of sins and exhibitionist fantasizing. More often than not, in spite of the confessions, truth sessions, weepings and conversions, the catharsis is a sham and the positive benefits non-existent. The glow lasts for the session and the novelty fades almost immediately. Then disillusion sets in, and a deep sense of the unreality of the whole set-up.

The gullible dupe of these empty ministrations feels ashamed that he has uncovered his body before strangers, has had a cheap sexual thrill, lived in an unreal world of hysterics and cranks, and all for nothing. No deep understanding is achieved, no lasting friendships are made, no shared love is experienced, and all his usual hang-ups come flooding back. For all the sentimentalism of the love-ins, say the critics, neither the quondam leader nor any of his erstwhile buddies would shed a tear if he himself literally dropped dead.

Books

Barnett, Michael, *People Not Psychiatry*, Allen & Unwin, London, 1973.

Bowskill, Derek, *Person to Person: a Survey of the Immediate Personal Confrontation Business*, Allen & Unwin, London, 1973.

Cartwright, D. and Zander, A., *Group Dynamics*, Tavistock Publications, London, 1960.

Egan, Gerard, *Encounter: Group Processes for Interpersonal Growth*, Wadsworth, Belmont, California, 1970.

Goffman, E., *Interaction Ritual: Essays on Face-toFace Behavior*, Anchor Books, New York, 1967.

Gustaitis, Rasa, *Turning On*, Weidenfeld & Nicolson, London, 1969.

Howard, Jane, *Please Touch: a Guided Tour of the Human Potential Movement*, McGraw-Hill, New York, 1970.

Liss, Jerome, *Free to Feel: Finding Your Way Through the New Therapies*, Wildwood House, London, 1974.

Mintz, Elizabeth, *Marathon Groups: Reality and Symbol*, Avon, New York, 1971.

Rogers, Carl, *Carl Rogers on Encounter Groups*, Harper & Row, New York, 1970.

Schutz, William, *Joy: Expanding Human Awareness*, Grove Press, New York, 1967.

Yalom, I. W., *The Theory and Practice of Group Psychotherapy*, Basic Books, London, 1970.

HERBALISM

The study of herbs, particularly their healing virtues. Strictly speaking a herb is a plant without woody stems, but the term popularly includes the soft parts of larger plants, like the leaves, flowers and roots, as also the sap of trees and the juice of fruits. The humble weed, everywhere despised and execrated by the gardener, has long been suspected of possessing wonderful curative properties. Ralph Waldo Emerson (d. 1882) described the weed as 'a plant whose virtues have not yet been discovered'. Certain herbs were treated as specifics and accordingly named after the ailment they healed or the organ they affected, thus: liverwort (Old English *wyrt*, 'root', or 'herb'), scurvy-wort, rupturewort, spleenwort.

Herbalism is probably the earliest of all healing systems, and herbs have been made into unguents, salves, philtres, perfumes, drugs and brews. They have the power to soothe, heal, calm, excite, sicken or kill. Primitive man observed the animals around him and noted that when sick they treated themselves by eating certain grasses and herbs. He did the same when he was ill, and by trial and error learned which herbs were best suited to the needs of particular ailments. The knowledge was handed down in families and tribes. In 1840 John Hoxley of Illinois discovered what he believed to be a treatment for cancer when a sick stallion with a cancerous hoof cured itself by eating certain kinds of herbs and weeds. Hoxley's grandson used the same remedy.

The Ebers papyrus (*c.* 1630 BC) of ancient Egypt contains many herbal medicines. Egyptian, Sumerian, Assyrian and Babylonian writings were enlarged on by the Greeks, who had a flourishing profession of herb collectors called rhizotomoi (Gk. *rhizo*, 'root') whose lore became the basis of herb-culling in medieval Europe. Culling is the all-important process of gathering herbs and plants in accordance with astrological times and seasons. From their herbs and roots the Greek rhizotomoi made drugs (Gk. *pharmakon*), which were preserved in special storerooms (Gk. *apothekē*). Thus these early compounders and dispensers of drugs were the direct forerunners of the modern apothecary and pharmacist.

Among the herbalists of the classical period were: Aristotle (d. 322 BC), who compiled a list of over 500 plants; Theophrastus (d. 285 BC), the first scientific herbalist and botanist; Dioscorides (d. AD 60), regarded as the father of medical botany, whose handbook provided the material for most of the items listed in the *materia medica* for the next 1,500 years; Galen (d. AD 201), physician and herbalist, whose 'galenicals' or simple combinations of herbs in unrefined form were used in Europe for centuries. The works of these writers translated into Syriac and Arabic were the foundation of Islamic herbal medicine.

There are many famous herbalists in European medicine, the best of the medieval authorities being the German abbess and mystic, Hildegard of Bingen (d. 1179), who wrote a giant herbal incorporating a great deal of current medieval European lore. Among English herbalists pride of place must be given to Nicholas Culpeper (d. 1654), who classified many hundreds of 'simples' or herbs, correlated with the astrological signs. Henry VIII (d. 1547) granted the herbalists a charter which is still in force.

The English philosopher Bishop Berkeley (d. 1753) came to regard resin as the last and quintessential product of the tree, exalted and enriched by the sun and containing, as it were, the 'vegetable' soul of the tree. During a visit to America he learned from the Amerindians the virtues of tar-water, made by mixing one part of dark pine or fir resin with four parts of water. This he believed to be a universal remedy, able to cure almost any disease.

Books

Arber, A., *Herbals: Their Origin and Evolution*, Cambridge, 1935.
Blythe, Peter, *Drugless Medicine*, Arthur Barker, London, 1974.
Budge, E. A. W., *The Divine Origin and the Craft of the Herbalist*, Society of Herbalists, London, 1928.
Crow, W. B., *The Occult Properties of Herbs*, Aquarian Press, London, 1969.
Culpeper, Nicholas, *The Complete Herbal*, Foulsham, London, 1965.
Hewlett-Parsons, J., *Herbs, Health and Healing,* Thorson, London, 1968.
Lucas, Richard, *Nature's Medicines: the Folklore, Romance and Value of Herbal Remedies*, Spearman, London, 1968.
Powell, Eric, *The Natural Home Physician*, 2nd edn, Health Science Press, London, 1975.

HOMOEOPATHY

A system of healing based on an ancient idea that disease can be cured by minute doses of a drug that normally causes symptoms like those of the disease. The homoeopathic principle was familiar to Hippocrates (d. 359 BC) and other Greek physicians, and was expressed in a famous saying attributed to the Delphic Oracle: 'The wounder heals.' It was later embodied in Latin maxims such as *similia similibus curantur*, 'like cures like' (first pronounced by Paracelsus), and *ubi venenum ibi remedium*, 'where the poison, there the remedy'. It is claimed that examples of this principle in operation are found in the fact that mild superficial burns are cured or eased by approaching fire; chilblains soothed by rubbing with snow; thighs chafed by horse-riding cured by foam from the horse's mouth; and in vaccine therapy for the prophylaxis and treatment of various diseases. The popular saying about taking 'a hair of the dog that bit you', was once literally interpreted, and a hair placed between two slices of bread and eaten. In emotional life, too, the people that have power to hurt have power to heal, like a mother or a loved one.

As a system of scientific therapy homoeopathy was discovered by the German physician Christian Samuel Hahnemann (d. 1843). While translating the *Materia Medica* of the English physician William Cullen (d. 1790) he came across the section on the curative powers of the cinchona bark. Experimenting with the drug himself, Hahnemann was amazed to find that when he took the drug he got all the symptoms of ague, which the drug was supposed to relieve. He continued his experiments for six years and found that drugs produced in healthy persons, conditions very similar to those which they relieved in the sick, and also that a drug that caused a sickness had the power to cure it, and this became the cornerstone of his system of cures.

He named his system homoeopathy (Gk. *homoeos,* 'same'), because it was a method of using drugs based on symptom similarity. Non-homoeopathic systems of medicines he called allopathy* (Gk. *allos,* 'different' or 'opposite'), based on treating diseases by giving opposite or contrary remedies to counteract the symptoms; for example, constipation is cured by a laxative. Allopathy is applied to the curing of disease by harsh drugs and surgery.

Hahnemann further held that violent cures were no good and he opposed blood-letting and other 'heroic' methods of treatment. He believed that for every condition requiring treatment there was one *simillimum* or single dose most like the disease that would exactly cure it. He therefore started using 'simples', that is, single drugs in their unadulterated and uncompounded form, as opposed to polypharmacy, where drugs were a mixture of a large number of medicines. In practice homoeopaths cannot always find the exact remedy and often prescribe a group of remedies instead.

In the course of homoeopathic history remedies have been taken from mineral substances, including gold, sand, anthracite, coal and gunpowder, from herbs and plants, and from animal substances. The latter have included bee stings, snake and spider venom, tears from a young girl (called *lacrimae filiae*), crushed live bedbugs (*cimex lectularius*), the secretion of skunk, powdered starfish, oyster-shells, uric acid obtained from human urine, snake excrement and spiders' webs. Hahnemann believed it was erroneous to think that some substances were naturally inimical to the body and were harmful. Reviving a maxim enunciated by Paracelsus he declared, 'No poison is inherently harmful; it is only the dose that makes it poisonous.'

This led to another fundamental postulate of homoeopathy set forth by Hahnemann, that the potency of drugs could be increased by diluting them. The 'homoeopathic dose' is proverbial. It is based on the belief that the more minute the dose, the greater its potency, for then, in a sense, the drug is 'dematerialized', and its quintessence emerges and its healing power is released from its limiting vehicle and it becomes a pure force.

It is widely known that a minute quantity of LSD, too small to be seen by the naked eye, and weighing only 1/200,000th of an ounce, can yet cause incredible reactions in the human brain. Pure penicillin is efficient in the unbelievable dilution of one part in 50 million parts of water. By spectroscopic methods the presence of one grain of salt dissolved in a cube of water one kilometer in length can be detected. The homoeopathic microdose is often so small that it cannot be detected even by spectroscopic analysis. Methods of reducing the mass of a drug and thus increasing its potency are variously termed dilution, minimization, potentization or dynamization.

A curious variant of homoeopathy was developed by the German physician Wilhelm Heinrich Schüssler (*c.* 1905). Analysis of the ashes of cremated persons showed him that twelve salts were the basic constituents of the human body. These same salts, he found, were also present in living tissues. His researches led him to develop tissue salt therapy, which he called bio-chemistry, though this should be distinguished from the orthodox study of the chemistry of living tissues.

Schüssler believed that disorders of the body arose from a deficiency of these salts, and that health could be restored by their assimilation. Like the microdose of homoeopathy, the biochemic tissue salts must be taken in minute doses to be effective in restoring the natural balance of the tissues and helping the assimilation of the essential mineral molecules. Although the twelve basic salts are still regarded as fundamental, subsequent therapists have added to their number, and today there are as many as 30 or 40 trace elements listed, some taken direct from standard homoeopathic remedies.

Books

Chapman, J. B., *Dr Schüssler's Biochemistry*, Thorson, London, 1960.
Hobhouse, Rosa, *The Life of C. S. Hahnemann*, Daniel, London, 1933.
Kent, J. T., *Lectures on Homoeopathic Philosophy*, Pal, Calcutta, 1957.
Lee, E., *Animal Magnetism and Homoeopathy*, London, 1838.
Leeser, Otto, *The Contribution of Homoeopathy to the Development of Medicine*, High Wycombe, 1969.
Powell, Eric, *Biochemistry Up To Date*, Health Science, Rustington, 1963.
Shepherd, Dorothy, *Magic of the Minimum Dose*, Health Science, Wellingborough, 1964.
Wheeler, Charles E., *Introduction to the Principles and Practice of Homoeopathy*, 3rd edn, Health Science, Wellingborough, 1974.
Wood, H. F., *Essentials of Homoeopathic Prescribing*, Health Science, Wellingborough, 1970.

HORMONE THERAPY

A form of organotherapy* based on the chemistry of the endocrine glands and of the cells of the nervous system, which manufacture hormones, power-ful substances that regulate the physical and mental functions.

Clinical analysis of the blood or urine can often indicate the quantities of hormones secreted. Many of the hormones can now be synthesized and intro-duced into the body orally or intravenously to make up for any deficiencies. So adrenalin manufactured in the laboratory can be administered to reinforce the action of the sympathetic nervous system. Certain hormones do not pass the blood-brain barrier and when introduced into the blood stream do not affect the nervous system. The endocrine glands and the main hormones secreted by them are briefly listed below.

Pineal, or epiphysis, situated at the base of the brain, and regarded by many as the point of contact between mind and matter. It is the brain of paraperception and the occult third eye. It manufactures melatonin, which responds to light and may be involved in circadian (day and night) rhythm. Melatonin is closely associated with the neurohormone serotonin.

Pituitary, or hypophysis, at the base of the brain, roughly above the roof of the mouth and behind the bridge of the nose. This is the master gland of the endocrine system, and consists of two parts. (a) The *anterior lobe*, which produces: somatotropin, also called the growth hormone because its activity during adolescence promotes growth; corticotropin (ACTH), which stimulates the production of hormones in the adrenal cortex (below); thyrotropin, which stimulates the thyroid gland (below); also other hormones controlling ovulation. (b) The *posterior lobe*, which produces: oxytocin, which stimulates the contraction of the uterus during labour, and the release of milk in response to sucking; and vasopressin, which inhibits urination, and tends to raise blood pressure. Stress results in an increased secretion of vasopressin.

Thyroid, on either side of the Adam's apple, associated with the release of energy in the tissues. Overactivity or hyperthyroidism results in enlargement of the gland (goitre) and excitability. Underactivity or hypothyroidism leads to mental dullness and apathy. Buried in the thyroid is the parathyroid, which controls the metabolism of calcium and phosphorus in the body.

Not far beneath, at the root of the windpipe, lies the thymus. The gland of youth, it regulates early development and shrinks after puberty. It plays an important part in the building up of immunities.

The adrenals, situated above the kidneys, consist of two main parts. (a) The *medulla*, which produces adrenalin (epinephrin) and noradrenalin (norepinephrin). (b) The *cortex*, which produces cortisone, aldosterone, androsterone and other corticosteroids, which provide the material for steroid therapy. Cortisone is used in the treatment of Addison's disease, arthritis, allergies and inflammations.

The pancreas (containing scattered cells called the islets of Langerhans) produces insulin which lowers blood sugar; and glucagon, which raises blood sugar. Insulin plays a part in diabetes as it controls sugar metabolism.

The gonads or sex glands differ in men and women. The male testes produce androgen (e.g. testosterone). The female ovaries produce estrogen, which regulates the general female functions; and gestogen (e.g. progesterone), which is involved in preparing the womb and maintaining pregnancy.

Psychologists have attempted a classification of people according to hormone types, which are presumed to occur as a result of the predominating endocrine activity of the individual. In esoteric physiology the subtle plexuses of the etheric body have roughly the same location as the endocrine glands (Walker, 1977, p. 221).

Neurohormone therapy is a branch of hormone therapy concerned specifically with the neurohormones, the chemical agents responsible for the transmission of impulses along the nervous system. Because of their function, the neurohormones are also known as 'transmitter substances', which are classed in three, not yet clear-cut and sometimes overlapping categories, namely: the catecholamines, the acetylcholines and the biogenic amines.

The nervous system, the central communications organization of the individual, controls thought, emotion and activity. It has two subdivisions. First, the central nervous system (CNS), which includes the brain and spinal cord, mainly under the control of the will. Second, the autonomic nervous system (ANS), also called the automatic, involuntary, ganglionic, visceral or vegetative nervous system, controlled principally by the thalamus and hypothalamus, and largely outside the control of the will. Neurohormone therapy is concerned more specifically with the chemical action and interaction of the ANS.

The ANS itself is divided into two parts:

(a) The *sympathetic nervous system*, whose activity is linked with the catecholamines or adrenalin class of hormones. This system is concerned with energy expenditure, as during stress, and stimulates the sweat glands, the roots of the hair, the dilation of the pupils, raises the heartbeat and blood pressure, inhibits the secretion of gastric juices and digestion.

(b) The *parasympathetic nervous system*, whose activity is linked with the acetylcholine class of hormones. This system is concerned with the rest, recuperation and nourishment of the organism, and stimulates the salivary glands, the sense of taste, slows the hearbeat, reduced the flow of air in the lungs, contracts the pupils, stimulates the evacuation of bladder and bowels and erection of the penis.

Neurohormone therapy is largely concerned with the effects of the catecholamines, the acetylcholines and the biogenic amines, together with certain related enzymes on the human organism. It should be noted that a number of the ANS neurohormones are also found in the CNS, but it is their activity in the ANS that is the special subject of psychophysical interest and research today. The action of the neurohormones is of great importance in understanding not only mood and emotion, but also how the psychotropic drugs operate.

The catecholamines are a class of hormones broadly regarded as the transmitter substances of the sympathetic nervous system. They include adrenalin (epinephrin) and noradrenalin. All stress situations cause the release of catecholamines. Drugs, hormones and enzymes that have the same effect as, or increase the activity of, the catecholamines are called adrenergic, 'adrenal energizing'. Since they stimulate the activity of the sympathetic nervous system, adrenergic drugs are known as sympathomimetic or sympathicomimetic. Adrenalin, ephedrine and amphetamine are adrenergic. So also are the mono-amine-oxidase inhibitors (MAOIs), used as antidepressants. The neurochemical action of the MAOIs is similar to that of drugs like LSD and mescaline.

Conversely, drugs, hormones and enzymes that inhibit the activity of adrenalin and certain other hormones, often leading to depression (e.g. phentolamine, propanolol) are called antiadrenergic. Mono-amine-oxidase (MAO), a group of enzymes that destroys an excess of certain transmitter substances in the brain, belongs to this class. These drugs that inhibit or block the activity of the sympathetic nervous system are called sympatholytic (e.g. tolazoline).

The acetylcholines are neurohormones broadly regarded as the transmitter substances of the parasympathetic nervous system. Drugs, hormones or enzymes that have the same effect as, or increase the activity of, the acetylcholines are called cholinergic, 'acetylcholine energizing' (e.g. muscarine, arecoline, pilocarpine). These drugs are parasympathomimetic, and stimulate the parasympathetic nervous system.

Anticholinergics are substances that have the opposite effect, they inhibit the activity of the acetylcholines and of the parasympathetic system; they are therefore parasympatholytic. These substances cause the sympathetic system to rise to the ascendant, so that the heart beats faster, the pupils dilate, etc. They include atropine, nicotine, hyoscine (scopolamine). They also include a class of enzymes known as cholinesterase (or acetylcholinesterase), which inactivates acetylcholine.

An ally of acetylcholine is a class of substances called anticholinesterase, or cholinesterase inhibitors, which are parasympathetic stimulants, delay acetylcholine decomposition and potentize acetylcholine action. These include pyridostigmine; physostigmine, found in the Calabar bean; neostigmine, endrophonium; tabune and various nerve poisons; parathione and many pesticides.

The biogenic amines include such substances as: histamine, the release of which gives rise to various allergies; dopamine, deficiency of which gives rise to parkinsonism; glutamic acid, believed to contribute to intellectual activity; serotonin, whose effect is heightened by the MAOIs (above); melatonin, found mainly in the pineal gland (above); tyramine, also found in cheese, and eating cheese seems to increase the output of adrenalin in the nervous system, which could be the reason why cheese at night disturbs the sleep of some people, and why patients taking antidepressive drugs are often advised to avoid cheese.

The overproduction or underproduction of hormones and neurohormones can radically alter an individual's physical appearance, character, and outlook on life. Many mental disorders, including schizophrenia*, cyclothymia*, anxiety* and stress*, are directly connected with disturbances of hormonal equilibrium.

It is believed that the control or increase in the activity of the endocrine glands and the neurohormones can be achieved by certain physical and meditative exercises practised in occult groups.

Books

Bajusz, E., *An Introduction to Clinical Neuroendocrinology,* Basel, 1967.
Eiduson, S. *et al.*, *Biochemistry and Behavior,* Van Nostrand, New York, 1964.
Ford, D. H. (ed.), *Influence of Hormones on the Nervous System*, Karger, New York, 1971.
Green, R., *Human Hormones*, Weidenfeld & Nicolson, London, 1970.
Pickford, Mary, *The Central Role of Hormones*, Oliver & Boyd, London, 1969.
Walker, Benjamin, *Encyclopedia of Esoteric Man*, Routledge & Kegan Paul, London, Stein & Day, New York, 1977.
Whalen, R. E., *Hormones and Behavior,* Van Nostrand, New York, 1967.
Young, W. C. (ed.), *Sex and Internal Secretions*, Williams & Wilkins, Baltimore, 1961.

HYDROPATHY

Hydropathy, or hydrotherapy (Gk. *hydōr*, 'water'), is a method of maintaining health and treating disease by using water, either internally or externally. Water possesses almost magical qualities and has always been regarded as the prime quenching, purifying and in some cases even creative agent. Water-cure was widely practised in ancient Egypt, Mesopotamia, India, China and other places, and was among the standard therapies prescribed by the Greek physician Hippocrates (d. 359 BC).

Herodotus (d. 425 BC) mentions the steam-bath of the Scythians who would throw water and hempseed on heated stones which produced intoxicating vapours. In Northern Europe the steam-bath, popular from early times, has survived as the banya in Russia and the sauna in Finland. Special cabins are built for the baths and both sexes bathe together. Water is thrown on heated stones to create steam and the body beaten with switches of birch, pine or juniper, which results in the skin becoming very heated and red. The bathers then douse themselves with cold water or roll in the snow outside.

Balneotherapy (Gk. *balaneion*, 'bath') or treatment by baths, as such methods were termed, can be pleasant, restful, energizing or soothing. The application of cold water to the skin stimulates the nerve ends, and the difference in temperature between water and body creates certain physiological reactions. Cold baths contract the small blood vessels, cause a rise in blood pressure, and thus stimulate the circulation and draw off heat from the surface of the body.

Cold-water treatment, used in many ancient and tribal societies, was reintroduced in modern times by a Silesian farmer, Vincenz Priesnitz (d. 1851), one of whose methods consisted in winding a cold, wet towel around the body and changing the wrapping about three or four times, every fifteen minutes. Another method, developed by Sebastian Kneipp (d. 1897), a Bavarian priest who was influenced by Priesnitz, consisted in douching the body with cold water. This, he claimed, cured him of a lung disease. He also recommended washing the feet in cold water every morning.

Warm baths 'open the pores', soothe the nerves and relieve pain. Hot fomentations relieve local pain and inflammation. Baths may also be taken in hot and cold water alternately. Wet packs and underwater exercises relieve muscular tension and are generally very beneficial. The sitzbath (German, *sitzen*, 'to sit') or hipbath, taken sitting in a small tub, is also regarded as excellent for certain ailments..

Water, one of the four great elements, becomes potentized as it flows through the earth, another of the great elements. Hence springs hidden in the earth's surface, especially if situated near the source of another element, that of fire, were eagerly sought for their almost magical virtues. Such was the mythical fountain of El Dorado, vainly sought by the Spaniards and other explorers.

Hermetics spoke of the *panacea aqua*, 'all-cure water', made by purifying (i.e. distilling) rain water several times in a special manner so that, having passed through the element of air, as rain, and been subjected to the influence of earth by filtering through clean sand, and the element of fire, by being boiled several times, it became colourless, tasteless and odourless and returned to its original pure 'watery' nature. This was supposed to be extremely beneficial to drink.

Many of the ancient springs were said to have been first found at sites where animals habitually came seeking healing waters. A number of such places later became famous as spas, named after the health resort of Spa in Belgium, whose mineral springs were discovered in the fourteenth century. Bath in England has hot springs, first developed by the Romans in AD 50, but like most Roman baths had a reputation for being 'a centre of wanton dalliance and a sink of iniquity', a reputation that lingered on until well into the nineteenth century. Other famous English spas include Buxton, Cheltenham, Harrogate and Matlock, the Matlock Hydro, established in the middle of the nineteenth century by John Smedley, high priest of hydropathy, being internationally famous. Similar resorts, whose names often have the suffix 'Baden' (from the German 'baths') in Germany, Austria and Switzerland, some known since Roman times, are popular for their hot saline or sulphur springs, especially suited for the treatment of gout and rheumatism.

If the water has mineral qualities, then, taken internally, it can give all the benefits of a powerful drug without the drawbacks. Various waters are said to be purgative (laxative), diuretic (promoting urine), phlegmagogic (promoting phlegm), carminative (reducing flatulence), diaphoretic (promoting sweat), and so on.

Water was believed to relieve internal congestion, restore vitality to a tired organism and dissolve waste matter in the tissues, and copious draughts were once given to patients to purify the system. Wiser counsels have since prevailed and in health resorts today only moderate quantities of the mineral waters are taken, supplemented by exercise and diet.

Books

Addison, William, *English Spas*, Batsford, London, 1951.

Alderson, Frederick, *The Inland Resorts and Spas of Britain*, David & Charles, Newton Abbot, Devon, 1973.

Graves, Charles, *Enjoy Life Longer: a Guide to the Sixty Leading Spas of Europe*, Icon Books, London, 1970.

Hartley-Hennessy, T., *Healing by Water*, Daniel, London, 1951.

Johnson, Edward, *The Domestic Practice of Hydropathy*, Simpkin, London, 1856.

Ramacharaka, Y., *System of Practical Water Cure*, Fowler, London, 1968.

Robins, F. W., *The Story of Water Supply*, Oxford University Press, 1946.

Trall, R. T., *The Hydropathic Encyclopedia: a System of Hydropathy and Hygiene*, 2 vols, New York, 1852.

Viherjuuri, M., *Sauna: the Finnish Bath*, Wyndham, London, 1969.

HYPNOSIS

(Gk. *hypnos*, 'sleep'), a state of mind in which the normal waking consciousness is put into a trance-like condition with a view to increasing and directing the natural suggestibility of a person. The person who reaches this induced trance state is called the *subject*, and the person operating on him is the *operator* or hypnotist. During the hypnotic state the subject is in rapport with the hypnotist, and accepts suggestions from him, or obeys his commands, all except those which conflict with his own instinct of self-preservation, or are opposed to his code of morality.

Certain types of people are more amenable to suggestion and can more easily be hypnotized, but in no case is there any question of a subject losing his identity and becoming a mere puppet, as the girl Trilby to the hypnotist Svengali in the novel by George du Maurier (d. 1896). Individuals as well as groups can be hypnotized. In the latter case it is called mass or collective hypnosis, and can be done through the recorded voice of the hypnotist and even over the television screen. For this reason the BBC has banned hypnotism from its television programmes as a result of a private test conducted in 1946, when a professional hypnotist sent some of his television viewers into a hypnotic sleep.

During hypnosis a man may revive lost memories; he may be induced to have positive hallucinations, that is, he may be made to see things that are not there; or negative hallucinations, when he will not see things that are actually there. He may be made insensible to pain or feeling, and carry out actions that he would normally be unable to perform when awake. Suggestions to perform actions can be given and carried out while the subject is entranced, or they can be *post-hypnotic suggestions*, made while the subject is under hypnosis, but carried out later when out of the trance state. He may, for example, be told that he will at noon on the following day walk three times around his chair. Although in his ordinary waking state at the time, he will do as directed, and if asked why will give as plausible a reason as he can for it. While under hypnosis a subject may be dehypnotized, or awakened from his trance at a command from the hypnotist to awake. But if left alone, he will normally sleep it off.

There are many methods of inducing hypnosis. These include drugs; breathing on the subject (insufflation); pressure on the carotid artery; staring at the space between the eyebrows; pressing the forehead of the patient; making 'passes'. These passes are slow, sweeping movements of the hand, from the head to the feet of the subject, which in earlier days were thought to cause the magnetic fluid to flow from the 'magnetizer' (hypnotist) via his hands into the patient's magnetic field, and so induce a 'hand-trance'.

Today the hypnotist uses a simple procedure. In a quiet room, with few distractions for eye or ear, the subject is made to recline on a couch or easy chair. The hypnotist stands or sits near the patient's head, and his suggestions are given in a firm, monotonous and not too loud voice. His whole manner must express confidence. The patient is told to breathe deeply, slowly and evenly, and to relax his body, starting from the heels and working upwards, particular attention being paid to the calves, thighs, stomach, back, neck and scalp. A small, bright object may be held up at a distance of about twelve inches from the subject's eyes, at such an angle that his gaze will be directed upwards in a slightly strained manner.

Then it is suggested that he is drowsy, and will soon be asleep. In time his expression will undergo a change: a far-away look will come into his eyes, the face will become expressionless, the eyelids will twitch spasmodically, and the pupils contract and dilate several times. The hypnotist continues his suggestions that the subject is sleepy, until the latter can no longer keep his eyes open, and in a short while his lids will close. The subject is now in a hypnotic trance, and in rapport with the hypnotist; he will not listen to what anyone says, and will react only to the hypnotist's voice.

Hypnotism differs from the mediumistic trance in two chief ways. The subject in a hypnotic trance is put into the state of hypnosis by an operator, but the medium enters it voluntarily. Again, in the mediumistic trance there is a form of 'possession' by another entity (a spirit or guide), whereas there is no possessing entity in the hypnotic subject. Hypnotic trance is also to be distinguished from sleep, for the subject under hypnosis is unlike a sleeping person both physiologically and psychologically. The knee-jerk or patella reflex that is absent in sleep, is present in the hypnotic trance. During hypnosis, as in the case of ordinary sleep, the sympathetic nervous centres are inhibited, and spontaneous thoughts and voluntary impulses are decreased. Hypnosis is, therefore, spoken of as 'brain-stem sleep'.

For thousands of years hypnotism has been practised as one of the most effective expedients of the priest, shaman, witch-doctor and thaumaturgist. It was used in ancient Egypt, Mesopotamia, Persia, India and China. The Gauls knew of it, and because the Druids were supposed to have been masters of the hypnotic art it was spoken of as 'Druidic sleep'. The early 'magnetizers' experimented with it, until Anton Mesmer (d. 1815) put it on a theoretical basis. Thereafter it was variously known as mesmerism or somnambulism.

Today hypnotherapy employs suggestion to cure or alleviate physical and psychological disorders. In a good subject hypnotic trance can be so deep and analgesia so complete that major surgical operations can be performed without the patient feeling any pain whatever. Many remarkable operations were carried out in this manner by the magnetizer James Esdaile (d. 1859) during his term of service in the government hospital in Calcutta in 1845. Hypnotherapy is particularly useful in getting to the bottom of hysterical disorders. As hypnoanalysis it is used in conjunction with psychoanalysis for mental ills. Several experiments have been tried in hypnotic age-regression, where a subject is made to remember an earlier period of his life.

Hypnotism is successful in dermatology; and is often used in dentistry and referred to as hypnodontics. It has also been successfully tried in childbirth to alleviate labour pains. The clinical applications of hypnosis are limited by the fact that complete anaesthesis can only be induced in deep trance, but only about 5 per cent of the population are deep-trance subjects; while about 35 per cent can be put into a medium trance; and nearly everybody into a light trance. Today the term 'hypnotism' is being increasingly replaced by the term 'psychosomatic sleep', to avoid the popular misconceptions associated with it.

Books

Cannon, Alexander, *The Science of Hypnotism*, Rider, London, 1947.

Cooper, L. F. and Erickson, M. H., *Time Distortion in Hypnosis*, Williams & Wilkins, Baltimore, 1959.

Dingwall, E. J. (ed.), *Abnormal Hypnotic Phenomena: a Survey of Nineteenth Century Cases*, 4 vols, Churchill, 1967–8.

Edmunds, S., *Hypnotism and the Supernormal*, Aquarian Press, London, 1961.

Esdaile, James, *Hypnosis in Medicine and Surgery* (originally entitled *Mesmerism in India*, published 1850), New York, 1957.

Gindes, B. C., *New Concepts in Hypnosis*, Allen & Unwin, London, 1956.

Haley, Jay (ed.), *Advanced Techniques of Hypnosis: Selected Papers of Milton M. Erickson, M.D.*, Grune & Stratton, New York, 1967.

Hammerschlag, H. E., *Hypnotism and Crime*, Rider, London, 1956.

Hull, C. L., *Hypnosis and Suggestibility*, Appleton-Century, New York, 1933.

Kline, M. V., *Freud and Hypnosis*, New York, 1958.

Kline, M. V. (ed.), *Hypnodynamic Psychology*, New York, 1955.
Le Cron, L. M. (ed.), *Experimental Hypnosis*, New York, 1952.
Marcuse, F. L., *Hypnosis, Fact and Fiction*, London, 1959.
Moll, A., *Hypnotism: Including a Study of the Chief Points of Psychotherapeutics and Occultism*, London, 1909.
Van Pelt, S. J., *Hypnotism and the Power Within*, Skeffington, London, 1950.
Wolberg, L. R., *Hypnoanalysis*, Grune & Stratton, New York, 1945.

HYSTERIA

(Gk. *hystera*, 'womb'), a nervous disorder long believed to be confined to women. According to the Greeks the womb when unsatisfied wandered around the body, causing great distress to the woman, who sought relief in raving, screaming, and the wild emotionalism known as 'hysterics'. Although hysteria frequently affects young women, it is now known to affect both sexes and all ages.

Some forms of hysteria, especially 'hysterics', can be contagious. If in a closed community, such as a nunnery, one person goes off the 'deep end' and gives way to unbridled emotionalism by screaming and weeping, it can easily spread and result in an 'epidemic' of hysteria. For example, in a girls' boarding school, one of the girls bursts into tears and has hysterics on receiving bad news from home. Her companions in sympathy follow suit and in a short while the whole school is in an uproar.

In the seventeenth and eighteenth centuries hysteria was often thought to be complicated by the *vapours*, or morbid exhalations from the wandering womb or from an excess of 'animal spirits' from the viscera, which clouded the mind and caused hypochondria and other ailments peculiar to young women. A woman with the vapours was in a state of mental imbalance and depression. A fit of the vapours was once quite fashionable among ladies.

In a more restricted context hysteria is applied to a psychoneurosis characterized by a wide range of symptoms, including dissociation and susceptibility to suggestion. As hysteria does not arise from any alteration of the nervous system or physical organism, it is classed as a functional nervous disorder and not an organic disease. Pathological or other symptoms may occur without defect in the associated organ: a hysterically blind person, for instance, has normal pupillary reactions to light; the reflexes and the electrical excitability of the muscles of a hysterically paralysed person are quite normal. Some authorities point out that hysteria and schizophrenia* are 'opposite'* diseases, hysteria being a disease of extraversion, schizophrenia of introversion.

Underlying hysteria is a 'will to sickness', a deliberately fostered desire to be sick, and to manifest symptoms of sickness for a specific purpose, mainly to attract attention and secure interest and sympathy, to avoid responsibility. It is a psychosomatic* defence mechanism designed by the patient, consciously or unconsciously, to protect him from his fears, imagined or real, to satisfy a repressed need. This self-protective sickness may take many forms and the symptoms have every mark of genuineness.

Thus a person faced with an unbearable situation and unable to meet the responsibilities of life, might attempt to escape from his intolerable situation

137

by simulating illness or disability. In what is called 'conversion hysteria', a mental conflict is converted into a physical symptom. Self-pity becomes a splitting headache; anxiety becomes nervous indigestion. Frequently the symptom points in a disguised and symbolical form to the original disturbing cause. Thus a person may become paralysed when called upon to meet danger, blind when he cannot bear to look at life, sick and helpless when called to action he cannot undertake.

Traumatic shock of some kind, especially if experienced at an early age, may bring on hysterical symptoms in later life. A painful childhood experience is buried in the unconscious and apparently forgotten so that the integrity of the ego might be maintained. But in fact it is not forgotten, only repressed, and continually seeks to surface and return to consciousness. Sigmund Freud said that 'the hysteric suffers from reminiscences'. The repressed emotion denied a normal outlet emerges into consciousness in a substitute form, as a separate independent phenomenon.

Another common cause is self-punishment, resulting from deep-seated feelings of guilt. Here symptoms may develop to help one out of an emotional problem whose solution is incompatible with the rest of the personality, or opposed to one's moral principles. Thus, a married woman who secretly wishes to have intercourse with another man but feels that it is wrong, may suddenly develop a pain in the back, thus drawing upon herself the painful consequences of her illicit wishes. This expresses both her frustration and expiates her sense of guilt.

Much of hysteria is connected with sexuality. According to the Greek physicians, the womb when sexually unsatisfied wandered about the body and caused the symptoms of hysteria (see above). Disorders of the uterus are still believed to create a climate favourable for the emergence of hysterical symptoms. So do psychological changes involving the sex life of the individual, such as puberty, pregnancy and the menopause. A related condition is 'womb starvation', resulting either from barrenness or sexual abstinence, which makes the victim seek this form of relief. According to Freud, 'The hysterical attack is an equivalent of coitus.'

Hysteria can produce incredible changes in the body cells and tissues. It creates modifications in the vasomotor system, and is a fruitful source of all kinds of symptoms. Such *pathomimesis*, 'disease imitation', is a characteristic feature of hysteria, which has been aptly described as 'a flight into disease symptoms'. Among the ways in which hysteria might manifest are: miscellaneous aches and pains; hyperaesthesia or excessive sensibility; anaesthesia or loss of sensibility; paralysis and invalidism; functional blindness and deafness; tremors, tics, spasms, muscular cramps, contractures of the limbs, convulsions*; hallucinations, both auditory and visual; xenophrenia* and dissociation; depersonalization*; amnesia; somnambulism; hypnotic or sleep-like states of consciousness; cataleptic stupor.

Still stranger symptoms are found among the hysterical stigmata. There is the pain or strange sensation that often starts in the lower abdomen, and spreads to the epigastrium, breasts and throat, and in the throat seems to increase in size and almost choke the patient so that he cannot swallow. This feeling of a choking ball lodged in the pharynx is known as the *globus hystericus*. Another curious symptom is the *clavus hystericus* (Lat. *clavus*, 'nail'), a sharp pain near the bregma, the centre top of the skull. Women sometimes suffer from *ovarie*, a painful sensation of pressure on the ovaries, and occasionally go through all the experiences of *pseudocyesis*, or false pregnancy.

Hysteria is the most dramatic and imitative of all illnesses. A hysteric's inventiveness (mythomania) is phenomenal. A hysterical subject does not always distinguish between his waking hallucinations and reality. He tends to embroider his experiences or his past, and will elaborate extensively on suggestions made to him. He believes his own tales to be absolutely true. Hysterics have excellent histrionic talents and a wonderful sense of drama. They will even resort to tricks of ventriloquism and legerdemain and similar acts of deception. They are able to create entirely new personalities by building on material in the subliminal self. An eminent physician, Sir Francis Walshe, once said that the hysteric was an actor who becomes more and more convinced by his own acting, and 'may ultimately come and join the audience'.

For these reasons hysteria is often invoked to explain various mystical and occult phenomena for which no other natural explanation is forthcoming. It is 'the sheet-anchor of the sceptic'. At one time or another all of the following have been attributed to it: the visions of the mystic; the marks and wounds of the stigmatist; the feats of the fire-walker; the long abstinence of the marathon faster; the morbid gluttony of the person suffering from bulimia; the prolonged coma of the person who sleeps for weeks; the sleeplessness of the insomniac; feats of suspended animation; the rapid healing of wounds by the wonder-worker; the incredible contortions of the convulsionary; the 'invasion' of the 'possessed'; the transfiguration of a person which gives him the appearance of a werewolf; the bloodlust of the vampire; the miracle cures of spiritual healing; all the manifestations of the séance room; the glossolalia of the man who 'speaks in tongues'.

But the fact is that the phenomena of hysteria still await adequate explanation. So far it remains an 'occult' disease. It is a convenient blanket term used in order to account for many kinds of complexes, philias and phobias. Although certain psychologists have stated that hysteria is an almost extinct disease, there are others who argue that it is now universally prevalent, since now more than ever before we display and react entirely to 'symptoms'. We are all repressed, on the defensive, histrionic and playing a part. We have all become, or desire to become, 'personalities'.

Books

Abricossoff, G., *L'Hystérie aux XVIIe et XVIIIe siècles*, Paris, 1897.
Althaus, Julius, *On Epilepsy, Hysteria and Ataxy*, London, 1866.
Babinski, J. and Fromont, J., *Hysteria or Pithiatism*, London, 1918.
Briquet, P., *Traité clinique et thérapeutique de l'hystérie*, Paris, 1859.
Cesbron, Henri, *Histoire critique de l'hystérie*, Paris, 1909.
Collie, John, *Malingering and Feigned Sickness*, Edward Arnold, London, 1917.
Eysenck, H. J., *The Dynamics of Anxiety and Hysteria*, Routledge & Kegan Paul, London, 1957.
Freud, S. and Breuer, J., *Studies on Hysteria*, Hogarth Press, London, 1955.

Hammond, W. A., *Nervous Derangement, Somnambulism, Hysteria, Hysteroid Affections*, Putnam, New York, 1881.
Janet, Pierre, *The Major Symptoms of Hysteria*, Macmillan, New York, 1929.
Kretschmer, Ernst, *Hysteria, Reflex and Instinct*, London, 1949.
Laycock, Thomas, *An Essay on Hysteria*, Philadelphia, 1840.
Owen, Alan R. G., *Hysteria, Hypnosis and Healing*, New York, 1969.
Robinson, Nicholas, *A New System of the Spleen, Vapours, and Hypochondriack Melancholy*, London, 1729.
Veith, Ilza, *Hysteria: the History of a Disease*, University of Chicago Press, 1965.

I

IATROGENICS

(Gk. *iatros*, 'physician'), the study of the factors underlying 'iatrogenic (physician-caused) illness' brought on by doctors themselves, by the medicines and drugs they prescribe, and by the methods of medical treatment. Popularly, iatrogenic diseases are called DOMP, 'diseases of medical practice'.

Illness and suffering are inflicted by wrong diagnosis, ignorance or negligence on the part of the physician in a number of cases. In the USA, for instance, about 25 per cent of all hospitalizations are due to injuries incurred by patients during medical treatment. Professional incompetence is compounded by lack of understanding and sympathy. Increasingly doctors represent an unresponsive, alien and sometimes hostile factor in the daily lives of people already beset by trouble. The presence of a doctor, or even the feeling that one should visit him, already sets in motion the internal chemistry bearing the seeds of stress and disease.

Medical institutionalization is a significant contributory ingredient in this set-up, and hospitals can in some cases do more harm than good. The depersonalization of modern medicine, X-rays, gadgetry, mechanical contrivances, computer diagnosis, potent drug therapy, are all unfavourable to the personal approach. 'The medical establishment', says Illich, 'has become a major threat to health.'

Some modern hospitals have been charged with having become highly efficient technocracies, with all the drawbacks of bureaucratic institutionalism. In the struggle between scientific efficiency and humanitarian considerations, the personal regard for the patient is beginning to recede in what is termed the management of illness, as distinct from the treatment of the person who has the illness.

Placing people in hospital, among strangers, with its routine of taking temperature, blood pressure, and so on, the hurried attentions of harassed staff and white-coated technicians, can add to the sense of insecurity and isolation, and aggravate the disorder, whatever it might be. The daily round of the senior doctor surrounded by juniors and teams of nurses and students, are not always calculated to reassure the patient. In spite of its efficiency, the impersonal atmosphere in the large hospital often promotes distress and in some cases even disease.

An investigation carried out in a teaching hospital in America showed that 20 per cent of all patients admitted to hospital contracted DOMP. At least 1 out of 10 patients suffers some adverse effects from hospital treatment in the UK. And 1 out of every 18 hospital patients actually contracts an infection while hospitalized. In the view of some psychiatrists, the hospital itself can be regarded as a sick organization.

During the middle of the last century, 1 expectant mother out of every 8 died in hospital of childbed or puerperal fever. In 1847 a junior Hungarian doctor, Ignaz Semmelweiss, demonstrated that this scandalous mortality was caused by doctors themselves, who examined women after they had touched other infected patients. For daring to make such an impious suggestion against the medical profession he was vilified and persecuted for several years.

Before the introduction of antiseptic surgery by Joseph Lister (d. 1912), conditions prevailing in the operating rooms of many hospitals were such that no surgeon even of the European Dark Ages would tolerate. Surgeons, some of the highest eminence, used to wear the operating coat they had first used as students, for it was a matter of pride to display the encrustations of filth it had acquired in the course of their career. In the lapel of the coat was a short length of ordinary whipcord for tying arteries.

The widespread and indiscriminate use of surgery is a danger that has to be noted even today. It has been said that surgery has advanced to such an extent that even a small talent is now adequate. And because of the development of antibiotics patients can be sent home even when their operation wounds are still suppurating.

The resort to surgery can sometimes be taken as an admission that medicine has failed. The tendency today is to remove troublesome organs rather than leave them to heal, albeit more slowly, by medication or natural process. Sometimes the mere suspicion that an organ might be the source of trouble is sufficient to prompt a surgeon to excise it, on the principle, 'If in doubt, cut it out.'

At the end of the last century the great fashion was for orificial surgery on the sexual organs or anus (*see* constipation). Up to the Second World War hundreds of thousands of now admittedly useless operations were performed to remove tonsils, gall-bladders, appendixes, even where there was no need to do so, because of the belief in 'focal sepsis' in these organs. More recently, after a study of 6,250 hysterectomies, an American survey concluded that one-third 'seemed to be unwarranted'.

There are critics in the profession itself who believe that recourse to extreme measures to effect more rapid cures may cause great damage in the long run. Earlier methods such as bleeding*, cupping*, purging, vesication, and other primitive devices, did not radically interfere with the human organism, and did not do harm, even if they did little good. Folk-medicines and nature-cures still depend on herbs and natural products, on osteopractic treatment and physiotherapy*.

But organ transplants, the tendency to use the knife to remove a trouble-some organ instead of healing it, blood transfusions, all can take a heavy toll of the human psyche. We still know too little about ourselves, they say, to be complacent about the long-term benefits of such procedures. In the USA, blood transfusions cause some 30,000 cases of hepatitis (inflammation of the liver) each year, of which more than 3000 are fatal. Eric Powell quotes the opinion of Dr John Wallace who says, 'Blood should be regarded as a danger-ous drug . . . there are now more than twenty viruses known to be trans-missible by transfusion.'

Frequent use of highly potent miracle-drugs, of mind-changing drugs, of tranquillizers, of sleeping pills, of pep-pills, of contraceptive pills, presents another possible danger whose long-term effects are as yet incalculable. Drug therapy*, like doctors and hospitals, can also be pathogenic, or 'sickness-making'.

Occultists point out that massive doses of antibiotics, and the widespread use of powerful synthetic compounds can be not only physically, but psy-chically, harmful. The human being is now being treated like a battery chicken. He is removed from healing human contact and put into a stream-lined, mass-curing machine, and dosed with synthetic products too harsh and dangerous for his constitution.

As though this alarming diagnosis were not enough, some indeed believe that the side-effects of modern treatment are already to be seen in the increase in mental sickness. Even more disturbing is the possibility that as a result of this crippling effect on body and mind, human development may be stultified on the psychical and spiritual planes as well.

The reassuring 'bedside manner' that released healing forces, both glandular and psychological, and that constituted a large part of the therapy* of more leisurely times, is today becoming increasingly rare. It used to be said that 'some people go to a doctor when what they want is an audience', and the family doctor of old, aware of the therapeutic value of sympathy, listened patiently and gave friendly advice. But few doctors today have the time to do more than give their patients a cursory examination and prescribe a proprie-tary drug.

Today the medical profession has expanded into a huge technocracy of specialists, paramedicals and ancillarists, who form a virtual industry, with a plethora of new ranks, grades, roles and duties. These include experts in haematology, biochemistry, histology, bacteriology, pharmacology, virology, neurology, endocrinology, anaesthesia, genetics, physiotherapy, orthopaedic surgery, radiology, not to mention the various laboratory technicians special-izing in ECGs, EEGs and other biotelemetrical aids. Each part and each func-tion of the body has its own range of specialists.

The nursing profession itself has proliferated into several ranges. Some nurses in the loftier ranks of the hierarchy are now almost as inaccessible to the patient as the consultant.

With the rapidly growing specialization in therapeutics it has been felt that the general practitioner is often only a filter, passing patients on to the specialist or the surgeon. He finds it very difficult to keep abreast of develop-ments when virtually every aspect of his work has expert practitioners. It is said that the old-style family doctor will soon be obsolete. His physical examination has been compared to the medieval laying on of hands, and the proprietary drugs of his prescriptions to the alligator saliva and powdered snake brain of the tribal medicine-man. But his usefulness is beyond dispute, and he has an important role to play if only he can be allowed to revert to his traditional function, 'to cure sometimes, relieve often, and comfort always'.

Books

Abse, Dannie, *Medicine on Trial*, Aldus Books, London, 1967.
Barton, Russell, *Institutional Neurosis*, John Wright, Bristol, 1959.
Branson, Roy, *The Doctor as High Priest*, Hastings Center Studies, New York, 1966.
David, M., *The Complications of Modern Medicine: a Treatise on Iatrogenic Diseases*, New York, 1963.
Dubos, René, *Mirage of Health Utopias, Progress and Biological Change*, Allen & Unwin, London, 1959.
Illich, Ivan, *Medical Nemesis: the Expropriation of Health*, Calder & Boyars, London, 1975.
Klein, Rudolf, *Complaints Against Doctors*, Knight, London, 1973.
Mair, George, *Confessions of a Surgeon*, Luscombe, London, 1974.
Malleson, Andrew, *Need Your Doctor Be So Useless?*, Allen & Unwin, London, 1973.
Maxwell, H. (ed.), *Integrated Medicine*, John Wright, London, 1976.
Meyler, L. and Peck, H. M., *Drug Induced Disease*, Royal Vangorcum Assen, Netherlands, 1962.
Moser, Robert H., *Diseases of Medical Progress: a Contemporary Analysis of Illness Produced by Drugs and Other Therapeutic Agents*, 2nd edn, Thomas, Springfield, Illinois, 1969.
Powell, Eric, *The Natural Home Physician*, Health Science Press, London, 1975.
Schindel, Leo, *Unexpected Reactions of Modern Therapeutics*, London, 1958.

INCUBATION

Incubation (Lat. *incubare*, 'to lie upon') is an old method of producing dreams by deliberate effort, usually as a result of sleeping in a temple or other sacred place, in order to obtain divine advice or assistance through the dream. 'Temple-sleep', as it is sometimes called, was frequently resorted to by the sick in the belief that the cure would be suggested to the patient or the priest-physician in the dream. Incubation was much practised in ancient times and is still popular in some parts of the world.

At the temple the inquirer performed certain preparatory rites: ablutions, a short fast, offerings and sacrifices to the deities. He then spent the night in a selected place in the temple, usually lying on the outstretched skin of an animal such as a goat or ram, in some cases one that had been specially sacrificed for the purpose. The following morning the dreamer related his dream to a professional oracle or dream-diviner who would interpret it. In Babylon a class of priests called the *shabru* specialized in inducing dreams in clients, while another class of priests, the *baru*, would interpret them.

In some places, like the Egyptian temples of Isis and Serapis in Memphis, there were priests who for a fee would procure dreams that revealed the future, gave guidance or advice in personal affairs, or brought good luck.

Some of these priests would themselves dream the dream for their clients. Herodotus (d. 425 BC) relates that at the temple of Bel in Babylon a priestess used to dream such divinatory dreams for her customers.

Besides temples, other hallowed places were frequented in order to obtain oracular dreams. Herodotus, writing of the Nasamonians of North Africa, says that for divination they went to the sepulchres of their ancestors, and after praying would lie down to sleep upon the graves, and by the dreams that came to them they guided their subsequent conduct. Incubation in the vicinity of burial places, cremation grounds, holy wells and sacred streams was common. The ancient Hebrews visited vaults or slept among tombs to get meaningful dreams.

Many other methods of forcing dreams were also current. Hypnosis and different forms of suggestion were certainly practised. Eating highly salted food without drinking water could make one dream, just as enforced wakefulness could be followed by sound dream-filled sleep. Physical discomfort was a reliable means of inducing dreams. Using a hard log of wood from a sacred tree, or a skull, for a pillow, and a hard lumpy bed were considered very effective.

The best attested cases of incubation come from Greece, especially from the temples of *Aesculapius*, the son of Apollo and a god of medicine. According to an ancient tradition he was a native of Memphis who lived about 1250 BC. From Egypt he emigrated to Greece and introduced the knowledge of medicine into that country. The serpent was especially sacred to Aesculapius, and also appears in representations of his daughter Hygeia, goddess of health. Harmless serpents, in whose touch healing powers were supposed to reside, were often kept in temples dedicated to them, and healed those they licked.

Many miraculous cures were recorded at the temples of Aesculapius. The most famous were at Athens and Epidaurus, in Greece, and Aegae, Colophon and Pergamum in Asia Minor, which were usually in charge of priest-physicians known as Asclepidae. The same general procedure was followed. The sick person spent the night in one of the *abatons*, or sleeping chambers, after the physician had suggested his cure. On awaking he related his dream to the priest and might even recommend his own means of healing. Frequently the patient dreamed that Aesculapius himself performed the operation or applied the treatment, and awoke to find himself cured.

After each successful cure the case history, with aetiology*, symptoms, prognosis and cure, was recorded in writing on tablets or carved on the temple walls. These *iamata* ('cures') or records of healing, provided a reliable archive in the course of centuries which was useful to later physicians. Hippocrates of Cos (d. 359 BC) the son of a midwife and a celebrated physician of antiquity, and reputedly a descendant of Aesculapius, was supposed to have been greatly indebted for his vast medical knowledge to the temple records of Cos, his native city.

Temple inscriptions show that among the ailments cured were barrenness, blindness, deafness, headaches, battle wounds, paralysis, often in a very extraordinary way: 'Nicasibule of Messene to obtain offspring slept in the sanctuary and saw a dream in which the god approached her with a snake which was creeping behind him, and with the snake she had intercourse. Within a year she had two sons.' In another case a partially paralysed man dreamed he was playing dice, and as he was about to cast the dice the god appeared, sprang upon the hand and stretched out his fingers. Another man suffered from a stone in his membrum. He dreamed that he was lying down with a fair boy and when he had a seminal discharge he ejected the stone. A lame man was brought to the sanctuary on a stretcher. He dreamed that the god broke his crutch, ordered him to climb a ladder, and chided him for cowardice when he got up only part of the way. At daybreak the man climbed the ladder.

Major contributory factors in healing were undoubtedly psychological. Many diseases were of a nervous or emotional nature and as such were more likely to be cured by dramatic means and the power of suggestion and faith. The long and exciting pilgrimage; the sight of the sanctuary usually situated high on the hillsides exposed to the sun and invigorating breezes; the stories of miraculous cures; the portentous dreams induced or suggested by the priests. It is possible that the patient was sometimes put under deep hypnosis and subjected to a minor operation.

With the advent of Christianity many Aesculapian temples were abandoned or taken over by the church, along with many of the curative procedures. Sleeping in holy places became common in the early Middle Ages, and several medieval churches became famous for their cures, with incubation quarters and priests and attendants on daily duty. The patrons of healing were the Archangel Michael, St Damien and St Hubert. Many places in Scotland and Ireland, Greece, Cyprus and Crete were used for incubation cures till the last century. Some suppliants still sleep in churches hopefully awaiting divine intervention and miracle cures.

Books

Caton, R., *The Temples and Ritual of Asklepios at Epidaurus and Athens*, London, 1902.

Dawson, G. G., *Healing: Pagan and Christian*, Macmillan, London, 1935.

Edelstein, Emma and Ludwig, *Asclepius: a Collection and Interpretation of Testimonies*, 2 vols, Johns Hopkins Press, Baltimore, 1945.

Hamilton, Mary, *Incubation or the Cure of Disease in Pagan Temples and Christian Churches*, London, 1906.

Herzog, Rudolf, *Die Wunderheilungen von Epidauros*, Dietrich, Leipzig, 1931.

Kerényi, Carl, *Asklepios: Archetypal Image of the Physician's Existence,* Thames & Hudson, London, 1960.

Leipoldt, J., *Vom Epidauros bis Lourdes*, Frankfurt, 1935.

Meier, C. A., *Antike Inkubation und moderne Psychotherapie*, Zurich, 1949.

Walton, A., *The Cult of Asklepios*, Boston, 1894.

INFECTION

The invasion of the body by micro-organisms, and the multiplication of those organisms, resulting in disease. Infections can be transmitted by air, water, food, by contact or by insect and animal carriers. The cure lies in attacking the micro-organisms responsible.

The mere presence of microbes does not necessarily lead to infection. Certain deadly bacteria are either normal inhabitants or temporary lodgers in our bodies, and we are constantly exchanging these with one another. We all have incipient throat, lung and digestive diseases. Many otherwise healthy people have patches on the lungs showing healed tubercular lesions. It is said that probably everyone has cancer once or twice in his lifetime (Ferguson, 1974, p. 43), but in most cases the tumour is destroyed in its early stages. Flea-infested rats are found in every city and numbers of these rats are potential plague carriers, yet very rarely do they cause epidemics like the Black Death. In the same way it is known that hundreds of people are carriers of mild infection, yet do no harm to themselves or to others, but can suddenly become dangerous foci of infection when time and circumstances are ripe.

For any invading bacteria to do harm they must find exactly the right ecological setting, which could be provided in a number of situations, such as: hereditary predisposition, cosmobiological factors, lowered physical resistance, and negative mental states like depression*, anxiety* and stress*. Where a proper foothold is secured, the body suffers sickness.

Recent studies of infections, and of the drugs used in dealing with them, have brought certain very significant facts to light: (a) that microbes* and viruses are becoming increasingly resistant to modern drugs; (b) that the effectiveness of these drugs is therefore being progressively diminished; (c) that the human body's natural resistance to disease has decreased because of the excessive use of chemotherapy for the prevention and treatment of infection; (d) that it is essential to have less recourse to drugs in order to restore the body's own natural defences in its fight against infection.

It has been pointed out that till well into the present century, until the arrival of the antibiotics, medicines effectively cured less than half a dozen infections. Except for mercury in syphilis*, quinine against malaria, and the anthelminthics for expelling worms, few specifics existed for any disease. It was believed from the time of Hippocrates (d. 359 BC) that the body has tremendous reserves of strength and resistance, and is able, with a little assistance, to overcome ordinary infections. In the past therefore the doctor relied mainly on the body's own resources, and prescribed simple remedies that gave the body itself a chance to deal with the malady.

Today's armoury of drugs includes many potent chemicals which seem to get to the source of infection, and attack the invading organism direct. Mass inoculations and vaccinations have made children resistant to the common diseases of childhood. Antibiotics and other drugs have greatly reduced the incidence of once deadly diseases. There has been a worldwide decline in TB and polio since the mid-1950s, and in measles since the early 1960s, while smallpox has been virtually wiped out since 1970.

Critics of modern drug therapy* do not object to it in principle, but to its widespread abuse by doctors. These drugs tend to undermine the body's natural resistance. Some drugs while killing the invading germs, exterminate useful bacteria in the body as well; some, like the immunosuppressives used in transplantation destroy the body's own defences; and some actually cause sickness.

Furthermore, as a result of their extensive use, microbes are becoming increasingly immune to the lethal effects of these drugs. Within bacteria there are certain genetic particles known as episomes, which can pass from one bacterium to another, so that resistance acquired by one can rapidly be transmitted to the rest, spreading resistance through the whole genera. Bacteria thus acquire a high degree of multiple resistance to the drugs we manufacture, which are becoming ineffective. And the growth of resistant microbial strains has consistently kept pace with new developments in antibiotics.

Soon after the sulphonamides came into use, certain types of pneumococci acquired resistance to them. By 1943 the sulphonamide-resistant bacteria became a matter of international concern. By the early 1950s bacteria of the throat, bowel and genital passages were mutating, to adapt to certain broad-spectrum antibiotics that were being used. At the end of the 1950s many strains of staphylococci had already developed resistance to penicillin. Drugs like dapsone and other sulphone drugs are successful against leprosy, but have to be taken regularly for two or more years, during which time the patient's microbes begin to develop resistance to them.

The micro-organisms responsible for venereal disease, both gonorrhoea and syphilis, were first successfully treated with sulphonamide drugs and antibiotics, but many new resistant strains have since evolved, so that their curative effects too are diminishing, and are not likely to last. It is becoming increasingly difficult to find new antibiotics to cope with the reinvigorated bacteria of other serious infections.

Malaria was, and still remains, 'the greatest single destroyer of mankind', as Sir William Osler (d. 1919), the famous physician and medical historian, once put it. Here, too, certain strains of the malaria parasite in some parts of Asia have evolved immunity to the drugs that were once effective. Now, resistant strains of mosquito are multiplying, according to reports from West Africa and South America, and new drugs are having to be sought. As the synthetic remedies fail, quinine, the natural drug, is once again returning to favour.

In the final analysis it would seem that the natural drugs, and the inbuilt defences of man, provide the chief line of defence in microbial infection. It is not unlikely that within the next few decades we shall be back where we were at the beginning of this century. We may have to go back to quinine for malaria, and the treatment of typhoid 'might be limited once more to diet and nursing' (Wade, 1973, p. 91).

In recent years, therefore, the optimism that greeted the promising new weapons of chemotherapy has been somewhat dampened. Microbes are countless in number, infinite in variety, capable of extraordinary metamorphoses, adapt remarkably to the most adverse conditions, and have an astonishing capacity for survival. And though we pride ourselves on having 'conquered' many deadly diseases, perhaps no illness is ever extinct.

As childhood and conventional diseases are ostensibly overcome, new and unknown diseases, and strange variations of the old ones, appear. Diseases of later life are often hang-overs from earlier infections. Bacteria and viruses, apparently killed, continue to 'smoulder' beneath the surface. In fact, we cannot be sure that we have rid the world of a single infectious disease known to man, and it is possible that before the end of this century, 'we may have lost much of our hard-won power over infections' (Taverner, 1968, p. 53), and many of the old diseases we imagined we had conquered will come flooding back.

For all we know, some of the great epidemic killers of the past have not disappeared, but as Dr Cartwright suggests, just gone into hiding. If this is so, the ineffectiveness of chemical drugs, combined with our diminishing natural resistance, could be catastrophic. Microbes could then mark a new swathe of destruction over mankind like another Black Death.

Books

Cartwright, Frederick, *Disease and History*, Hart-Davis, London, 1972.
Ferguson, Marilyn, *The Brain Revolution*, Davis-Poynter, London, 1974.
Norton, Alan, *The New Dimensions of Medicine*, Hodder & Stoughton, London, 1968.
Smith, Geddes, *Plague on Us*, Commonwealth Fund, New York, 1941.
Taverner, Deryck, *The Impending Medical Revolution*, Hodder & Stoughton, London, 1968.
Wade, O. L., *Adverse Reactions to Drugs*, Heinemann, London, 1973.

INFERTILITY

The male or female condition of being sterile or unable to produce offspring. When applied to women, the term implies barrenness or absence of fecundity, which may be due to some defect in the structure of her reproductive organs or deficiency in her hormone balance. In theory the fertile period begins at menstruation. But young girls can be infertile even after menstruation begins, and can menstruate without being able to be fertilized, since their ova are sterile for about six months to a year after the onset of puberty.

In times past the responsibility for unfruitfulness was almost always laid at the door of the woman, her barrenness being ascribed to a divine curse. It was also believed that a sorcerer could make a woman barren by ligature or knotting, that is, by tying knots in a piece of string while uttering the appropriate spells, which resulted in the channels and tubes of the woman's reproductive organs getting blocked or knotted up.

Since a wife's fertility was of supreme importance to the husband, assuring the continuance of his line, numerous tests were devised to find out if a woman was barren. According to Hippocrates (d. 359 BC), barrenness was often due to an impediment in the subtle canals that ramify through the body. To detect this, an ointment made with galbanum should be applied inside the vagina at bedtime; if in the morning the woman's mouth lacks a perfumed smell, she is sterile.

Even more numerous were the methods devised for removing the blight of barrenness. In ancient Egypt, for instance, the woman placed an onion in her rectum for a whole day and night to clear the internal passages. Celsus (fl. AD 50), Latin physician, recommended mixing lion's fat with oil of roses and inserting it into the vagina. Suppositories of a similar nature for the rectum and vagina continue in use in many parts of the Middle East.

In man, infertility generally implies impotence, which is the incapacity for sexual intercourse. It includes his inability to achieve erection or to sustain erection till his own or his partner's climax (impotence proper); premature ejaculation, or the inability to withhold orgasm before penetration;

the inability to emit sperm; and sterility, or the inability to produce motile sperm. Lack of desire in the woman, or female frigidity, is no hindrance to her fertility, but lack of desire on the part of the male makes penetration, intercourse and hence impregnation of the female, impossible.

Young boys can ejaculate without being able to fertilize, and during the period of adolescent sterility the boy's semen does not contain sperm cells. Again, male sperm is not formed in the testes until the temperature is several degrees below that of the body. Frequent warm baths or warm-water washing of the testes is therefore harmful to the sperm. After a fever or warm bath a man is temporarily sterile. On the other hand, according to Aristotle (d. 322 BC) cold douching of the testes restores vigour, but will cause baldness, because it produces a transient chill in the brain which loosens the hair roots.

Impotence sometimes has a physical cause, but to a large extent it is psychogenic or mind-produced. The following are among the many reasons given for impotence: immaturity, senility, physical weakness or disability of some kind; an attack of mumps during puberty may give rise to inflammation of the testicles (orchitis) with resulting impotence and infertility; chickenpox in adult life can also lead to a shorter or longer period of infertility; certain other diseases can also have the same effect, and many diabetics are impotent; overindulgence in eating, drinking, smoking, drugs, masturbation, sexual intercourse; psychological blocks created by childhood threats of punishment by castration or sexual mutilation; guilt feelings such as accompany adultery or rape; youthfulness and inexperience in the other partner, or again, the greater experience of the partner; shyness and confusion; lack of desire, or again, too violent an infatuation for the partner; fears and inhibitions of various kinds, such as fear of being disturbed while in the act, fear of venereal disease, of impregnating the woman, of failure to satisfy her and acquit oneself worthily in her eyes, of loss of sperm which might result in weakness.

After castration, impotence is one of the great masculine phobias, and lack of virility or the fear that one might become impotent has sometimes led men to suicide. Among the stresses to which the male is subjected today is the stress of having to cope with what he believes to be a more aggressive female, whose constant demand for sexual satisfaction must be met, for this determines his status with her. Modern sexologists state that the belief that such a demand exists is largely imaginary, found mainly in novels, films, television, plays and pornographic magazines, and has little relation to the real situation. Women do not demand or expect marathon performances from their mates; they usually have moderate sexual appetites, are content with normal satisfaction, and where love is present are usually patient and understanding. In any case, during temporary loss of potency, there are other ways, such as clitoral stimulation, oral sex or digital manipulation that can satisfy a woman.

Impotence fears have haunted men from earliest days, and a great deal of primitive and medieval magic has been devoted to measures for counteracting impotence by aphrodisiacs*, or removing the cause by rituals and spells. Impotence caused by magic was usually attributed to ligature or knotting to prevent erection or ejaculation. Medieval writings contain many accounts of ligature and its remedies. Indeed, belief in the possibility of inducing impotence and impeding consummation of the sexual act by such acts of witchcraft is not dead yet.

Barrenness in women and sterility in men, which have been important problems in their own way for centuries, have begun to assume a totally different aspect in our own day. Within the lifetime of most people living now, the population problem will become virtually insoluble. It has been estimated that some 20,000 infertile women in Britain, 250,000 in Europe and 1,000,000 in the USA have been helped in one way or another to reproduce. In the light of the demositic nightmare facing us some people would question whether this represents a step in the right direction. The alleviation of infertility is one of the most insignificant problems with which the world is confronted today.

Books

Buxton, C. L. and Southam, A. L., *Human Infertility*, New York, 1958.
Hammond, W. A., *Sexual Impotence in Male and Female*, Detroit, 1887.
Hastings, D. W., *Impotence and Frigidity*, Little, Brown, Boston, 1963.
Huhner, M., *The Diagnosis and Treatment of Sexual Disorders in the Male and Female, Including Sterility and Impotence*, F. A. Davis, Philadelphia, 1946.
Kleegman, S. J. and Kaufman, S. A., *Infertility in Women*, Davis, Philadelphia, 1946.
Runeberg, A., *Witches, Demons and Fertility Magic*, Helsinki, 1947.
Vecki, Victor G., *Sexual Impotence*, Saunders, Philadelphia, 1915.

INFLUENZA

An infectious virus disease, among the great killers of mankind. Evidence of severe recurrent respiratory epidemics found in the records of the ancient Egyptians, Babylonians and Chinese, and a virulent chest ailment described by Hippocrates (d. 359 BC) that regularly broke out at the time of the winter solstice, suggest the prevalence of influenza in antiquity. Many of the epidemics and plagues of the Middle Ages could have been the same disease.

In 1580 two astrologically-minded Italian historians, Domenico and Pietro Buoninsegni, believing that the disease that ravaged Italy at the time was due to the 'influence' of the stars, gave it the name by which it is still known, influenza. In 1892 Richard Pfeiffer, a German bacteriologist isolated a haemophilic (blood-nourished) bacillus in influenza patients, but the real culprit, a virus, was not discovered till 1943, with the aid of an electron microscope. It is incredibly small, so that 30 million of them could be placed on the head of a pin.

The great pandemics of recent times occurred in 1836, 1847 and 1899. In October 1918, just before the end of the First World War, a strange type of influenza reached Europe. Its place of origin was unknown but since the first cases were reported from Spain it was generally called the Spanish plague, or the Spanish flu. But it had other names as well: Bolshevik disease (in Poland), black whip (Hungary), Flanders grippe (British troops), wind disease (Persia), cold disease (India), great cold fever (Thailand), wrestlers' fever (Japan), blitz katarrh (Germany), Ispanka (Spanish lady) (Russia).

The symptoms of this disease varied to such an extent that throughout the duration of the epidemic there was no unanimity about its nature. Seasoned doctors frankly expressed themselves perplexed, worried, even panicky. Diagnoses differed, aetiology* was in doubt. Besides all the usual signs there were others, which made it difficult to determine its nature. It was neither wholly respiratory nor gastrointestinal. It resembled a score of other diseases of the skin, eyes, heart and brain. Sometimes the body took on a heliotrope shade, showing that the blood was hungry for oxygen. The venous blood became dark and thick, sometimes clotting in the syringe when being drawn out. These symptoms could be accompanied by loss of sight, hearing and other senses. The sexual organs could be affected; the spleen was often hugely enlarged.

As in all disastrous epidemics, speculation about the nature of the disease took on an aura of the bizarre, with science and superstition vying for sway in the popular imagination. Some said the disease was caused by unseasonal winds blowing from the wrong direction; by miasma from the Flanders battlefield; by insects, silkworms, bedbugs. Astrologers said that the electromagnetic vibrations from Jupiter caused a new and lethal type of germ to develop and breed; others attributed it to a planetary conflict between Saturn and Neptune in the house of Leo.

How it spread is easily explained: by physical contact, by the breath and by the sneeze. It is estimated that a single sneeze can distribute more than 86 million bacteria at supersonic speeds up to a distance of 12 feet, and these remain suspended in the air for about 30 minutes. In a matter of weeks the contagion had spread to five continents.

The suggested cures were often quaint, contradictory and mostly of no avail. Some recommended copious draughts of alcohol; some advocated smoking; opening doors and windows to let in fresh air; shutting them tight to exclude noxious air; enemas; ice-cold packs; fumigations; castor oil; camphor injections; asphyxiation; cupping*; emetics; bleeding*; quinine; aspirin; opium; garlic; a plentiful diet; starvation; immersing the feet in ice-cold water for several hours; immersing the feet in near-boiling water. Reviving a medieval fallacy, drugs were prescribed in large combinations, in the hope that one of them might be the right one. It was polypharmacy run riot.

Primitive beliefs held the day. Sacred pebbles were sucked; holy water drunk; homage offered to ancestral spirits; poultices of stinking ingredients applied around the neck; the smell of latrines inhaled; urine drunk. Chicken feathers, cucumber slices, potato peel, onion skin and dead men's nails were carried in the pocket.

Omens and auguries were rife, some reminiscent of those that prevailed at the time of the Black Death. Owls were heard hooting on the windowsills; the sign of the cross was seen in the sky; statues of the Virgin shed tears; roses faded and died on the bush; apparitions were common. People had visions and hallucinations, deliriums and delusions. Prophetic utterances were made of the imminent end of the world. People pounded drums and cymbals to drive off evil spirits. Ouija boards and spiritualist séances flourished. Voodoo charms, amulets, talismans, verses from the scriptures were all brought into action. Polish Jews revived ancient rituals. Norwegian villagers performed an old Viking ceremony. Spanish peasants sprinkled graveyard dust over the threshold. No community or culture was immune to the pull of ancient beliefs.

The majority of victims were those between the ages of 15 and 40. In the early days an attempt was made at isolation. Houses with the disease bore a red or yellow flag, or had a large white 'I' (for influenza) painted on the door or wall. Tradesmen left provisions at the gate. Pedestrians crossed over to the opposite side of the road.

Patients who were nearly dead and even pronounced dead miraculously revived, and apparently healthy persons died in minutes. Some collapsed as they walked. In Cape Town during a three-mile journey the city train stopped five times to deposit five passengers on the pavement to be collected by the death carts. According to contemporary accounts the disease struck like a bolt of lightning; men fell as if pole-axed; it spread like a bushfire. The routine entry in hospital.administration books for most of the patients was BID (brought in dead).

The hospitals were soon overflowing. Patients slept two in a bed, and on the ward floors. Conditions were such that going to hospital meant almost certain death. An Alberta hospital was described as 'an inferno of sick and suffering'. In Philadelphia over 500 died in one day. In one town in South Africa patients were treated in the post office tucked up in mail bags. Some places could only provide a heap of hay for patients to die on. The sick in Sweden were housed in stables; in Arizona in jails; in Wellington in dance halls.

Added to this was a desperate shortage of doctors. Retired physicians of 85, medical students still learning the rudiments of their craft, even dentists and veterinary surgeons were recruited to help out in hospitals and homes. Boy Scouts and the Salvation Army did service as orderlies and porters. Necessary equipment was either not available, or inadequate. In rural New Zealand dairy thermometers one foot long and as thick as a finger, meant for testing cream, were used on patients. Nurses were in dreadfully short supply, and typists were hurriedly put through a few first-aid lessons and made to stand by in case of emergencies. In most hospitals medical supplies ran out. Needless to say many of the sick received no treatment at all.

The effect on social and economic life was devastating. Throughout the Western world about half the schools, public libraries, theatres, dance halls, bioscopes (cinemas) and other places of entertainment closed down. In some countries all parliamentary and public meetings were suspended, because so many members were sick. Churches were often shut or services shortened. Hymns and audible prayers were prohibited so as not to spread the contagion. Over 10,000 men of the British fleet were sick. Army regiments in all countries were decimated.

In places like Rio de Janeiro and Cape Town, trade was temporarily at a standstill. In Poland the potato crops rotted; the Guatemala coffee crop was lost; in the Ganges valley the rice was not harvested; in Malaya the rubber plantations closed down. The frontiers between states were often closed and train services suspended. It seemed, in the words of Richard Collier, that 'the world was dying'.

Then, as suddenly as it began, the epidemic came to an end in the first weeks of 1919. It had lasted for approximately 120 days, and in that period, in one way or another, had directly affected the lives of over 1,000 million people, or half the population of the world at the time. It had made an estimated 100 million people sick; and killed more than 21 million, double the number of all men killed in the four years of fighting on all fronts. It ranks with the plague of Justinian and the Black Death as 'one of the three most destructive outbreaks of disease that the human race has known'.

The cause of the epidemic is still unknown. The particular virus that started it has never been identified. Though the bodies of some of the victims have been exhumed in an effort to track down the virus, no trace of it has survived.

In spite of the devastation it brought, the great epidemic of 1918 has left little impress on the popular memory and today is virtually forgotten. Perhaps the shock was too sudden, its duration too brief, and the extent of the disaster too vast for it to be fully appreciated.

The problem now facing scientists is whether such a disaster can recur. Experts have identified three groups of influenza virus, each with literally hundreds of strains. Animals and men carry viruses all the time. The Spanish virus seems to have resulted from the conjoint activity of the mild virus of the hog flu and the Pfeiffer bacillus. It had a short life and a lethal effect. It died out within four months. But the chief danger in micro-organisms and viruses is that inoculation does not provide permanent immunization. They easily acquire resistance, are extremely versatile, mutate and adapt with remarkable facility. Thus, two comparatively mild variants produced the Hong Kong flu of 1957, and the Mao flu of 1968, each of which killed off several thousand people. Sir Christopher Andrewes believes that viruses 'go underground' and persist without causing outbreaks, but can sometimes become active and epidemic, 'when the time is ripe'.

Books

Ackerknecht, Erwin, *History and Geography of the Most Important Diseases*, Hafner, New York, 1955.

Beveridge, W. I. B., *Influenza: the Last Great Plague*, Heinemann, London, 1977.

Collier, Richard, *The Plague of the Spanish Lady: the Influenza Pandemic of 1918–1919*, Macmillan, London, 1974.

Cummins, S. L. (ed.), *Studies of Influenza in Hospitals of the Armies in France, 1918*, Medical Research Committee, London, 1919.

Graves, Charles, *Invasion by Virus*, Icon Books, London, 1969.

Hare, Ronald, *Pomp and Pestilence*, Philosophical Library, New York, 1955.

Hoehling, A. A., *The Great Epidemic*, Little, Brown, Boston, 1961.

Jordan, E. O., *Epidemic Influenza: a Survey*, American Medical Association, Chicago, 1920.

Newman, George, *Report on the Pandemic of Influenza, 1918-19*, HMSO, London, 1920.

Smith, Geddes, *Plague on Us*, Commonwealth Fund, New York, 1941.

KINESIOTHERAPY

Kinesiotherapy (Gk. *kinēsis*, 'movement'), earlier known as somatherapy (Gk. *sōma*, 'body'), entails training in the correct use of the body in posture and movement. It is to be distinguished from physiotherapy*, in which a person is usually in actual need of treatment, as for a slipped disc, and is the passive recipient of the treatment. Physiotherapy has a basically physical objective; kinesiotherapy is concerned with psychophysical dysfunction. Physiotherapy deals with injury to the body; kinesiotherapy with misuse of the body.

The principle behind kinesiotherapy is that mental, as well as physical, energy is tied up in wrong postures and slipshod actions. This blocked energy is freely released in animals, which accounts for their grace and ease of movement. Man, particularly modern man, is fixed in bad habits of posture and movement from childhood. It is as important to train a child to sit, stand and walk properly, as to eat, dress and talk. The long hours spent sitting on badly designed chairs and motor-car seats, and the lack of normal exercise like walking and running, put a great strain on the muscles, creating bundles of trapped energy crying for release.

Kinesiotherapy corrects tense muscles, bad posture, a humped back, contracted vertebrae, depressed neck. It goes on to eliminate injurious bodily movements, through proper use of the limbs in sitting, standing, walking and all physical activities, and also during work, to reduce stress* and avoid fatigue and tension.

There is a series of progressive exercises, ranging from passive to active, for toning up the muscles, lubricating the joints, and stimulating the heart, lungs, liver and other internal organs. These include massage* and stretching, and variations of what was once known as succussation, 'shaking', in which a patient is shaken up to stir up the body in order to bring out phlegm and 'humours'. Swinging and swaying in various gentle forms of rhythmic movement, gymnastics and dancing are also included.

It also deals with the proper use of the body during repose, and thus recommends relaxation exercises for the key tension areas like the neck, shoulders, belly, buttocks and thighs. Breathing exercises and meditation are taught in certain schools.

Kinesiotherapy dates back to very ancient times in Egypt, Babylonia and Greece. From the latter comes the term eurhythmy (Gk. *eu*, 'right'; *rhythmos*, 'rhythm'), meaning a system of harmonious and ordered movements as in dancing, gymnastics and acrobatics. Certain features of the sacred dances of Turkestan, Tibet, Afghanistan and Central Asia, similarly suggest an acquaintance with the fundamental occult principles underlying body movement.

Rudolf Steiner (d. 1925), founder of anthroposophy, studied Eastern dance patterns during his early years as a theosophist and taught a form of eurhythmy as a means of uniting the cosmic and mundane principles within the individual. At about the same time the Russian-Buriat mystic, George Gurdjieff (d. 1949) combined certain central Asian dance modes and temple rituals, and introduced them to Europe. Another contemporary mystic Aleister Crowley (d. 1947) taught a kind of eurhythmy that was also an amalgam of several schools, along with techniques of his own devising.

A famous variation of dance therapy was developed by Rudolf Laban (d. 1958), son of an officer in the imperial Hungarian army. He studied as an architect, and later, following his interest in the dynamics of motion, became a dancer and choreographer. He was fascinated with the problem of dance notation, and in the 1920s while in Germany invented a notation based on space, force, form and time, which is now internationally used. The parts of the body, the poses, movements and sequences are allotted certain symbols, and these are written as musical notation. Laban went on to study human movements in general, in work, fighting and ritual. The Laban method enjoyed great popularity and was widely used in schools and factories, and in therapy.

The next step forward in kinesiotherapy came through the Australian, Frederick Matthias Alexander (d. 1955). Use, said Alexander, affects functioning; ill-use distorts and misshapes the body and interferes with its free functioning. His pioneering studies laid the foundation of most of the later work on the subject. Among his followers were G. B. Shaw, Aldous Huxley, Professor John Dewey, Sir Stafford Cripps, Archbishop William Temple. When in 1973 Professor Tinbergen was awarded the Nobel Prize for medicine, he devoted the best part of his Nobel oration to Alexander's work.

The Austrian-born American psychiatrist, and disciple of Freud, Wilhelm Reich (d. 1957) spoke of certain horizontal bands and tension zones that exist in the body, which act like armour blocks and unconsciously influence character. These are situated across the forehead and eyes, throat and shoulders, chest and heart, waist and small of the back, pelvic and sexual areas. His system of bioenergetics, elaborated further by his pupil Alexander Lowen, provided a means of releasing these blocks.

Among the still more recent developments are the two systems of Rolf and Ichazo. Ida Rolf of California, who developed her techniques in the 1930s, is concerned not so much with posture as with structure, not only with movement but with mechanics. Children grow up with imbalances and dislocations because the body is not aligned with respect to gravity but battles constantly with gravity to the detriment of physical stability and mental health. Her system, known as 'rolfing', helps to untie the energies that are locked up in hard-set muscles by deep massage and other exercises, and so achieves better 'structural integration'.

The Chilean, Oscar Ichazo, who runs a development centre in Arica, Chile, has a system combining physical culture and mysticism, largely influenced by the teachings of Gurdjieff. The course includes meditation, mantras, prayers, astrology, exercise, gymnastics (yoga and akido), dynamic tension, exhaustion techniques and dance. He uses the music evolved by sufis, with notes 'placed' in the belly, chest and head to induce special states of consciousness.

Books

Barlow, Wilfred, *The Alexander Principle*, Gollancz, London, 1973.
Birdwhistell, R. L., *Introduction to Kinesics*, University of Kentucky Press, 1952.
Broer, M. R., *Efficiency of Human Movement*, Saunders, Philadelphia, 1960.
Duvall, E. N., *Kinesiology: the Anatomy of Motion*, Prentice-Hall, Englewood Cliffs, New Jersey, 1959.
Gardiner, M. D., *The Principles of Exercise Therapy*, 3rd edn, Bell, London, 1973.
Laban, Rudolf, *The Mastery of Movement*, 3rd edn, Macdonald & Evans, London, 1971.
Schultz, J. H. and Luthe, W., *Autogenic Training*, Grune & Stratton, New York, 1959.
Scott, M. G., *Analysis of Human Motion*, Appleton-Century, New York, 1963.
Thornton, S., *Movement Perspective of Rudolf Laban*, Macdonald & Evans, London, 1971.
Wells, Katharine, *Kinesiology: the Scientific Basis of Human Motion*, Saunders, London, 1971.

L

LEPROSY

An awesome disease inspiring an almost occult dread, very common in antiquity. The semi-mythical Chinese emperor Shen Nung (2700 BC), who compiled the earliest known pharmacopoeia, recommended chaulmoogra oil, obtained from an evergreen Himalayan tree, as a cure, a remedy that was rediscovered in modern times, and is now used in purified form as antileptol.

Leprosy is mentioned in Egyptian texts dating from 1350 BC, and in the early Indian epics. In Hindu legend a number of famous kings were afflicted with leprosy, which was cured by eating the fruit of the kalao tree and devotion to the gods, usually the sun god. From earliest times it seems to have been regarded as an affliction imposed by the deities and its cure was a matter of divine grace.

The Greeks described several kinds of disfiguring skin diseases. One variety, known as the 'Herculean psora' (Gk. *psōra*, 'itch'), was said to have been contracted by the great hero during his adventures on the African coast. More specifically it was known as *elephantiasis graecorum*, because the induration (hardening) of the skin on the legs exactly resembles elephant hide. Another variety was called the scaly disease (Gk. *lepis*, 'scale'), from which we get the word leprosy. The fact that these scales resembled fish-scales, later linked it with the Christian attitude to leprosy. Among the early remedies for the disease in the Mediterranean world was powdered gold in potions, and bathing in human blood, especially of virgin girls and boys, a few drops in the bathing water being enough. The neo-Platonist philosopher Plotinus (d. AD 270), and the Byzantine emperor Constantine (d. AD 337) were among those who contracted an unsightly skin disease which may have been leprosy.

In all parts of the ancient Middle East, the victims of the disease were segregated in special enclosures outside the confines of the town, and were expected to fend for themselves. The philanthropic people of the town usually sent food and clothing. The pagan peoples of Europe also dealt very cruelly with leper victims. Hector Boece (d. 1536) records that it was customary among the ancient Scots to castrate men suffering from all inheritable diseases, including leprosy.

The disease is frequently mentioned in the Bible, often in a symbolical context. In the earliest allusion, God gave leprosy to Moses (Ex. 4:6) and then healed him as a sign of his consecration. Miriam, the sister of Moses, was smitten with it as a punishment for murmuring against the patriarch. The Syrian captain Naaman, also a leper, was advised by the prophet Elisha to wash in the Jordan seven times to be healed. Under Jewish law leprosy had to be diagnosed by the priests, after which lepers were segregated.

With Christianity the symbolical character of leprosy was brought to the fore; leprosy became more a type of spiritual malady than a condition of the flesh. In the parable of Jesus, Lazarus the beggar is a leper, but after his death is carried into Abraham's bosom, while the rich man is made to suffer in hell (Lk. 16:22). Christ made his disciples 'fishers of men', so that they might heal the scaly souls of those cursed with this dread disease. It was in the house of Simon the leper that the woman with the alabaster box anointed the head of Christ as a symbolical preparation for His work of redemption on the Cross.

The early ecclesiastical authorities, especially the Greek church fathers, notably Gregory of Nazianzus (d. 389) and John Chrysostom (d. 407), termed leprosy the 'sacred disease'. It was a trial imposed by God, which singled out the sufferer as an object of divine preference and Christian example. Christian saints humbly cleansed the wounds of lepers with their own hands and some were known to kiss the open sores as if they bore the living stamp of the divine chastisement.

The Hebrew term (TsR'ATh) for leprosy used in the Bible, is related to the word (TsR), which means anguish, affliction, distress, almost in the modern sense of angst*. It is a psychic rather than a bodily disorder, a disfigurement of the soul caused by spiritual neglect and moral uncleanliness. In this latter sense, it has been said that leprosy, that most ancient of diseases, is rampant in contemporary society, and the healing touch of Christ means as much to the afflicted today as to those lepers whose sores were cleansed on the shores of Galilee.

Books

Burgess, P., *Who Walk Alone*, rev. edn, London, 1962.

Hude, Carolus (ed.), *Aretus* (Cappadocian physician of the first century AD), Teubner, Leipzig, 1923.

Keenan, Mary Emily, 'St Gregory of Nazianzus and Early Byzantine Medicine', *Bulletin of the History of Medicine*, 9, 1941, 8–30.

Temkin, O., *The Falling Sickness,* 2nd rev. edn., Johns Hopkins Press, Baltimore, 1971.

Weymouth, A., *Through the Leper Squint*, London, 1938.

MAGNETOTHERAPY

A method of healing based on the principle of a magnetic energy distributed throughout the universe and inherent in all things, including the earth, inanimate objects and man. The ancients were well aware of the lines along which the magnetic forces moved through the earth, and set up stones along these *ley*-lines, as they were called in Britain, and built temples at important junctions to mark the alignment.

Until the end of the last century, it was popularly believed that the magnetic currents streaming north and south between the poles had an effect on the nervous system, and that it was beneficial to sleep while they flowed in a straight line through the length of the body, though some benefited with the body aligned differently. Each person could discover the best direction with a little practice.

Charles Dickens invariably slept with his head to the north, and during his tours, when staying at hotels, he would locate the north with a pocket compass he always carried, and move his bed accordingly. On the other hand, Michael Faraday maintained that the body was most comfortable in an east—west direction.

There is a widespread superstition that changing the position of one's chair, and thus one's alignment relative to the earth's magnetic flow, can change one's luck at cards. It is also a commonplace observation that if one changes direction while walking, one will change the flow of one's thoughts. In order to see something from a different point of view, therefore, one is advised to go for a walk along roads that turn in as many directions as possible.

The magnetism of the earth is the ultimate source of life itself. The earth's magnetic field activates the enzyme system in fruit and vegetables, and causes them to ripen. If placed within the field of an artificial magnet, seeds will germinate at many times their normal rate. It has been found that even very weak magnetic fields, if vibrating, will lower the level of cholesterol and white-cell count in the human body.

On the principle that ordinary magnets themselves possess to some degree the properties of the earth's magnetism, Paracelsus (d. 1541) applied magnets to diseased organs and then buried the magnet. This he said did not harm the soil for the earth was easily able to neutralize the disease carried by the magnet. The magnet was withdrawn after a few days, washed clean, given a week's 'rest', after which it was used again for the next patient. Until the seventeenth century, it was believed that any wound inflicted by a metal object could be cured by applying a magnet to the wound, or if that were not possible, to the weapon that caused the wound.

A curious method of magnetotherapy was introduced in the eighteenth century by James Graham (d. 1794), an enterprising Edinburgh physician and advocate of the earth-bath (*see* geotherapy). In a converted room in his London house, which he grandiosely called the Temple of Hygeia, he installed a specially designed Magnetic Bed, 'to exalt the faculties of the human species'. This bed, resting on six transparent pillars, had its mattresses stuffed with stallions' hair to give vigour to the male, and was perfumed with oriental scents and fragrant herbs. The bedclothes were of satin, the decor purple and sky-blue, and through innumerable glass tubes and cylinders came a healing stream of 'magnetic effluxion', fed by hundreds of lodestones and artificial magnets, while soft music from hidden organs, flutes and strings soothed the ear. The privilege of sleeping in this 'celestio, medico, magnetico, musico, electrical bed' was £50 sterling. Progeny were assured. Emma Lyon, one of the 'half-naked wenches' who served in Graham's establishment, was later to become the wife of Lord Hamilton, and mistress of Horatio Nelson.

Healers in France preferred to apply magnets direct to the body. Among them, the Abbé Lenoble (d. 1798) had a large stock of magnets of various shapes and sizes adapted for use on the pulse, thorax, stomach, genitals, back and legs. The Société Royale de Médecine reported favourably on the many cures allegedly effected by this mode of treatment. In more recent times Jean Charcot (d. 1893), one of the teachers of Sigmund Freud, experimented with the influence of magnets on hysterical patients, but did not find this method of treatment satisfactory. Magnetotherapy, depending on the fields of artificial magnets, is to be distinguished from animal magnetism, which is based on the so-called 'magnetic' powers of human healers.

Books

Barnothy, Madeleine F. (ed.), *Biological Effects of Magnetic Fields*, Plenum Press, New York, 1964.

De la Warr, George and Baker, Douglas, *Biomagnetism: the Effects of Magnetic Fields on Living Tissues and Organs of the Human Body*, Delawarr Laboratories, Oxford, 1967.

Halacy, Daniel, *Radiation, Magnetism and Living Things*, Holiday House, New York, 1966.

Pressman, A. S., *Electromagnetic Fields and Life*, Plenum Press, New York, 1972.

White, G. S., *The Finer Forces of Life*, Mokelumne, California, 1969.

MANIA

A mental disorder in which a person's mood is one of uncontrollable excitement and hyperactivity. The term is used for many psychological states suggesting obsession, compulsion, delusion and monomania*.

The word is derived from the Greek root meaning 'madness', which recurs in the Latin *manes*, the spirits of the dead. The Romans thought that a mad person was possessed by the household goddess Mania, and became so afflicted because he had failed to fulfil some domestic duty. The popular term 'maniac', as applied to a person who is emotionally unbalanced and violent, retains this usage. In earlier times mania was also classed as a furor*, manifesting in ecstasy, prophecy, poetry, eroticism and war.

In modern psychology mania is often treated as a bipolar illness, representing the upward phase in cyclothymia*, or manic-depressive insanity. But mania can also be unipolar, where the manic type of insanity is characterized by a frequent shift of mood from the normal to one of hyperelation.

In this upward swing a person exhibits symptoms of progressive excitement from hypomania, or mild mania, through hyperthymia (Gk. *thymos*, 'emotion') or acute emotionalism, to mania proper. Thus, he starts with signs of cheerfulness, and an increased capacity for physical acitivity. He feels good, and begins to be active and busy. His mood is one of optimism, general expansiveness, euphoria and buoyancy. The tempo then shifts to one of exaggerated elation, agitation, restlessness and physical activity (hyperkinesis), accompanied by increased sexual activity. He is uninhibited in behaviour, spends money lavishly, gets by with a minimum of food and sleep, but shows no signs of fatigue. .His thought processes are accelerated though lacking in critical judgment. He talks endlessly, gets hilarious about nothing at all, is full of ideas and grandiose schemes, skipping from subject to subject without coherence or relevance.

His speech is marked by elements of echolalia, the senseless reiteration or rhyming of words; or polylogia, random talk or gibberish. He becomes more and more boisterous, shouting and bursting into fits of maniacal laughter and senseless raving. He is extremely irritable and suspicious, resents criticism and violently opposes interference. Often he attempts to attack others or to inflict injury upon himself by cutting himself or hitting his head against a wall. By now his judgment is thoroughly impaired; he becomes subject to delusions and ungovernable frenzy.

Mania has the same aetiology* as cyclothymia and modern therapy is usually confined to the administration of tranquillizers. In occult theory the disorder stems from an imperfect alignment or periodic dislocation of the second body.

Books

Abraham, K., *Selected Papers*, Hogarth Press, London, 1927.
Kraepelin, E., *Manic-Depressive Insanity and Paranoia*, Livingstone, Edinburgh, 1921.
Lewin, B. D., *The Psychology of Elation*, Hogarth Press, London, 1951.

MASSAGE

Massage (Gk. *massein*, 'to knead'), also known as shampoo (Hindi, *chāmpnā*, 'to squeeze'), was an art greatly favoured by the ancient Egyptians, Chinese (taoist specialists were famous), Greeks and Indians. In some primitive cultures it was and still is used as a kind of exorcism*. Thus, in Melanesia where it is very popular, the movement is centrifugal, outward towards the extremities, to drive off any disease demons. In most other places the motion is inward, towards the heart.

Since the time of Homer (*c.* 800 BC), who tells of Greek women massaging the bodies of battle-weary warriors, its popularity has never waned.

Hippocrates (d. 359 BC) prescribes massage for dislocations, and a Hippocratic dictum goes: 'Hard rubbing binds, soft rubbing loosens.' Oribasius (d. AD 403), physician to Julian the Apostate, describes methods still in use. Medical rubbing, as it was once known, was widely practised all over Europe for centuries, though till the early part of the present century most massage parlours had an unsavoury reputation because so many also operated as brothels.

Massage as a form of therapy was not officially recognized in Britain till 1920, with the establishment of the Chartered Society of Massage and Medical Gymnastics, which in 1943 changed its name to the Chartered Society of Physiotherapy.

Today massage is a standard adjunct of the technique of physiotherapy*. It has proved to be very beneficial in certain cases that respond to no other treatment. This was amply demonstrated by Sister Kenny (d. 1952), an Australian nurse who devoted her attention to the victims of infantile paralysis and by means of massage and hot, moist applications helped many to walk again and live near-normal lives. It has been claimed for massage that it promotes the circulation, loosens stiff joints and muscles, tones up the skin and tissues, invigorates the nerves, and both relaxes and vitalizes the whole system. It is invaluable for all athletes, as well as for tired businessmen. The foremost exponents of massage are the Swedes and the Japanese.

The chief movements of massage are: (a) *effleurage*, 'stroking', where the hand is moved in one direction, using fingers and palms, with greater or lesser friction according to need; (b) *petrissage*, 'kneading', that is, rubbing, squeezing and rolling, by using the whole hand, and knuckles; this relaxes and conditions the muscles; (c) *tapotement*, 'tapping', a brisk, vibratory chopping movement with the flat or side of the hand; it usually ends the treatment.

Pressure while massaging may be firm or gentle, and different effects are believed to be achieved in this way. The American, Ida P. Rolf, of California, uses the hard touch, employing fingers, knuckles and elbows to massage the deepest fascia or muscle-bundles and joints of the body. Mrs Gerda Boyesen, originally from Oslo, teaches 'dynamic relaxation' or soft-touch therapy, which includes abdominal respiration and massage by gentle circular strokes. As the muscles loosen the patient becomes aware of the 'vegetative streamings', currents of warm buzzing feelings running through the body.

Books

Ackerknecht, Erwin H., *Therapeutics: From the Primitives to the Twentieth Century*, Hafner, New York, 1973.
Downing, George, *The Massage Book*, Wildwood House, London, 1973.
Gunther, Bernard, *Massage*, Academy Editions, London, 1971.
Knutson, Gunilla, *Book of Massage*, St Martin's Press, New York, 1972.
Mennell, J. B., *Physical Treatment by Movement, Manipulation and Massage*, 4th edn, London, 1940.

MASS HYSTERIA

An expression of crowd psychosis in which a great upsurge of enthusiasm, fear*, exhilaration, panic, sex mania and violence grips the minds of people. It may start on a small scale, be felt by one or two persons, and then be transmitted by pathemic contagion to others around them. Once sparked, the blaze spreads with great rapidity among those who happen to be in the vicinity, engulfing large numbers of people, all of whom get caught up in the prevailing state of highly charged emotionalism.

Several types of mental disorder seem to carry such contagion, and those near the victim become affected to a greater or lesser extent. The sight of a person in an epileptic* fit, for instance, can give a sensitive onlooker a mild attack. In one condition, known as *folie-à-deux* (Fr. 'madness of two', or 'madness together'), a normal person living in close proximity to a patient suffering from paranoid delusions, can develop paranoid delusions himself; he usually recovers when they are separated.

During mass hysteria people seem to be deprived of their senses; they talk and behave quite irrationally. In many cases the symptoms resemble those of possession*, and would be regarded as incredible were it not for the first-hand accounts of dispassionate witnesses. Often the infection spreads from participants to spectators, and those who come to scoff may, in the midst of their derision, be caught up in spite of themselves.

Records both ancient and modern are filled with instances of mass hysteria, from the orgiastic excitement of the corybantes of ancient Greece, and the frenzies of the Roman bacchantes, to the no less unbridled capers of religious and social enthusiasts of Christian Europe.

Religious wars have always been a prolific source of mass hysteria. Thus, during the First Crusade (1096), the crusading army was made up of many thousand men, women and children, who were roused to zealous fervour by fanatical preachers. Most of them were either slain or sold into slavery long before they reached the Holy Land.

Eleutherian sects, preaching and practising free love, have been prominent among the dissidents of the church, and have aroused a great deal of hysterical zeal, as we find in the history of the thirteenth-century eleutherians known as the Brethren of the Free Spirit.

There were several phases of dance mania in medieval Europe, when a violent and uncontrollable impulse to jump and dance took possession of large crowds of people. Notable among them were the outbreaks of Kolbig (1027) and Erfurt (1237), followed by others at intervals of about 50 years. During the great epidemic of 1380 the streets of Metz were filled with 11,000 dancers, who seemed totally oblivious of their surroundings. Another kind of dancing mania called tarantism was rampant in Italy from the fourteenth to the seventeenth centuries. It was said to be caused by the bite of the tarantula spider (whence the name), and even in the present day, attacks are said to be due to possession by the spirit of a spider.

From about 1210 the flagellant craze spread over Europe, starting in the south. Men, women and children marched in winding procession through the streets of towns and villages, whipping themselves, weeping and praying for forgiveness of sins. As in the case of the dancers, many were naked or half naked. Each phase of mania lasted about two or three months, and then died down, but the craze persisted for about 150 years.

Between the fifteenth and eighteenth centuries the social and religious history of Europe is marked by hysterical disorders in convents, which neither civil authority nor ecclesiastical censure was able to control, and the witchcraft mania, in which thousands of people were convicted after cruel tortures, and then burned to death. The witch hunts spread across the Atlantic to America, culminating in the terrible trials and executions of Salem (1692). A more curious manifestation of mass hysteria was seen in an epidemic outbreak of tulipomania in the middle of the seventeenth century, when the craze among the Dutch for tulips, newly introduced from Persia, became so great that fantastic prices were paid for a single bulb. All classes of society took to tulip cultivation, and it seemed that the whole of the regular trade and commerce of Holland would be brought to a standstill. Then as suddenly as it began the demand ended, and thousands of families were ruined.

Other examples of mass hysteria include the so-called Popish Plot (1678) during the reign of Charles II; the mad financial speculation that culminated in the South Sea Bubble (1721); the ecstatic religious revivals of the eighteenth and nineteenth centuries in Kentucky, England, Ulster and Wales. Then there were the various gold and diamond rushes that started from the middle of the last century; the anti-Bolshevik Red Scare in England in 1919; the Florida Real Estate Boom in 1920. The political rallies of the Nazis (c. 1937-9) produced some extraordinary scenes of mob neurosis.

A unique case of mass hysteria occurred in the USA on the night of Hallowe'en, 1938, when the actor Orson Welles, broadcasting a radio version of H. G. Wells's *The War of the Worlds*, so vividly narrated the invasion of the earth by Martians, that over 1 million listeners prepared for fight or flight in the ensuing panic.

It was once thought that outbreaks of mass hysteria could be attributed to a prevailing sense of apprehension, bewilderment and despair, among poor and oppressed populations, usually in time of danger, want, pestilence, uncertainty, persecution and general helplessness. But observers of the modern scene find that they continue to take place when stomachs are full and security assured, as can be seen in the screaming and fainting fits among teenagers at pop festivals; the wild rampage of youthful gangs like the Mods, Rockers, Leatherjackets, Hells Angels and Skinheads; the hooliganism of football fans; the mass contagion that gives sudden rise to cults like the Beatniks and Hippies. All forms of mass hysteria would appear to be manifestations of the prevailing sociopsychosis.

Books

Backman, E. L., *Religious Dances in the Christian Church and in Popular Medicine*, Allen & Unwin, London, 1952.

Cantrill, H., *The Invasion from Mars: a Study in the Psychology of Panic,* Princeton University Press, 1940.

Clark, E. T., *The Psychology of Religious Awakening*, New York, 1939.

Cooper, W. M., *A History of the Rod: Flagellation and Flagellants,* John Hotten, London, 1887.

Davenport, F. M., *Primitive Traits in Religious Revivals*, Macmillan, New York, 1905.

Hecker, J. F. C., *The Epidemics of the Middle Ages*, Sydenham Society, London, 1844.

Mackay, Charles, *Extraordinary Popular Delusions*, London, 1956.
McLoughlin, W. G., *Modern Revivalism*, Ronald Press, New York, 1959.
Murray, R. K., *Red Scare: a Study in National Hysteria, 1919-20*, University of Minnesota Press, 1955.
Pollock, J., *The Popish Plot*, Cambridge University Press, 1944.

MEDICAL MATERIALISM

A term used by William James (d. 1910) for the attempt to explain all spiritual, altruistic and creative experience in terms of morbid states of body and mind. Thus, mother love arises from gratitude to the sucking infant for easing the swollen milk glands; charity is an investment against the fear of one's own possible ill-luck; constipation is responsible for the vision of saints; sexual libido underlies the desire for spiritual union.

The professions, artistic and otherwise, have been particularly vulnerable to the diagnoses of medical materialism. Thus, a painter smears faeces (paint) because of strict bowel-training in infancy. A dancer wants to seduce the audience to sexual intercourse. An actress is an exhibitionist, a surgeon a sadist, a gynaecologist a voyeur. A lawyer is a momphomaniac (Gk. *momphē*, 'complaint'), obsessed with quarrels. A priest is a peccatophobic subject (Lat. *peccare*, 'to sin'), obsessed with sins. A doctor has nosophilia (Gk. *nosos*, 'illness'), an unhealthy preoccupation with diseases. A teacher is a pederast. The choice of zoology as a profession shows leanings towards bestiality. A couturier is a fetishist. A pathologist suffers from necrophilia (Gk. *nekros*, 'corpse'), and so on.

To take a few specific examples. The 'pantings', 'breathings', and 'roarings' in the Biblical writings point to the respiratory ailments of the Psalmist, of Amos, Isaiah, Jeremiah and other prophets. St Paul's experience on the road to Damascus was of epileptic* origin. The voices of Joan of Arc (d. 1431) were due to tinnitus. Martin Luther (d. 1546) had a bad liver, and St Ignatius of Loyola (d. 1556) had worms, accounting for the Reformation and Counter-Reformation. The erotic experiences described by St Teresa of Avila (d. 1582), St Veronica Giuliani (d. 1727) and other female saints suggest nymphomania.

Some literary critics of this school scarcely make any distinction between the philosophy of Blaise Pascal (d. 1662) and his migraine; the poetry of John Keats (d. 1821) and his tuberculosis; and the career of Napoleon Bonaparte (d. 1821) and the functioning of his pituitary gland. The spastic colon of George Fox (d. 1690) was responsible for his social mysticism. The powerful eruptive style of Thomas Carlyle (d. 1881) sprang from gastric ulcer. The misogyny of August Strindberg (d. 1912) was due to his syphilis.

A Freudian analyst adjudicating on the work of Goethe (d. 1832) found evidence of pre-genital fixations, depressive-manic disorder, paranoia, fetishism, obsessions*, and so on, explaining his struggle for beauty and spiritual values as an attempt to overcome the problem of premature ejaculation.

Those who do not go so far, none the less point out the clear relationship between genius and its physical correlatives. Sensory hallucinations, dislocation of space and time perception, trances and visions are often hysteric*, psychotic, oneiric or hypnagogic in origin. One of the curious concomitant factors of an epileptic or migrainous* attack is a 'kinking' of the optic nerves, leading to the condition known as scotoma, the malfunctioning of the retina. The effects of scotoma can be quite extraordinary. Common objects may become greatly enlarged or greatly reduced in size; the flowing movement of things may be distorted or slowed down (cinematographic vision), or appear like a 'flicker of stills', one frame at a time. Things may flare up in bright cascades of colour, or break up into crystalline or polygonal mosaics, or grainy and dotted pointilliste figures, or cubist, abstract patterns. A convincing case could, in fact, be made out to explain much of modern surrealist and impressionist painting in terms of scotomic vision.

The psychoanalyst is perhaps more guilty than most of trying to find a morbid interpretation for even the most commonplace occurrence. Thus, if a person comes late to work, it is because he is hostile; if he comes early, he is anxious; if he comes in time, he is compulsive. It appears that one can never win with an analyst.

While it is true that musicians, writers, mystics and creative people are physiologically predisposed to imaginative experience, it is also true that their physical shortcomings cannot entirely explain the genesis of their creative or mystical instinct. It would be as unreasonable to dismiss a Trappist monk as a dumb eunuch because he is a celibate under a vow of silence, as to account for the writings of Plato in terms of humoral pathology or gastritis.

The physiological event can only become productive within the context of a prepared consciousness, ready and receptive to the influence of a supreme experience that has nothing to do with the physical network through which it is relayed. The disease might condition but does not create; it might modulate but not direct the inspired mood.

Books

Clissold, Augustus, *The Prophetic Spirit in Genius and Insanity*, Longmans, London, 1870.
Custance, John, *Wisdom, Madness, Folly*, Gollancz, London, 1951.
Hyslop, T. B., *The Great Abnormals*, London, 1925.
James, William, *The Varieties of Religious Experience*, Longmans, Green, London, 1941.
Walter, W. Grey, *The Neuro-Physiological Aspects of Hallucinations and Illusory Experience*, Society for Psychical Research, London, 1960.

MELANCHOLY

(Gk. *melan*, 'black'; *cholē*, 'bile'), a mood of sadness, depression and gloom, sometimes classed with the furors*. According to the theory of humoralism, melancholia results from a noxious degeneration of black bile, and this, said Galen (d. AD 201), 'darkens the seat of reason'. Astrologically, melancholics are ruled by the planet Saturn.

According to students of the subject, the melancholic is usually tall and swarthy, or at least darker in complexion than other members of his family.

He is lean and angular in appearance, although his face seems to be puffy. His veins are prominent, his body emits a stale odour. He has strong sexual urges but is sexually weak and often impotent.

As a rule melancholics are also hypochondriacs, morbidly concerned about their health, especially their bowels. Many are convinced that their intestines are blocked up. They are liable to heartburn and ulcers, may develop spasms and tics, and are prone to paralysis and phobias. But melancholy is most closely associated with epilepsy*. In fact, say the ancients, melancholy and epilepsy are two facets of the same disease, the first attacking the mind, the second the body.

It is said, furthermore, that the melancholic is secretive and silent. He often clenches his fists, not from aggressiveness, but out of a desire to keep to himself, which unconsciously expresses itself in this way. By nature avaricious and misanthropic, he is not given to charitable works. He hates to enter the rough and tumble of life, loves solitude and prefers to live apart from the rest of mankind. He cares little for the opinion of others and goes the way he chooses without concern for what they think of him. Plato (d. 347 BC) classed the melancholic with the lover and the drunkard. Above all he cannot endure restraint. In the words of Immanuel Kant (d. 1804), 'From the courtier's golden chains to the heavy irons of the galley slave, all fetters are abhorrent to the melancholic.'

Deep study and research come easily to the melancholic for he is studious by nature, has a good memory and an excellent mind. He prefers books to people, and his library to the theatre. When he walks he looks down at the ground, deeply absorbed in his thoughts. He can think ahead of most people, and because of the speed of his thought tends to stammer when engaged in conversation. Since the spleen, which generates black bile, is also the seat of laughter, the melancholic is given to fits of laughter, which is often very unpleasant to hear.

He is full of deep unaccountable fears and anxieties, even when financially well off and suffering from no real ailment. He suffers long periods of sleeplessness, disordered mental functions, and sometimes has moods of the blackest despair. But the number of suicides among melancholics is remarkably small, as they seem to be able to live with their depressions without succumbing.

He has true dreams, that is, his dreams are often undisguised so that he sees things as they are, or as they will be. He has fantastic nightmares of dark abysses and horrible tortures, lonely endless corridors behind which lurk nameless horrors. Sometimes he is obsessed with the feeling that he is inanimate or only partly animate. One delusion frequently cited in Greek writings is that the melancholic imagines that he is a jar or that he has no head.

According to Aristotle (d. 322 BC), the melancholic has the gift of prevision and can 'prophesy as if from hidden books'. He has an intuitive insight into occult matters and is a man of deep understanding and profound but impractical wisdom, which although it appears to other men to be useless, strikes at the very bedrock of the human situation. He has a brooding spirit and restless blood; and intenser yearnings and wilder longings consume him than trouble ordinary men. Few men understand as he does the significance of grief and despair, and see in life's shocks and reverses the naked reality behind all things.

This 'dark genius' is himself capable of great suffering, and in fact seems to thrive on suffering. The Renaissance scholar, Marsilio Ficino (d. 1499) said, 'Saturn seldom takes over ordinary characters and destinies, but watches over those set apart from the common run of mankind.' These men are unique and unrepeatable. All outstanding men, whether philosophers, statesmen or poets, are to a certain degree, melancholic. Aristotle said that the gods are jealous by nature, and implant in men of great talent an overdose of black bile.

The Greeks prescribed the following treatment in the case of melancholics whose affliction needed relief. The diet must not be rich, and should contain fresh fish, honey and fruit, but not vegetables, especial care being taken to avoid onions and garlic. Moderation should be observed in food and the drinking of wine. The room where he lives should be cheerful and should face east. Also very beneficial are early morning walks, sea voyages if possible, soothing music (not loud music with a harsh beat), baths, massage, flagellation, cautery. If one can induce fever* in the melancholic, it assists cure. Relief for insomnia should be obtained by being rocked to and fro, or by the sound of running water. All drugs should be avoided.

Renaissance scholars recommend attracting the beneficent influences of the Sun, Jupiter, Venus and Mercury to counteract the baleful influence of Saturn in all cases of melancholy. The Solarian virtues were drawn down by a 'planetary rite' in which the victim robed himself in a gold or yellow mantle, strewed the ground with heliotrope, played on a lute, sang a hymn to the Sun, burned frankincense and drank a small quantity of wine. This was best done when the Sun was in Leo, and when the day and hour were appropriate for its full benefits to be received.

In the early writings the following were listed among the great melancholics: Priam, last king of Troy; his eldest son the Trojan hero Hector; the Trojan prince Aeneas founder of the Roman people; the Greek heroes Hercules, Ajax and Bellerophon; the philosophers Thales of Miletus (d. 550 BC), Anaxagoras (d. 428 BC), Empedocles (d. 425 BC), Socrates (d. 399 BC), Plato (d. 347 BC) and Lucretius (d. 51 BC).

Among the moderns we have: Albrecht Dürer (d. 1528); Martin Luther (d. 1546); Isaac Newton (d. 1723); Jonathan Swift (d. 1745); Johann Sebastian Bach (d. 1750); David Hume (d. 1776), who described himself as 'a strange monster unfit for human society'; Jean-Jacques Rousseau (d. 1778); Wolfgang Amadeus Mozart (d. 1791); Robert Burns (d. 1796), who spoke of 'the deep incurable taint of melancholy which poisons my existence'; Lord Byron (d. 1824); Johann Wolfgang Goethe (d. 1832); Edgar Allan Poe (d. 1849); Robert Schumann (d. 1856), who once threw himself into the Rhine but was rescued; Arthur Schopenhauer (d. 1860), 'the prophet of pessimism'; Thomas Carlyle (d. 1881); Piotr Tchaikovsky (d. 1893), who died of cholera after deliberately drinking unboiled water; Otto von Bismarck (d. 1898); Leo Tolstoy (d. 1910); Virginia Woolf (d. 1941), who drowned herself during a phase of depression.

The melancholic temperament is basically, though not always, depressive. In modern medical practice melancholy is treated as depression*, although a distinction can be made between the two. Depression may be a passing phase of cyclothymia* or an organic and curable condition, whereas melancholy is a feature of the character and is unalterable in the individual. Melancholy, like insanity, is often associated with genius*.

Books

Babb, Lawrence, *The Elizabethan Malady: a Study in Melancholia in English Literature*, Michigan College Press, 1951.
Bandmann, Günter, *Melancholie und Musik*, Cologne, 1960.
Binswanger, L., *Melancholie und Manie*, Pfullingen, 1960.
Bright, Timothy, *Treatise of Melancholie*, London, 1586.
Burton, Robert, *Anatomy of Melancholy*, London, 1621 and many subsequent editions.
Dreyfus, G. L., *Die Melancholie*, Jena, 1907.
Flasher, Helmut, *Melancholie und Melancholiker in den medizinischen Theorien der Antike*, De Gruyter, Berlin, 1966.
Harrison, G. B., *Essay on Elizabethan Melancholy*, London, 1929.
Hopewell-Ash, E. L., *Melancholie in Everyday Practice*, London, 1934.
Klibansky, R., Panofsky, E. and Saxl, F., *Saturn and Melancholy*, London, 1964.
Kraepelin, E., *Manic-Depressive Insanity and Paranoia,* Livingstone, Edinburgh, 1921.
Wittkower, R. and M., *Born Under Saturn,* Weidenfeld & Nicolson, London, 1963.

MENTAL ILLNESS

Whether mild or serious, mental illness is characterized by abnormal patterns of mood and behaviour. Its study is the province of psychopathology, psychiatry, psychoanalysis and other forms of psychotherapy*. The normalcy of man is so precariously balanced, that judged by the strictest standards we are all abnormal at times. 'Men are so necessarily mad,' wrote Blaise Pascal (d. 1662), 'that not to be mad must be another form of madness.' From infancy to senility man exhibits deviations from the normal standard. In some degree dreams, drunkenness, hysteria*, inspiration, sickness, ecstasy and other xenophrenic* states can all be described as aberrant conditions of mind.

But, strictly speaking, mental illness refers to the more marked abnormalities, which extend from the lesser ranges of neurotic fancies to the more serious forms of insanity. The stress of modern life has brought about a great increase in mental disorders. Nearly half the hospital beds in Britain, and the developed countries generally, are occupied by mental patients. A well-known psychologist has said that a child born in Britain today stands a ten times greater chance of going to a mental hospital than to a university.

In the USA a large proportion of the adult population is suffering from an anxiety state or mental depression, and more people are locked up for mental illness than for criminal offences. In the view of one American psychologist, 'the whole population of the US is getting more emotionally and mentally disturbed by the day' (Rogow, 1971, p. 166). The victims come from all levels of society, ranging from those in the well-to-do professions, like doctors, lawyers and psychiatrists, to those that are not so well educated or so well off.

More alarming still is the fact that mental illness is rapidly overtaking the younger age groups. A survey of New York school children carried out in 1969 showed that 12 per cent suffered from marked to severe psychiatric impairment of the kind that afflicted Lee Harvey Oswald (assassin of President John Kennedy) and Sirhan Sirhan (assassin of Robert Kennedy); 34 per cent were moderately impaired; 42 per cent were mildly impaired; and only 12 per cent were in good mental health. The number of patients under 15 years of age in American mental hospitals was 325 per cent higher in 1962 than in 1956. It shows a comparable increase in 1976.

Identifying and classifying a mental disease is extremely difficult, and the methods confused even in defining the major ones. 'In England,' says Dr Flach of Cornell University, 'the diagnosis of manic-depressive reaction is frequently used for patients who in the United States would be diagnosed as schizophrenic.' Many crucial questions concerning the aetiology*, prognosis and therapy* of mental illness are still largely unanswered. Treatment continues to be rather drastic, consisting principally of brain surgery, shocks, and drugs of high potency. In the final analysis the healing process in all mental illness, except those cases that are organic, remains a moral, and some would say, a religious, one.

Broadly, mental disorders are considered in three major divisions, namely: psychoses, neuroses and psychopathy. *Psychoses* include the more serious types of what is known in sociolegal terms as insanity, covering cyclothymia* or manic-depression, and schizophrenia*. Psychotics usually need care in an asylum or other institution. *Neuroses** are milder forms of mental illness, and cover many kinds of obsessions*, compulsions, monomanias*, often stemming from fear*, anxiety* and stress*. Even otherwise normal people have mild neurotic phases from time to time. *Psychopathy** is characterized by antisocial behaviour, and in many ways reflects the current sociopsychosis* or malaise afflicting society itself, and the prevailing angst* underlying it.

The causes of mental illness cover practically every item listed in the aetiology of disease in general. It may result from mental deficiency, congenital or otherwise, as found in the idiot with a mental age of a 2-year-old child, in the imbecile with a mental age of a 7-year-old child and in the moron with a mental age of a 12-year-old child. It may be due to brain injury or brain tumour; to drugs, toxins or alcohol, as in alcoholism, or Korsakov's syndrome; to syphilis*, terminating in GPI or general paralysis of the insane; to ageing, leading to senile dementia; to metabolic, glandular or hormone dysfunction; to sickness following infections of various kinds. Occultists believe that the root causes arise from a pathological condition of the etheric body. Others would add cosmobiological factors such as the disposition of the stars, the recurrence of sunspots and even the phases of the moon.

The term lunacy (Lat. *luna*, 'moon') preserves the age-old belief in the strange influence the moon has on the minds of men and women. It was said that the fuller the moon, the greater the degree of insanity, since 'the brain is a microcosmic moon'. In England, the Lunacy Act of 1842 defined a lunatic as a demented person 'afflicted with a period of fatuity in the period following after the full moon'.

Lovers through the ages have felt the deep surge of emotion and desire coursing through them on full-moon nights. Many perfectly normal people, it would seem, are apt to 'go over the edge' at these times. Policemen, bartenders, taxi-drivers, fire-station superintendents, nurses in hospitals and even psychiatrists have reported an increase in odd and erratic behaviour during the full moon. Instances of drunkenness, false fire-alarms, wife beating, theft, arson, kleptomania, fights, rash driving, automobile accidents, epilepsy*, hysteria, post-operative haemorrhaging, all seem to show a marked rise.

A significant feature about mental illness, is that it is often found in association with great intellectual and artistic abilities. Genius*, it appears, is particularly vulnerable in this respect.

Books

Eaton, J. W. and Weil, R. J., *Culture and Mental Disorders*, Free Press, Chicago, 1955.
Flach, Frederic, *The Secret Strength of Depression*, Angus & Robertson, London, 1975.
Kraepelin, E., *Manic-Depressive Insanity and Paranoia,* Livingstone, Edinburgh, 1921.
Linton, Ralph, *Culture and Mental Disorders*, Thomas, Springfield, Illinois, 1956.
Rogow, Arnold, *The Psychiatrists*, Allen & Unwin, London, 1971.
Sullivan, H. S., *Schizophrenia as a Human Process*, Norton, New York, 1962.
Szasz, T., *The Myth of Mental Illness*, Secker & Warburg, London, 1962.

MENTICIDE

'Mind murder', the systematic disorganization and destruction of a person's individuality and way of thinking, followed by the substitution of another set of values and opinions foreign to his free conscience, through physical and mental duress or coercive persuasion. More commonly called 'brainwashing'.

It is a method used in totalitarian states, both of the extreme right and the extreme left, chiefly against political opponents and those who oppose the régime. The tactics include: imprisonment; enforced sleeplessness; starvation; isolation; sensory deprivation; subjection to excessive heat or cold; total darkness; blinding light; noise; drugs; torture; surgical operations; and various anxiety, stress and fear situations. Also, the threat of applying such methods to loved ones.

Sooner or later the inevitable result is a total breakdown of the victim's will and power to resist. He passes through a period of confusion, crisis, mental blankness. The required behaviour patterns are then imprinted on the mind, leading to depersonalization*, an alteration of personality, and a complete reversal of values originally held. He will report on relatives and friends; bear false witness; disclose any secrets entrusted to him; alter his political, moral or religious views. In Nazi concentration camps, the victims of menticide became conditioned to accepting the values of the SS. They became their willing underlings, and to all intents and purposes were on the side of their Nazi tormentors, helping in the extermination of their own kith and kin.

Such mind-bending has an old history. It was adopted in many ancient communities in their treatment of enemies, though mostly carried to the point of death. In Christendom the Inquisition, in close collaboration with the church organization and dedicated to the propagation of the faith (which gave us the word propaganda), frequently resorted to methods that had all the features of modern dictatorial régimes.

To a lesser extent people are constantly being subjected to indoctrination and manipulation by the press and other media. In particular, advertising is a subtle form of manipulation, which in its worst forms works on the greed, envy, discontent, insecurity, fear and sensuality of the public, and is thus opposed to human dignity and freedom. Psychology has also been debased, some people believe, in the service of certain forms of publicity (including public relations) which, in its more unpleasant manifestations, has been classed as a black art.

Many forms of modern psychological persuasion represent the practical application of behaviour therapy*, stemming from experimental work on monkeys, dogs, cats, geese and other animal species both wild and tame. There is obviously some danger in indiscriminately applying to human beings the result of work on animals in laboratory or even in their natural surroundings, as is evident in the case of the eminent Konrad Lorenz, who was led from the 'goosification' of human beings to approval of certain Nazi ideologies.

Books

Bandura, A., *Principles of Behavior Modification,* Holt, Rinehart & Winston, New York, 1969.
Beech, H. R., *Changing Man's Behaviour*, Allen Lane, The Penguin Press, London, 1969.
Biderman, A. D. and Zimmer, H., *The Manipulation of Human Behavior,* New York, 1961.
Brown, J. A. C., *The Techniques of Persuasion*, Penguin Books, Harmondsworth, 1963.
Cohen, E. A., *Human Behaviour in the Concentration Camp*, Jonathan Cape, London, 1954.
Lifton, R. J., *Thought Reform and the Psychology of Totalism*, Gollancz, London, 1961.
Lorenz, K., *Evolution and Modification of Behaviour*, London, 1965.
Meerloo, J. A., *Mental Seduction and Menticide*, Jonathan Cape, London, 1957.
Schein, E. H. *et al.*, *Coercive Persuasion*, New York, 1961.

METALLOTHERAPY

The healing of sickness by bringing the patient in contact with metal specifically indicated for the cure, is based on the alleged qualities that are said to inhere in different metals, which exercise an influence on mind or body by causing the brain, nerves, blood and tissues to vibrate gently in response to the impulses sent out by the metal.

According to Aristotle (d. 322 BC), metals are specialized substances created by the exhalations arising from the earth. Dry or 'smoky' exhalations cause minerals to be produced; and steamy, wet or 'vaporous' exhalations result in metals, giving them their malleable, shiny and fusible qualities. A distinction was sometimes made between metals, which were regarded as 'male', and stones (gems), which were 'female'.

Those who have made a life-long study of metals believe that they may, indeed, have more energy-potential in them than we suppose, and even a latent mind, in elementary form. Under prolonged and arduous use they show definite signs of 'stress', a word used by scientists themselves. They appear to have a distinct life-span, after which they disintegrate rapidly. Medieval alchemists believed that metals could be energized by some process akin to growth, and that in the course of the operation, while the metal was in a molten state, vitalic forces could be infused into them. Sorcerers were said to imbue statuettes and other metal objects with evil emanations in this manner.

Metals have been used in therapy from early times. Certain metallic elements, such as mercury, arsenic and antimony, were taken internally. Paracelsus (d. 1541) was chiefly responsible for the use of metallic compounds from the sixteenth century onwards. Some metals, although they did not form part of the pharmacopoeia, were worn in contact with the body as protective and therapeutic amulets and ornaments. The chief metals used for this purpose were those traditionally associated in astrology with the heavenly bodies, and were worn in accordance with astrological indications. Gold, the metal of the Sun, was the perfection of metals, and the others were graded in descending hierarchical order, thus: gold, silver, mercury, tin, copper, iron and lead.

When used as amulets, these metals were supposedly beneficial for the following physical and mental ailments. Gold (Sun), general debility, eye troubles, depression. Silver (Moon), digestive and alimentary complaints, lack of imagination. Mercury (Mercury), bladder and skin troubles, shyness. Tin (Jupiter), lung and respiratory complaints, mental sluggishness. Copper (Venus), sexual weakness, poor concentration. Iron (Mars), bad circulation, feeble will. Lead (Saturn), heart troubles, mania.

One of the foremost metallotherapy exponents was Dr Elisha Perkins (d. 1799) of Connecticut, who claimed to have discovered what happens when living tissue is brought in contact with metal. He stated that when a metal touches the skin near an affected organ, the nerves in the area contract, relieving the pressure and assisting healing. He invented what he called tractors, made of two metal rods each three inches long; one a copper-zinc compound with a little gold, the other an iron-silver compound with a little platinum; and with these he stroked the affected part to draw away the pain towards the extremities. Perkins sold his tractors to many notables including George Washington, whose entire family used them. His son Benjamin Perkins continued his work.

The magnetizers of the eighteenth and nineteenth centuries believed that certain metals could absorb and store the magnetic fluid of the healer, and then, acting as conductors, could transmit the energy to the person wearing the metal. Gold, silver, copper and nickel were considered good conductors; and tin, pewter and zinc poor conductors.

In spite of the claims made by healers, many occultists regard metals on the whole as being inimical to man. Some people are sensitive to metals and can distinguish them by touch alone from the vibrations they give out, and many of them report being conscious of the generally harmful influence of metallic radiations. It has often been noted that men of saintly character shrink from the touch of metallic objects, and are repelled by contact with metallic coins.

Sensitives declare that many of the complaints of civilization are due to the great increase in the use of metals today, in buildings, cars, factories, and in beds, desks, chairs, shelves and other domestic and office furniture. The indiscriminate use of certain metals, especially when brought in contact with heat and moisture, can be highly injurious, as in metallurgical industries. Some even deplore the use of metals like aluminium for cooking utensils.

The proximity of metals affects the character of localized electromagnetic fields. It is believed that the environment of urban areas is depressing and disturbing because of the concentration of so much metal in a comparatively small compass. Most of the metals used are alloys, which often bring into combination two or more metals that are not naturally in harmony, and this creates a confusing resonance in the human mind. Many neurotic problems can be laid at the door of the ever-increasing use of metals in modern life.

Books

Andree, Richard, *Die Metalle bei den Naturvölker*, Leipzig, 1884.
Clement, Mark, *Aluminium: a Menace to Health*, Health Science Press, London, 1965.
Pagel, Walter, *Paracelsus: an Introduction to Philosophical Medicine in the Era of the Renaissance*, Karger, New York, 1958.
Perkins, Benjamin, *The Influence of the Metallic Tractors on the Human Body*, Boston, 1798.
Rickard, T. A., *Man and Metals*, McGraw-Hill, London, 1942.
Tomlinson, H., *The Divination of Disease*, Health Science Press, London, 1953.

MICROBES

Microbes comprise all organisms of microscopic or submicroscopic size, and include bacteria, 'germs' and viruses, although it is not clear whether all viruses are strictly living organisms or not.

The presence of viruses can be determined by X-ray processes, or they can be photographed by means of an electron microscope. They are specks of nucleic acids, and have distinct non-living features. For example, they can be constituted out of inorganic chemicals and can be produced in crystalline form, but will still multiply and grow like any other microbe. Many scientists still do not believe that viruses are alive; so they are treated as a borderline case, between animate and inanimate, living and non-living, between biology and chemistry.

Viruses are responsible for many diseases of plants, animals and men. For example, in *plants*: tobacco mosaic disease. In *animals*: foot and mouth disease (in cattle), myxomatosis (in rabbits), psittacosis (in parrots) and swine-fever (in pigs). In *human beings*: certain cancers, the common cold, chicken pox, dengue, encephalitis, glandular fever (infectious mononucleosis), hepatitis, herpes, infective jaundice, influenza, measles and German measles, multiple sclerosis, mumps, pneumonia, poliomyelitis, rabies, sandfly fever, smallpox, tick fever, trachoma, typhoid, typhus and yellow fever.

Today molecular biologists can breed new species of viruses, even deadly ones. Scientists are also aware of the possibility of a deadly type of virus being accidentally created during experiments. Such a virus, having a serological character different from any known to us, possibly with an exceptionally high degree of virulence, might be of a kind to which we have no natural resistance, and for which antibiotics would be of no avail. 'The devastation caused,' says Alan Norton, 'could rival that of the more talked-of thermonuclear catastrophe.'

All microbes multiply with great rapidity, as a rule asexually. It is estimated that if their reproduction were not checked by various adverse counterbalancing conditions, such as limited food supply, bacteria-eaters, poisons and lack of moisture, the progeny of a single microbe, if allowed to reproduce uninterruptedly, would exceed the total bulk of the earth in a month.

Bacteria are responsible for the processes of fermentation and decomposition, the conversion of dead organic matter into soluble food for plants, the fixation of atmospheric nitrogen and the biological cycle responsible for soil fertility. In the human body they provide important and essential vitamins for the body's survival and wellbeing.

Microbes are extremely resistant, adapt to the most adverse conditions, and have an incredible tenacity for survival. Within a few generations they mutate and evolve, and are ready to face changed contingencies. There are anaerobic bacteria that can live without free (atmospheric) oxygen; others can tolerate high vacuum and extreme temperatures; they can survive in springs of boiling water, and flourish in a refrigerator. They can remain quiescent in deep-freeze conditions. Single-celled micro-organisms trapped and frozen in the icy wastes of Antarctica for millennia, have revived with the entry of man.

Bacteria find lodgment in atomic reactors, unaffected by radiations of more than 500 times the dose that would kill any other living thing. Today there are germ strains that need streptomycin in order to flourish. Others thrive on cyanide and similar deadly poisons. Microbes are probably more fitted to survive than any other biological species. They have developed resistance to every drug, antibiotic and poison used by man to exterminate them.

Many bacteria are pathogens, or disease-carriers, and responsible for all the great epidemics that have beset mankind. One can say that they have played a more significant role in the making of human history than Alexander, Genghis Khan, Napoleon and Hitler combined. If the plan to use germs in warfare were sanctioned and brought into operation at any future time, it could well mean the end of the human race.

Microbial infections communicated by animals, or animal-communicated diseases, are termed *zoonoses*. For example, blood-feeding arthropods and parasitic insects are notorious vectors or carriers of disease: the mosquito (yellow fever and malaria), the fly (cholera), the louse (typhus), the flea (plague), the tick (relapsing fever), the sandfly (kala-azar) and the tsetse fly (sleeping sickness). The larger animal species are also responsible for numerous infectious diseases: sheep (anthrax), the dog, fox, wolf and vampire bat (hydrophobia or rabies), the rat (plague), the goat (undulant fever), the parrot (psittacosis), the horse (glanders) and the rabbit (tularaemia).

It is to be noted that, although these animals might communicate the disease, they themselves are only carriers and not the cause of the disease, for it is the micro-organisms that bear the actual malignancy. Thus, the rat harbours the flea (*Pulex irritans*), which itself carries the bacillus (*Pasteurella pestis*) which causes the plague.

It has been suggested that ultimately all disease is microbial in origin. If so, then every disease is an infection*, but on a level far beyond the merely physical. In the case of the plague, the big flea (man) is tormented by the lesser flea (the rat), which has a still lesser flea (the pulex) which carries the still tinier culprit (the bacillus); and for all we know that is not the end of the series. Bacilli themselves can be hosts to viruses, and viruses may be concatenations of biotoxic particles, which are generated, as it were, in a 'field' of infection. And this field may be etheric, psychic, perhaps cosmic.

There appears to be a certain 'destiny' element in the incidence of disease* as it affects individuals, and in the incidence of epidemics* as they affect communities. They are linked not only with germs, but with a wider series of events and processes. Germs, then, are not the ultimate cause, but only the precipitating factor, and can only come into action when conditions are right for them. Certain dangerous micro-organisms are the normal inhabitants of all healthy bodies, but do not cause epidemics. Not everyone in contact with a contagious disease becomes infected.

Louis Pasteur (d. 1895) said on his death-bed, 'Claude Bernard was right: the microbe is nothing, the terrain is everything.' The great cellular pathologist, Rudolf Virchow (d. 1902) said, 'If I could live my life over again, I would devote it to proving that germs seek their normal habitat – unhealthy tissue – rather than being the cause of unhealthy tissue.' In 1925, Léon Vannier, the doyen of French homoeopaths, suggested that 'the toxin precedes the microbe'.

And the 'terrain' of Pasteur, the 'habitat' of Virchow, the 'toxin' of Vannier, is the milieu that includes more than the physical system, more than cosmobiological factors, important as these are. It is the milieu created by the psychological predispositions of the individual, and the social environment in which he lives. Physical disease is often a direct product of a wider field of sociopsychosis*.

Books

Castellani, Aldo, *Microbes, Men and Monarchs*, Gollancz, London, 1956.
Dubos, R. J. and Hirsch, J. G. (eds), *Bacterial and Mycotic Infections of Man*, 4th edn, Lippincott, Philadelphia, 1965.
Ford, Brian, *Microbe Power*, Macdonald & James, London, 1976.
Norton, Alan, *The New Dimensions of Medicine*, Hodder & Stoughton, London, 1969.
Rivers, T. M. and Horsfall, F. L., *Viral and Rickettsial Infections of Man*, Pitmans, London, 1965.
Rosebury, Theodor, *Life on Man*, Paladin Books, London, 1972.
Smith, W., *Mechanisms of Virus Infection*, Academic Press, London, 1963.
Stanley, W. M. and Valens, E. G., *Viruses and the Nature of Life*, Dutton, New York, 1961.

MIGRAINE

Migraine (Gk. *hēmi*, 'half'; *kranion*, 'skull'), also called megrim, sick, nervous or psychosomatic headache, is a severe periodical pain in the head usually on one side only, hence the name. It sometimes runs in families, and there are more female than male victims of the affliction. It has been known from earliest times, and is mentioned in the Ebers papyrus (*c.* 1630 BC) of ancient Egypt as 'a sickness of half the head'.

Even before an attack the sufferer experiences an 'aura' or foreboding of its coming, before the pain actually reaches the point at which it is centred. There may be a feeling of pins and needles in various parts of the limbs; a ringing in the ears; a growing sensitivity to light and severe eyestrain, followed by pain in the eyes. Coloured flashes appear before the vision, and dancing bright lights with jagged or zig-zag patterns. Black spots constantly obscure the vision; often one suddenly sees only half of what one is looking at. A feeling of tightness grips the epigastrium and there is a sensation of nausea, which may bring on vomiting. The mental faculties become blurred, the victim cannot think clearly; words are mispronounced, or forgotten, or are said backwards or jumbled. At some stage during these symptoms comes a headache of varying severity. The migraine attack may last for anything from an hour up to two days.

Doctors speak of the migrainous personality and the migrainous temperament. Victims of this affliction are usually sensitive, imaginative, intelligent, serious and ambitious. They are keen in whatever they undertake, tend to be perfectionists, and worry if what they aim for is not attained. They may suffer from moods of depression. Each person is affected in a different way.

Some specialists regard migraine as an entirely psychosomatic*, almost occult, disease. To start with, no one knows the cause. Its origins have been sought in the physiological system and attributed to such factors as brain tumours or congestion of the cerebral blood vessels, but the symptoms emerging from such conditions differ from migraine. An attack is commonly set off by humiliation, anger, insecurity, lack of love, nervous stress*, emotional conflict or general angst*.

Many medical authorities believe that migraine and epilepsy* are related diseases. Both an epileptic and migrainous attack may be ushered in by an aura, that is, a warning of its approach, with a feeling that it is travelling up towards the region of the head. Its manifestations often parallel those of epilepsy. Campbell says, 'Like epilepsy migraine can produce altered states of consciousness.'

There is sometimes a sense of awe or even rapture, as at some mystical revelation. Some authorities, indeed, feel that certain kinds of religious experience could be explained in terms of this affliction. The psychic sensitivity is heightened and strange new experiences may be presented to the consciousness. The victim feels that time has stopped or that it 'mysteriously recapitulates itself'. There is an uprush of forgotten memories, a peculiar feeling of déjàism. He has a sense of clairvoyance, a rising above the self, even a moving outside the self, amounting at times to depersonalization*, so that he feels a stranger to himself.

The history of art, literature, philosophy and public life is filled with the names of those who have suffered from acute nervous headache. Religious mystics, too, have added their quota to the list. Oliver Sacks, discussing the visions of St Hildegard of Bingen (d. 1179), a woman of great intellectual ability, who described and also drew her visions, says that they are 'indisputably migrainous'.

Michelangelo (d. 1564) suffered from bouts of giddiness, blackouts and nervous prostration. Throughout his life Blaise Pascal (d. 1662) was the victim of agonizing headaches bordering on epilepsy. Alexander Pope (d. 1744) was deformed, sickly and frail from birth, and suffered from migraine. Edward Gibbon (d. 1794) had attacks of migraine from his childhood. Immanuel Kant (d. 1804) too was periodically afflicted. Napoleon (d. 1821) and Thomas Jefferson (d. 1826), the author of the American Declaration of Independence, were both subject to this ailment. Ludwig van Beethoven (d. 1827) suffered from hypochondria and blinding pains in the head that left him depressed for days. Sir Walter Scott (d. 1832) suffered from paralysis and apoplexy, and his severe headaches kept him awake at night for hours on end. William Wordsworth (d. 1850) was likewise a victim. Count Cavour (d. 1861), the Italian patriot, when afflicted with migraine gave way to paroxysms of rage that often led him to try to take his own life. Thomas Carlyle (d. 1881) was a martyr to dyspepsia, neurasthenia and migraine. Charles Darwin (d. 1882), who was always a sick man, suffered from giddiness and swimming in the head, and at times could hardly stand owing to the severe pain he suffered. Lewis Carroll (d. 1898) was another constant sufferer. In the case of dozens of other eminent men and women, the migrainous attacks developed into fits of epilepsy, and at times their condition bordered on insanity.

Books

Campbell, Anthony, *Seven States of Consciousness*, Gollancz, London, 1973.
Gowers, W. R., *The Borderland of Epilepsy: Faints, Vagal Attacks, Vertigo, Migraine, Sleep Symptoms, and Their Treatment*, Blakiston, Philadelphia, 1907.
Hanington, Edda, *Migraine*, Priory Press, London, 1974.
Klee, A., *A Clinical Study of Migraine*, Munksgaard, Copenhagen, 1968.
Leyton, Nevil, *Migraine*, Foyle, London, 1962.
Sacks, Oliver W., *Migraine*, Faber & Faber, London, 1972.
Smith, Robert, *Background to Migraine*, Heinemann, London, 1969.
Sperling, Melitta, 'A Psychoanalytic Study of Migraine and Psychosomatic Headache', *Psychoanalytic Review*, 39, 152–63.
Temkin, O., *The Falling Sickness*, 2nd rev. edn. Johns Hopkins Press, Baltimore, 1971.

MIND CURE

A system of healing through healthy-mindedness or right-thinking. The philosophy underlying mind cure has been known and practised in many parts of the world from ancient times, but its principles were first systematically formulated in the nineteenth century in the USA, where it came to be known as Menticulture, New Thought, Free Thought, Mental Healing, Higher Thought and Divine Science.

One of its pioneers was Phineas Parkhurst Quimby (1802–66), the son of a New Hampshire blacksmith, who was apprenticed to a clockmaker and received little education. At the age of 36, following a lecture on mesmerism given by a French mesmerist, Charles Poyen, then touring New England, Quimby was inspired to start out on his own as a professional mesmerist. He began practice in Portland, Maine, in 1859, basing his methods on the magnetic-fluid theory then in vogue. The 'Portland healer' used to lay his hands on the patient's head and abdomen and allow the 'healing rays' to flow into the sick body. But he soon abandoned this for a new system of curing by right-thinking. He frequently referred to it as the Science of Health, or Christ Science, because, he said, it was based on the teachings of Jesus. He recruited many disciples, among them Mrs Mary Baker Eddy (d. 1910), who came to him for treatment and stayed as his disciple. Her own movement, Christian Science, was largely adapted from Quimby's theories, although in later years she did her best to repudiate her indebtedness.

Mind cure rests on the belief that the infinite God alone fills the universe, and that we are all partakers of the life of God, and are in a sense divine, although wrong-thinking has shut out the flow from the divine source. Disease* is a delusion, an error of the mind. Evil thoughts cause fevers*, cancer* and tumours. Right-thinking is constructive, creative and healing. A good thought is worth a dozen tonics. The mind is the basis of our selves and we should ensure that it is stocked with the right principles. We are what we think we are.

Unhealthy thoughts should, therefore, be expelled at all costs. We should never allow them to enter our mind, or give verbal expression to them. We should banish all negative emotional attitudes: fear*, worry, anxiety*, fretfulness, pessimism, lack of faith, hatred, contempt, complaint, blaming, meanness, greed, passion, anger, lust and wantonness. We should not even complain about the weather, or of having missed the train. What we think is a dis-appointment may be God's re-appointment with us for a higher purpose. We should reject even from our vocabulary words like hate, envy, disease, jealousy, pain, doubt, fear. Giving expression to our woes, merely 'increases the total evil of the situation'.

The best way to avoid pessimistic, sick and poisonous thoughts is to fill the mind with healthy thoughts. Good thoughts drive out bad. Loving thoughts integrate, bind, hold and heal. We should think curative and health-inspiring thoughts, and fill the mind with courage, confidence and love. We should learn to relax, and let go and let the goodness of God take over. We should let our expectations be high and know that they will be fulfilled as is best for us. All good things are divine, and all things are divinely good.

A contemporary form of mild cure is termed Concept Therapy, or healing with ideas. Here positive ideas are formulated and held in the mind to effect a cure.

Books

Braden, C. S., *Spirits in Rebellion*, Dallas, 1963.
Cutten, G. B., *3000 Years of Mental Healing*, London, 1910.
Dresser, H. W. (ed.), *The Quimby Manuscripts*, London, 1921.
James, William, *The Varieties of Religious Experience,* Longmans, Green, London & New York, 1902.

Stocker, R. D., *New Thought Manual*, New York, 1906.
Towne, E., *Joy Philosophy*, New York, 1903.
Trine, Ralph Waldo, *In Tune With the Infinite*, Bell, London, 1956.
Wolff, William, *Psychic Self-Improvement for Millions*, Bell, New York, 1967.
Woodbury, J. C., *Quimbyism, or the Paternity of Christian Science*, New York, 1909.
Zweig, Stefan, *Mental Healers*, London, 1937.

MOLECULAR BIOLOGY

Molecular biology studies the cellular ultrastructure of the living process at its most basic level, or more specifically, the chemistry and biology of the molecules in the cell. It is an offshoot of genetics and biochemistry, and embraces cellular biology and microbiology. Great strides were made after the 1940s, when advances in electron microscopy, crystallography and X-ray diffraction greatly enlarged the scope of research in cytological (cellular) organization.

Cellular biology examines the precise chemical nature of the cell, the chromosome or genetic molecule, and the gene. Each genetic molecule is made up of nucleic acids, namely, DNA (deoxyribonucleic acid) and RNA (ribonucleic acid), in the shape of two complementary, ladder-like bands which interlink to form a double helix, or double spiral. The difference between a human being and a plant is traceable to the difference in the order and arrangement of these molecules.

Several thousand DNA components go to form a gene, which might be described as a specialized arrangement of the nucleic acids at a particular place in the coiled DNA strand. Here, again, the specific qualities of a gene lie in the arrangement rather than in the composition of its constituents. The gene is the biochemical unit which transmits hereditary 'genetic' characteristics.

Several hundreds of genetic molecules make up a chromosome. The chromosome can be seen under a microscope, individually identified and analysed, its character and weakness detected, and it can be manipulated and interfered with. Molecular biology (or 'genetic engineering') consists both of a large-scale manipulation of the gametes (sperm and ova) for purposes of artificial generation and selective breeding, and on a smaller scale of manipulation of chromosomes and genes with a view to altering species.

So far experiments in this field have been for ostensibly useful purposes. For example, molecular biology makes it possible to diagnose geneoses in prospective parents before marriage; and in the pre-natal stage of the foetus. Mental abnormality, mongolism and other genetic defects, and the predisposition to certain diseases (and even, it is claimed, asocial traits such as sexual deviation) can be spotted, and sometimes corrected. Eugenists* see in it a wonderful new instrument for selective mutations and the control of genetics and heredity.

For example, in amniocentesis, in which the cells of the amniotic fluid are analysed, the sex of the foetus can be determined, and a foetus of the unwanted sex can then be aborted. Experiments have also been carried out to enrich the male chromosome or Y-sperm in order to raise the ratio of male births or to produce better male children. Conversely, by suppressing Y-sperm, girl births may be increased.

It is further claimed that molecular biology is useful in what is called gene therapy or cell therapy, where the cell or gene itself can be modified to cure disease. Defective groups of cells or even individual cells in a diseased organ, as well as genes in sperm and ovum can be traced, and replaced by healthy or normal cells and genes. Many kinds of bodily cells could be grown in culture in the laboratory, like microbes, so that defective cells could be removed, the defect eliminated, and the cured cell replaced in the body.

Molecules of DNA have already been synthesized in the laboratory. It is also hoped that the same will be done with genes, and that such synthesized genes will be planted in the body in place of transmissible defective genes. Scientists hope eventually to achieve a synthesis of a complete set of genes and incorporate such genes into the cell where they will divide and grow naturally. This would make it possible for the molecular biologist to synthesize organisms of any type in the laboratory. Yet another and more far-reaching objective is the growing of human genes and reproductive cells (sperm and ova) in tissue culture, which would greatly advance research in human breeding, cloning, parthenogenesis, androgenesis, test-tube babies and other experiments in artificial generation*.

Even now scientists can alter the genetic make-up of viruses, bacteria, chromosomes and animal cells, including reproductive cells. They are altering genetic material to produce new species, or to breed special characteristics into existing species. Experiments in genetic crossing, in which the DNA chemical substances are crossed with whole bacteria, have produced 'transformed' progeny-bacteria, having one or more genes from the added DNA. Experiments have also been tried with human cells and mouse cells in culture, producing hybrid cells made up of both human and mouse genetic material.

Such research is the province of teratogenesis (Gk. *teras*, 'monster'), the artificial creation of living monstrosities. Even in the current state of scientific knowledge the molecular biologist can create biological aberrations. Scientists have, indeed, claimed success in teratogenic experiments by inducing congenital abnormalities in animals at the early stages of their development.

The birth of monsters has been recorded in the past, but this has come about in the natural course of things and not through scientific tampering. Babies born with severe deformities were said to be so created as a result of unnatural copulation between human beings and animals or demons, or because of sorcery or divine curse. Many examples are mentioned in a curious work known as *Aristotle's Problem* or *Aristotle's Masterpiece*, a medieval treatise which has nothing to do with the philosopher.

A teratoid birth was called a monster (Lat. *monstro*, 'to show'), or a prodigy (Lat. *prodigium*, 'a portent'), because it was a prophetic sign of something ominous coming; or a freak (or prank) of nature, or more eruditely, a *lusus naturae,* 'a sport of nature'.

In more recent times there have been instances of babies born with two heads, or four arms, or with some organ missing. Also pisciform or molluscous births, suggesting arrested development at an early ontogenic stage. A Polish lady living in the seventeenth century gave birth to two small creatures that were said to be two fish without scales. An American girl was alleged to have been brought to bed of an octopus, presumably a baby with eight legs. None of these children survived more than a few days.

Today such abnormalities may result from geneosis in the parents, from drugs taken by the mother, from radioactive fall-out affecting the gametes or the genes, or from deliberate scientific interference with the genes. What is more, scientists have been able to keep alive aborted foetuses and severely malformed babies for several days in an artificial environment, and in theory could keep them alive until they were grown up.

The scientific value of such experiments in molecular biology is open to question. Many stress the moral undesirability of biological interference at such a profound level as the genetic substructure of life itself. Even in gene therapy we cannot be sure that the genetic material will not be harmed in the manipulation process. There are also ethical and religious problems involved in genetic crossing and artificial generation*.

Again, tampering with the genetics of a virus is bound to be fraught with danger. In spite of controls, there is always a chance that some zealous scientist might tamper still further with the mechanism to see the worst that could emerge from his experiments. He might create a new type of deadly germ for which we will have no natural immunity (*see* microbe). Even now, under state auspices, some of the best brains in molecular biology are concentrating on new types of bacteria and viruses for BW (bacteriological warfare), perhaps the most devastating weapon in the armoury of modern destruction.

In view of all this, Nobel prize winner, Sir Macfarlane Burnet, Australian biologist, frankly admitted that 'molecular biology may be an evil thing'.

Books

Abse, Dannie, *Medicine on Trial*, Aldus Books, London, 1967.
Bloch, R., *Les Prodiges dans l'antiquité classique*, Paris, 1963.
Hamilton, Michael (ed.), *The New Genetics and the Future of Man*, Eerdmans, Grand Rapids, Michigan, 1972.
Harrington, Alan, *The Immortalist*, Panther, London, 1973.
Jones, A. and Bodmer, W., *Our Future Inheritance: Choice or Chance?*, Oxford University Press, London, 1974.
Leach, Gerald, *The Biocrats*, Jonathan Cape, London, 1970.
Penrose, L. S., *The Biology of Mental Defect*, Sidgwick & Jackson, London, 1949.
Ramsey, Paul, *Fabricated Man: the Ethics of Genetic Control*, Yale University Press, 1970.
Rostand, Jean, *Can Man Be Modified? Predictions of our Biological Future*, Basic Books, New York, 1959.

MONOMANIA

A term largely obsolescent in modern psychology, but still popularly used, for a mental abnormality in which a person is under the domination of a single idea, good or bad. Any morbid, unreasoning and irresistible interest in or aversion to an object or situation can amount to a monomania, and this includes all obsessions*, compulsions, furors*, delusions, idiosyncrasies, eccentricities*, likes, dislikes and fears* disproportionate to the demands of the occasion. The cause of monomania is not clear, but it is said to result from childhood trauma, hormonal imbalance and even allergy.

A monomania normally manifests only when the stimulus situation presents itself, and is therefore sometimes distinguished from the *idée fixe*, 'fixed idea', which is the persistence in a person's mind of any notion that dominates his life and is always present in his consciousness, as when he has delusions of grandeur or of persecution.

A monomania is regarded as an obsessional neurosis*, beyond voluntary control, but usually innocuous, which does not as a rule amount to a psychosis, although many forms of persistent monomania are symptomatic of schizophrenia*.

Literally hundreds of monomanic forms have been listed. They are designated by the operative word followed by the suffixes *-phobia* (Gk. 'fear'), *-philia* (Gk. 'love') or *-mania* (Gk. 'madness') as the case may be. Thus we have nosophobia, fear of disease; necrophilia, love of corpses; kleptomania, an irresistible impulse to steal.

In trying to bring order into the confused scheme, some psychologists have attempted to classify the various monomanias under certain broad categories, such as those connected with situations (heights, open spaces), with animals (snakes, cats, spiders), illnesses (syphilis, disease in general, poisons), with people (doctors, dentists, hairdressers), with society (theatres, crowds, parties), with the unknown (strangers, travel, darkness).

A brief list of the commonest operative prefixes in the textbooks on psychology is given below:

acro- (Gk. *akros*, 'top'), heights
aero- (Gk. *aēr*, 'air'), draughts of air, fresh air, foul air
agora- (Gk. *agora*, 'market-place'), open spaces
aichmo- (Gk. *aichmē*, 'point'), sharp objects
ailuro- (Gk. *ailouros*, 'cat'), cats
algo- (Gk. *algos*, 'pain'), pain
andro- (Gk. *andros*, 'man'), specifically the male sex (cf. anthropo-)
Anglo- things English
antho- (Gk. *anthos*, 'flower'), flowers
anthropo- (Gk. *anthrōpos*, 'man'), people; thus, anthropophobia is the fear of
    people
aqua- (Lat. 'water'), water (see hydro-)
arachno- (Gk. *arachnē*, 'spider'), spiders
asteropo- (Gk. *asteropē*, 'lightning'), lightning (see bronto-)
bacterio- bacteria
batho- (Gk. *bathos*, 'depth'), deep places
biblio- (Gk. *biblion*, 'book'), books
bronto- (Gk. *brontē*, 'thunder'), thunder (see kerauno-, and asteropo-)
cardio- heart disease
clasto- (Gk. *klasis*, 'breaking'), clastomania, a mania for destruction
claustro- (Lat. *claustrum*, 'an enclosed place'), confined places; thus, claustro-
    phobia, fear of enclosed spaces; claustrophilia, urge to seek small enclosing
    space

copro- (Gk. *kopros*, 'dung'), dirt, especially faeces

cyno- (Gk. *kynos*, 'dog'), dogs

demento- (Lat. *dementis*, 'mad'), insanity

demo- (Gk. *dēmos*, 'people'), crowds, mobs

demono- devils

dermato- (Lat. *derma*, 'skin'), skin disease

dipso- (Gk. *dipsa*, 'thirst'), commonly as dipsomania, a periodical craving for alcoholic beverage

dora- (Gk. *dora*, 'skin or fur'), the touch of the skin or fur of an animal

dromo- (Gk. *dromos*, 'running', or 'a course'), dromophobia is the fear of crossing streets, or fear of travel; dromomania is wanderlust, a desire to travel and to be on the move

dysmorpho- (Gk. *dysmorphia*, 'ugliness'), ugliness

ego- (Lat. 'I'), self; thus, egomania is a pathological preoccupation with one-self

elephanto- elephants; thus, elephantophobia, fear of elephants

equino- (Lat. *equus*, 'horse'), horses

ergo- (Gk. *ergon*, 'work'), work

eroto- (Gk. *erōs*, 'love'), making love (*see* erotomania)

erythro- (Gk. *erythros*, 'red'), blushing

felino- (Lat. *feles*, 'cat'), cats

femino- women

Franco- things French

Gallo- things French

gano- (Gk. *ganos*, 'marriage'), wedlock

Germano- things German

grapho- (Gk. *graphein*, 'to write'), writing

haemo- (Gk. *haima*, 'blood'), blood; thus, haemotomania is the pathological craving for blood

hagio- (Gk. *hagios*, 'holy'), holy things

haphe- or hapho- (Gk. *haphē*, 'touch'), touching or being touched; thus, haphephobia, fear of being touched by someone

helleno- (Gk. *Hellēn*, 'a Greek'), things Greek

heresio- (Gk. *hairesis*, 'choice'), choosing or deciding; thus, heresiophobia is the fear of making a choice; also the fear of heresy or dissent

herpeto- (Gk. *herpeton*, 'a creeping animal'), lizards, reptiles, crawling things

homo- (Lat. 'man'), mankind; homicidal mania is the pathological urge to kill

hydro- (Gk. *hydōr*, 'water'), hydrophobia is a horror of water, a symptom of rabies

hypno- (Gk. *hypnos*, 'sleep'), sleep

hypso- (Gk. *hypsos*, 'height'), heights; thus, hypsophobia is the fear of falling from a high place

kerauno- (Gk. *keraunos*, 'thunder and lightning'), keraunophobia is the fear of these phenomena

klepto- (Gk. *kleptein*, 'to steal'), stealing; thus, kleptomania is a compulsion to steal

lysso- (Gk. *lyssa*, 'rage'), lyssophobia is the fear of angry people

martyro- as in martyromania or persecution complex

megalo- (Gk. *megalē*, 'big'), megalomania is the delusion of power and greatness

miasmo- (Gk. *miasma,* 'defilement'), dirt and defilement

micro- (Gk. *mikros*, 'little'), small things; thus, microphobia, or more specifically, microbobphobia, is the fear of germs

mompho- (Gk. *momphē*, 'complaint, or quarrel'), quarrels

mono- (Gk. *monos*, 'alone'), monomania is obsession with a single thing; monophobia is the fear of loneliness

muro- (Lat. *murmus*, 'mouse'), mice

myso- (Gk. *mysos*, 'defilement'), dirt, uncleanliness, contamination

necro- (Gk. *nekros*, 'corpse'), death, corpses (*see* necrophilia)

negro- (Lat. *niger,* 'black'), Negroes, or black people

neo- (Gk. *neos*, 'new'), innovation, change, novelty

noso- (Gk. *nosos*, 'sickness'), disease

numero- numbers, or a specific number

nycto- (Gk. *nyktos*, 'night'), night or darkness (see also scoto-)

nympho- (Gk. *nymphē*, 'girl'), *see* erotomania

ochlo- (Gk. *ochlos*, 'crowd'), crowds

onio- (Gk. *ōnios*, 'buying'), buying things

ophido- (Gk. *ophis*, 'snake'), snakes

pano- (Gk. Pan, Greek god who caused panic), panophobia is a causeless fear*

panto- (Gk. *pantos*, 'all'), fear of everything, as found in conditions of pathological fear*, anxiety*, stress* and angst*

patho- (Gk. *pathos*, 'suffering'), pain and disease

peccato- (Lat. *peccare*, 'to sin'), committing sin

pharmaco- (Gk. *pharmakon*, 'drug'), drugs, medicines, poisons

phobo- (Gk. *phobos*, 'fear'), being afraid; phobophobia is fear of one's own fears

phono- (Gk. *phōnē*, 'voice'), sounds

photo- (Gk. *phōtos*, 'light'), light, especially strong light

porio- (Gk. *poreia*, 'journey'), poriomania is the desire to wander, to run away

porno- (Gk. *pornē*, 'prostitute'), *see* erotomania

psycho- all psychological questions

pyro- (Gk. *pyr*, 'fire'), pyromania is a morbid compulsion to set things on fire

Russo- things Russian

scoto- (Gk. *scotos*, 'darkness'), the dark

sexo- *see* sexophobia, and erotomania

sito- or siteo- (Gk. *siteō*, 'to feed'), food and eating

syphilo- syphilis*

tapho- (Gk. *taphos*, 'burial'), taphophobia, fear of being buried alive

thalasso- (Gk. 'sea'), the sea

thanato- (Gk. *thanatos*, 'death'), dying and death (*see* thanatomania, and thanatophilia)

theo- God, *see* theomania

topo- (Gk. *topos*, 'place'), places and localities

toxico- (Gk. *toxicon*, 'arrow-poison'), poisons

tricho- (Gk. *trichos*, 'hair'), trichomania is a fetishistic preoccupation with hair

venero- (Venus, goddess of love), venereal diseases
xeno- (Gk. *xenos*, 'stranger'), strangers
zoo- (Gk. *zōon*, 'animals'), animals

Books

Frampton, Muriel, *Overcoming Agoraphobia*, Thorson, London, 1974.
Julier, D., *Agoraphobia in Man*, University of London, 1967.
Marks, Isaac, *Fears and Phobias*, Heinemann, London, 1969.
Rachman, S., *Phobias: Their Nature and Control*, Thomas, Springfield, Illinois, 1968.

MULTIPLE PERSONALITY

The state in which the waking consciousness of an individual is apparently under the temporary control of a personality different from the normal self, so that he or she seems to be possessed at different times by different persons. The subject sometimes behaves like one person, and sometimes like another, entirely different person, and the two or more personalities concerned act differently, speak differently, each in its own voice and with its own distinctive vocabulary and pronunciation; each has its own moral standards and its own patterns of behaviour. Often the intrusive personality is not aware of the existence of the other, and if it is, is likely to be hostile or antagonistic to the other. Alternative terms for the condition are: alternating, dissociated, plural, dual or split personality.

Robert Louis Stevenson (d. 1894), in his famous story about Dr Jekyll and Mr Hyde, was the first to use this theme as the basis for a novel. Instances of genuine multiple personality are not at all common, only about 70 cases having been recorded by psychologists. Usually there are two or three distinct personalities, but some patients have shown as many as seven.

A classic case occurred in the year 1900 when a Miss Beauchamp, a student nurse, consulted Dr Morton Prince of Harvard, who worked as a specialist in nervous diseases at the Boston City Hospital, about her headaches and insomnia. Miss Beauchamp was 23 years old, physically healthy and a pious and gentle creature, but during treatment she began manifesting another character calling herself 'Sally', and behaving in a manner which was the direct antithesis of her usual self. The young woman was not aware of Sally's existence, but Sally was of Miss Beauchamp's, and made the latter's life miserable with her pranks. For instance, knowing that the nurse was afraid of spiders, she would, while she had possession of their common body, collect spiders and place them in Miss Beauchamp's desk, where she would find them. In the course of treatment a third, and later a fourth, personality emerged, and it was only after about six years that Dr Prince was able to force the invading characters out of the girl's life for good.

Another interesting case concerned Mollie Fancher (1849–1915) of Brooklyn, who suffered two serious accidents at the age of 17 as a result of which she became blind, paralysed and bed-ridden. She took practically no food for nine years and at times her pulse could not be felt and her body would turn cold. During these periods she appeared to be possessed by an alien personality who was able to execute delicate fancy work with her crippled hands, read books and letters clairvoyantly, and help in tracing lost articles. Her original personality returned after nine years, but for the next three years she remained subject to epileptic seizures, and in between would be possessed by several new personalities who discussed various matters and often quarrelled among themselves. Mollie Fancher became quite normal again in 1912 and passed away quietly in her sleep three years later.

Dr Walter Franklin Prince, a research officer of the American Society for Psychical Research (not to be confused with his contemporary Dr Morton Prince, mentioned above), found in his investigation of a young spirit medium, Doris Fischer (c. 1924), that she also exhibited two separate and distinct personalities, joined later by three others. With the aid of hypnosis he was able to get rid of the aliens and restore Miss Fischer to her normal self as an integrated person.

The phenomenon of multiple personality has received a great deal of interest as a result of the publication of a book called *The Three Faces of Eve* and a film of the same title, telling the story of a girl who exhibited different personalities.

Demon or spirit possession is sometimes invoked to explain this strange phenomenon, but this theory is not generally accepted today. Psychologists attribute the manifestations to hysteria*.

Books

Azam, E., *Hypnotisme, double conscience et altération de la personnalité*, Paris, 1887.
Dailey, A. H., *Mollie Fancher*, Brooklyn, 1894.
Lancaster, Evelyn and Boling, J., *Strangers in My Body, or The Final Face of Eve*, Secker & Warburg, London, 1958.
Prince, Morton, *The Dissociation of a Personality*, New York, 1906.
Schreiber, F. R., *Sybil*, Regnery, Chicago, 1973.
Smith, A. J., *The Three Sally Beauchamps*, New York, 1940.
Thigpen, C. H. and Cleckley, H. M., *The Three Faces of Eve*, Secker & Warburg, London, 1957.

MUSIC THERAPY

Music therapy was widely practised in many ancient communities because of the curative and soothing powers believed to be inherent in harmonious sounds. In general music was thought to be especially good for frayed nerves and the troubled spirit. The Bible records that the shepherd lad David cured the madness of King Saul by playing the harp to him (1 Sam. 16:23). In the same way, nearly three thousand years later, the songs of the castrato singer Carlo Farinelli (d. 1782) allayed the malady of Philip V of Spain during the final months of his madness.

Aesculapius, the Greek god of healing, ordained that fevers and mental disorders could be cured with song, and many mythical musicians of Greece were reputed to have healed the sick with their music or singing. The paean, the Greek song of triumph and thanksgiving, was originally a charm against sickness and insanity. The *Iliad* relates that during the Trojan War a paean was sung to banish the plague, and when some centuries later a plague ravaged Sparta, the rulers appointed Thaletas (d. 650 BC), a Cretan musician, to sing paeans to the accompaniment of his lyre, as a result of which the pestilence ceased. Similar public recitations by professional rhapsodists like Homer and Hesiod were performed in ancient Greece as a spiritual salve.

According to Pythagoras (d. 500 BC), music has definite value in alleviating certain illnesses and in helping to maintain health, through what he calls 'soul catharsis'. He prescribed it to treat those with spiritual or mental afflictions, making use of the musical mode appropriate to their illness. Iamblichus (d. AD 333) the neo-Platonist records that Pythagoras composed certain melodies against the passions of the soul, and others as remedies against despair, rage and furor*.

The philosopher Democritus (d. 361 BC) also recommended music therapy, in particular the melodious notes of the flute, which he declared suffused the nerves and caused them to distil a harmonious energy throughout the body. Asclepiades (*c.* 70 BC), physician of Bithynia who founded a medical school in Rome, had a trumpet blown to relieve the pain of sciatica, because its penetrating and prolonged notes caused the fibres of the body to become violently agitated and, as a consequence, the 'stings' of sciatica to be dispersed. The Greek writer Athenaeus (*c.* AD 180) wrote that patients with sciatica could be cured if one played the pipe in the Phrygian mode over the affected part.

In the highly developed Arabic *maqāmāt* or modal system of the eleventh century, different modes were required to be played and sung for different ailments: the *rāst* for eye diseases, the *irāq* for dementia, *isfahān* for colds, *zangula* for heart trouble, *buzurg* for colic, *shirāz* for venereal disease, and *rahāwi* for headache.

In medieval Europe the Swiss-German physician Paracelsus (d. 1541) said that the sound of the flute would cure epilepsy* and melt the pains of gout. Another advocate, the Jesuit physician Athanasius Kircher (d. 1680), following the principle that music had the quality of drawing out disease, especially of the temperament, improvised an ingenious instrument for the purpose, consisting of a row of five tumblers of very thin glass, filled respectively with mature wine, new-made wine, brandy, oil and water. By striking the edge of the tumblers gently with the finger-nail, a melodious sound emerged, drawing forth from the patient his diseased biomagnetic* waves, which streamed out to meet the music, and the disease vanished as the music and waves blended and dispersed.

Franz Mesmer (d. 1815) the 'magnetizer', after whom 'mesmerism' is named, often had music as part of his treatment, a practice continued by his followers for certain ailments. William James (d. 1910) introduced the use of music in hospitals. In our own day Fritz Kreisler (d. 1962), the Austrian violinist and composer, firmly believed in the benefits of music therapy and used to send unemployed musicians to hospital to play to patients. Today music therapy, in rehabilitating, educating and treating people, both children and adults, who are mentally or physically ill, has more advocates than ever, and is used extensively in hospitals and institutions.

How music effects cures is not clear, but among the suggestions put forward by exponents, both ancient and modern, are the following: it promotes the flow of stagnant 'humours' and removes obstructions; it opens constricted blood vessels and dissipates 'noxious vapours'; it unknots the fibres of the brain and dispels melancholy; it restores the equilibrium of the disturbed etheric double; it causes the nerves to 'vibrate' responsively and thus assists the healing process; it pleases the ear and diverts attention from the disease.

Whatever it may be, the undoubted influence of sound on the psyche has also brought to the fore a better understanding of the harmful effects of certain kinds of music, which, far from having soothing or therapeutic value, can do a great damage to one's physical and mental health.

Though both Plato (d. 347 BC) and Aristotle (d. 322 BC) advocated music as a therapeutic aid, both warned against its indiscriminate use, since it could do as much harm as good. The famous physician Soranus of Ephesus (c. AD 100) said that people who imagined that the power of disease could be dissipated by music and melody were stupid.

To be effective music requires no abstract thought, no intelligence, and no concentration on the part of the listener, for the mind is easily and effortlessly captivated by its spell. It operates not on the upper ranges of consciousness, but at a more profound level, and it therefore becomes imperative that the right sort of music be played at all times.

Music is not a tranquillizer, although it is often thought of as such. It can be a very powerful and heady stimulant. After wide-scale experimental studies, experts agree that care should always be exercised before prescribing this form of therapy for the sick. Many factors have to be taken into account, such as the temperament of the patient, whether child or adult, male or female, the physical and mental condition, the nature of the illness.

The predominating instruments are equally important. In the old tradition: the flute is the lunatic's instrument, the lyre the harlot's, and the drum the barbarian's. In other words, wind instruments tend to stir the mind, stringed instruments stimulate the sexual feelings, and percussion instruments affect the savage instincts.

The manner of performance and the technique used are of the greatest significance. High pitch, loud volume, a strong compulsive beat, rapid rhythm, dissonance, abrupt contrasts, sudden accelerations of tempo, can start uncontrollable reflexes that create both physical and mental disturbance in sensitive subjects. All these appeal to the lower faculties, and a fascination for music that employs these devices indicates an unhealthy craving for stimulation that characterizes the degenerate, and is a sign of insecurity, immaturity and mental instability. This was fully realized and, therefore, condemned by the ancient Greeks as well as the early Church Fathers.

The effects of music cannot be overstressed. They are felt on the physical, physiological, nervous, mental and psychical levels. To begin with, there is an intimate connection between musical beat and the bodily pulse. It has been found that music has an effect on the secretions of the sweat glands, and on the involuntary pupillary reflexes. It can bring about changes in the even flow of blood circulation, raise blood pressure, accelerate the breathing rate, cause constriction of the respiratory passages, interfere with digestion and, occasionally, trigger convulsive reflexes, cortical discharges and myoclonic seizures. Instances of 'musicogenic epilepsy', fits caused by music, have been established beyond doubt.

Music stimulates physical reactions, and people tend to hum, sing, clap, stamp, dance or participate in some form of vigorous physical activity. Fear and embarrassment are overcome and inhibitions thrown overboard. Certain kinds of music can arouse the instinctive forces of sex and aggression, leading to promiscuousness and violence, especially in the adolescent. The simultaneous rise of venereal disease and the appearance of pop music in the 1960s, says Ivor Felstein, 'may now be considered less fortuitous than on first observation'.

Some feel that the wrong kind of music has a destructive effect on the etheric body. Music arouses deep and intense emotions. And many pop rhythms have a deleterious effect on the mental and psychical systems. Plants exposed to hard rock rhythms have been known to shrivel up and die.

Music works directly on a person's mood and behaviour. It can make people agitated, turbulent, excited, furious. For this reason some people are instinctively suspicious of music; they freeze up, as it were, because they are reluctant to submit to its influence and let themselves go, regarding it as demeaning in some way to be so strongly moved by it.

For these reasons music therapy, unless the music is of a very gentle kind, is not considered desirable for the weak-minded, for adolescents and the mentally disturbed. It is contraindicated in the case of schizophrenia* and the manic phase of cyclothymic* insanity, since the activity of the imaginative faculty in cases where the imagination is already overwrought, might aggravate rather than mitigate the abnormal condition. The most that can be said for music therapy is that a gentle, soothing type of music, played quietly in the background, is sometimes, and in moderation, helpful in convalescence.

Books

Alvin, Juliette, *Music Therapy*, Hutchinson, London, 1975.
Brocklesby, Richard, *Reflections on Ancient and Modern Musick with Application to the Cure of Diseases*, Cooper, London, 1749.
Felstein, Ivor, *Sexual Pollution*, David & Charles, London, 1974.
Gaston, E. T. (ed.), *Music and Therapy*, Collier-Macmillan, New York, 1968.
Guilhot, J. *et al.*, *Musique, psychologie et psychothérapie*, E.S.F. Paris, 1964.
Licht, Sidney, *Music in Medicine*, New England Conservatory of Music, Boston, 1946.
Nordoff, Paul and Robbins, Clive, *Music Therapy in Special Education*, John Day, New York, 1969.
Podolsky, E. (ed.), *Music Therapy*, Philosophical Library, New York, 1954.
Priestley, Mary, *Music Therapy in Action*, Constable, London, 1975.
Savil, Agnes, *Music, Health and Character*, John Lane, London, 1923.
Schullian, D. M. and Schoen, M. (eds), *Music and Medicine*, Schuman, New York, 1948.
Sigerist, Henry E., 'Disease and Music', in *Civilization and Disease*, University of Chicago Press, 1943.
Soibelman, D., *Therapeutic and Industrial Uses of Music*, Colombia Univeristy Press, 1965.
Stebbing, Lionel, *Music: Its Occult Power and Healing Virtues*, New Knowledge Books, London, 1958.
Teirich, H. R. (ed.), *Musik in der Medizin*, Stuttgart, 1958.

N

NATUROPATHY

Naturopathy relies entirely on natural methods for maintaining good health and treating disease. It is founded on the dictum of the Greek physician Hippocrates (d. 359 BC), later adopted by the Roman physicians as *vis medicatrix naturae*, 'the healing power of nature', or the body's own ability to maintain the proper functioning of the organs and to recuperate from illness. Thomas Sydenham (d. 1689) known as 'the English Hippocrates', believed that illness itself was a form of therapy, for during illness the body mobilizes its resources to control the disorder and restore its lost equilibrium.

Basically the body is a remarkable vehicle of self-cure and one that runs with incredible efficiency. Many ingenious parallels have been drawn between body and machine. Its bony framework is an extraordinary compromise between' strength and weight. The muscles are pulleys worked by fuel cells. The lungs are bellows. The veins hydraulic pipes. The heart, the world's most efficient pump. The blood a better transport system than any we have devised. The brain, an electric computer beyond compare. The skin is waterproof, germicidal and more versatile than any material yet invented by man. As a unit the body has an unbeatable and irreproducible system of homeostasis (feedback control and self-correction).

Naturopathy believes in the power of the body to cope with almost any emergency. Illness is regarded as a struggle between body and disease, and the naturopath's aim is to help the body to resist, and not to concentrate on the disease, for which the body's own resources are quite adequate. While accepting the mechanical analogy of the human organism, it is emphasized that man is not a machine. Computer diagnosis and institutionalized treatment are not the best methods of keeping him in health or curing his ills. Nor is man a chemical contrivance, and modern drugs are not the best answer. Naturopathy is strongly opposed to artificial aids like chemotherapy and surgery except in emergencies, and to all forms of allopathy*.

It advocates its own daily regimen of physical exercises, including deep breathing in the open air, massage, and heliotherapy (Gk. *hēlios*, 'sun') or regular exposure of the nude body to sunshine. In earlier times exposure to the sun was practised as a ritual device by Chinese taoists and Hindu tantrics. Heliotherapy was once popular in treating tuberculosis of the bones and joints, its efficiency being due to the ionizing ultraviolet and actinic rays emanating from the solar spectrum. A similar effect can be obtained from ultraviolet lamps, though natural sunlight is better; neither should be carried to excess.

Naturopathy also lays great stress on natural foods, unprocessed and simply cooked (*see* diet), as well as periodical fasts. Also regular natural sleep, without drugs; cold baths if possible (but in any case never hot baths); regular bowel movements without the aid of purgatives.

In the case of sickness or setbacks, mind-cure and herbal remedies are prescribed. Many naturopaths accept homoeopathy*, hydropathy*, osteo-practic*, and similar therapies* as natural aids in treating certain ailments.

Books

Benjamin, Harry, *Everybody's Guide to Nature Cure*, Health for All Publishing Co., London, 1961.

Blythe, Peter, *Drugless Medicine,* Arthur Barker, London, 1974.

Gallert, Mark, *New Light on Therapeutic Energies*, Clark, London, 1966.

Inglis, Brian, *Fringe Medicine*, Faber & Faber, London, 1964.

Powell, Eric, *The Natural Home Physician*, Health Science Press, London, 1975.

Rollier, Auguste, *Heliotherapy*, London, 1923.

Shackleton, Basil, *The Grape Cure*, Thorson, London, 1969.

NECROPHILIA

(Gk. *nekros,* 'corpse'; *philia,* 'love'), any excessive preoccupation with corpses. In a wider sense it implies a morbid interest in death and decay, murders and suicides, funerals and festivals of the dead; in the worship of ancestors and relic-homage. It is found in necromancy or conjuration of the dead, of zombies and revenants; in therianthropy, vampirism and cannibalism; in fascination with graveyards, morgues, cremation grounds, dissecting rooms, cadavers and skeletons. It crops up even in the highest circles of civilized society, as we find in the case of Jeremy Bentham (d. 1832), English philosopher and apostle of utilitarianism. At his own request his body was dissected after death, and his skeleton, dressed in his accustomed garb, presided at University College, London, for many years.

Many graveyard ceremonies are necrophilic, even those with religious intent. Concentration on the subject of death and the personal enactment of the dying process is taught in a number of religious cults. The neophyte has to lie down and assume the position of a cadaver. He thinks of various fatal diseases that afflict mankind, imagines their symptoms, or the accidents that lay men low, and realistically acts out the part, visualizing in every agonizing detail the moments of dying and the final extinction. In the terrifying *chod* rite of the Bon sect of Tibet, a hierophant offers up his own astral body for spirit entities to devour. The purpose behind all such rituals is to teach the transience of life, to subdue and banish carnal desire and the lusts of the flesh.

More specifically, necrophilia refers to sexual congress with cadavers. The first recorded instance of coition with a corpse occurred in ancient Egypt, when an embalmer violated the body of a beautiful woman brought to him for embalming. He was suitably punished, and it became customary thereafter never to hand over the bodies of beautiful women or females of high class to embalmers, until three or four days had elapsed after death. In the Middle Ages in Europe the duty of keeping vigil over the dead bodies of persons of high estate was entrusted to monks, but after several cases were reported of monks abusing dead women to appease their sexual hunger, the custom had to be stopped.

Greek mythology tells how Achilles committed an act of necrophilia upon the body of the Amazon queen Penthesilea, after he had slain her. Herodotus records that Periander (d. 585 BC), tyrant of Corinth and one of the seven wise men of Greece, committed an offence on the body of his wife Melissa after he had, perhaps accidentally, killed her. The practice of intercourse with a corpse frequently took place at black magical ceremonies that were once regularly observed in certain primitive communities. Rollo Ahmed states that in some parts of Asia and Africa necrophilia was performed on the bodies of women during a rite in which the necromancer's assistant had intercourse with a female cadaver 'as a preliminary means of animating it'.

Sometimes a necrophilic act is enjoined as a religious duty, since it was regarded as inimical to the state of the soul after death if a girl were unmarried when she died, as it made her spirit restless. Thus, among the Kachin of upper Burma and among the Nambudri of India, post-mortem marriage rites were performed to give peace to the soul, and the dead virgin was married to a man, who then had intercourse with her. In central Europe, until about two centuries ago, if a betrothed girl died before marriage, the prospective bridegroom solemnized the rite by congress with the body.

The erotic attraction of a complaisant sexual partner may to some extent explain the prevalence of necrophilic customs in modern Europe. In the more select brothels of Paris arrangements were made to cater for the tastes of those who sought such titillation. Catafalque, bier, black pall, were all part of the funereal décor of the room. A woman was laid out like a corpse, and made no movement but lay exactly as she was arranged by the client, offering no resistance to intercourse in any fashion he desired. This was regarded as the last word in erotic finesse and had a number of eminent devotees.

Medically, necrophilia is regarded as a pathological symptom, and those who indulge in it are to a certain degree insane. Many cases of criminal necrophilia are noted in the police records of all countries.

Books

Ahmed, Rollo, *The Black Art*, John Long, London, 1936.
Licht, Hans, *Sexual Life in Ancient Greece*, Routledge & Kegan Paul, London, 1932.
Spoerri, T., *Nekrophilie*, Basle, 1959.
Summers, Montague, *The Vampire: His Kith and Kin*, Kegan Paul, London, 1928.

NEUROSIS

A term introduced in 1780 by William Cullen for a broad category of mental illnesses known since the days of ancient Greece. It commonly describes a functional, as distinct from a structural, disorder of the nervous system. It is psychologically and not physically caused, and may range from the threshold of normality to actual mental derangement. A neurosis does not usually deprive a person of contact with reality, and is thus to be distinguished from psychosis, which is a more severe mental illness, often requiring care in an institution. According to a medical witticism: 'The psychotic says, two and two make five; the neurotic says, two and two make four, and I just can't stand it.'

There are a number of related conditions which overlap the neurotic state. The term psychasthenia, 'mental weakness', introduced by Pierre Janet (d. 1947) and now rarely used, refers to the mild mental disorders covering obsessions* and anxieties*. Another related condition is neurasthenia, 'nerve weakness', manifesting in fatigue, loss of energy, poor concentration and general debility. These symptoms are not as a rule due to malnutrition, infection or anaemia, or any other recognizable physical cause. The neurasthenic is usually a valetudinarian, worrying constantly about his health, which is often good. Malingering, or pretending to be ill, is also a symptom of depressive neurosis. Yet another related condition is hypochondria, an exaggerated concern with the bodily functions, and a morbid fear of disease. The term is derived from the zone* of the body called the hypochondrium, which lies somewhat beneath the nipples, on either side of the epigastric plexus. It was once believed that disaffections of this region caused morbid depression, with anxiety about one's health. It was once regarded as a male affliction, and the opposite* of hysteria*, which afflicts women. Hypochondria or hypochondriasis was classed as one of the characteristic features of melancholia*, though the term is now in disuse in psychology.

Neurosis may have a number of physical symptoms, but these cannot always be readily identified. Broadly, when a person's response to an individual or a situation is abnormal or unhealthy, he is neurotic about it. It has been said that one man's tidiness is another man's neurosis. The accompanying manifestation are wide-ranging, and cover monomanias* (phobias, philias, manias), paranoia (sometimes leading to aggression), various forms of depression*, anxiety, hysteria, emotionality and obsession. It may show itself in morbid oversensitivity and suspicion, excessive preoccupation with trifles, in meticulous cleanliness of one's person. A person can be neurotic about anything: growing old, noise, young people, parents, children, religion, work, disease, sex. What is called anorexia nervosa is a neurotic loss of appetite, usually affecting adolescent girls and young women, and interpreted by Freudians as a rejection of the burden of adult sexuality.

The causes of neuroses are variously listed: childhood trauma, sexual repression, inhibitions, shock, self-conflict, guilt. As a rule there is always some personal, family, social or moral maladjustment. According to Ledermann, neurosis is not a scientific but a moral phenomenon, and 'for its understanding a moral philosophy must be found'.

Neurosis is a very widespread, even universal type of mental illness which has probably afflicted everyone at some time or other, in varying degrees of severity and with varying symptoms. The neurotic is not feeble-minded; he is often a person of high intelligence. Some, indeed, find a correlation between neurosis and genius*. The world's history, it is said, has been made by men of neurotic stock, and neurotics have been called the torch-bearers of civilization.

Books

Eysenck, H. J. and Rachman, S., *The Causes and Cures of Neurosis*, Routledge & Kegan Paul, London, 1965.

Fenichel, O., *The Psychoanalytical Theory of Neurosis*, Routledge & Kegan Paul, London, 1945.

Horney, K., *The Neurotic Personality of Our Time*, Norton, New York, 1937.

Kubie, Laurence, *Neurotic Distortion of the Creative Process*, University of Kansas Press, 1958.

Ledermann, E. K., *Existential Neurosis*, Butterworth, London, 1972.

Pickering, George, *Creative Malady*, Allen & Unwin, London, 1974.

Ryle, Anthony, *Neurosis in the Ordinary Family*, Tavistock Publications, London, 1967.

NIGHTMARE

A terrifying dream, often of an encounter with a being, supernatural, human or animal, of great strength and energy, accompanied by various symptoms of fear* and oppression. These symptoms include a feeling of great weight or pressure on the chest, a consciousness of suffocation and difficulty in breathing, and a sense of powerlessness to move or speak, although the victim may occasionally sigh, moan, groan or murmur as if in the jaws of death.

An ordinary terror dream is not as a rule accompanied by any such feelings of weight or helplessness, and the fear may be sufficient to awaken one. But in the true nightmare one has to endure the terrifying dream for some considerable time and it is only with the utmost effort and exertion, or some external help, that one escapes out of that dreadful torpid state.

As soon as he is able to move, the victim is affected by strong palpitations and a rise in blood pressure, a feeling of languor and listlessness as though physically and emotionally exhausted, an indescribable depression, uneasiness and anxiety, and all in all a general reaction as though from an actual experience. In a nightmare there is an acute impression of a real encounter with terror.

In the term, the derivation of the suffix '-mare' indicates that it was once believed to have a demonic origin. The Old High German *mara*, a cognate term, meant an incubus. The Old English *mare* (quite distinct from the Old English *mere*, for a female horse) means demon or spectre. The French word for nightmare, *cauchemar*, means an oppressive demon. Robert Macnish gives a vivid description of the traditional *mare*, or nightmare demon: 'A monstrous hag squatting upon the breast — mute, motionless, and malignant; an incarnation of the evil spirit — whose intolerable weight crushes the breath out of the body, and whose fixed, deadly and incessant stare petrifies the victim with horror.'

In medieval times the term *mare* was used interchangeably with incubus. By the fifteenth century the nightmare began to be associated, through false derivation, with the horse. It was believed to be a dream that attacked horses, and Sir Thomas Browne (d. 1682) tells how a stone hung up in the stable prevents the disease. Before long the nightmare began to be pictured as a snorting wild-eyed horse, with its two forelegs pressing heavily upon the victim and suffocating him with its weight.

Among the many explanations put forward to account for the occurrence of nightmares, the earliest was that of an actual visitation by a night demon whose presence rendered the sleeper powerless and who sought to drive terror into him. In medieval times a number of strange theories were current. According to one authority, nightmares were due to 'incongruous matter mixed with the nervous fluid in the cerebellum'. Another said they resulted 'from a thick phlegm which intercludes the vital spirits and makes us think there were some unnatural burden holding us down'. Occultists explain a certain class of nightmare as an occult attack on the astral body by an evil entity, experienced by the sleeper on one of the lower planes. Such nightmares can be dangerous since, if the attack is successful, the sleeper's spirit may be subjugated, and he may be found dead.

A more rational approach sought their origin in a disorder of the internal organs, pressure on some vital part of the body during sleep, overeating and indigestion. Some scholars believed that nightmares had a sexual origin, and that they were a predominantly female oppression. Physiological malfunctioning, female disorders, particularly irregular or painful menstruation, and repressed sexual desires, were the chief factors contributing to their occurrence.

Freudians state that nightmares result from sexual repression, and are perverse manifestations, in dream imaginings, of sexual congress, particularly in the passive form characteristic of women. Hence we have the pressure on the breast (as when the man 'mounts' her), self-surrender and a feeling of powerlessness, palpitations and sweating, fear such as often accompanies coitus.

Nightmare eroticism, it should be noted, may take a form alluring to men, also resulting from repressed desire. There may be vivid sexual experiences accompanied by voluptuous sensations. These sexual dreams, however, are not necessarily of a pleasant character, since the female concerned may be an old, decrepit and ugly crone. Nightmares, it has been observed, usually come to people sleeping on their backs, a position conducive to erotic thoughts.

Books

Bond, John, *An Essay on the Incubus or Nightmare*, London, 1753.
Burton, Robert, *Anatomy of Melancholy*, London, 1621.
Hadfield, J. A., *Dreams and Nightmares*, Penguin Books, Harmondsworth, 1954.
Jones, Ernest, *On the Nightmare: Nightmares, Witches and Devils*, Hogarth Press, London, 1949.
Macnish, Robert, *The Philosophy of Sleep*, London, 1830.
Waller, John, *A Treatise on the Incubus or Nightmare*, London, 1816.

OBSESSION

Obsession (Lat. *obsidere*, 'to haunt'), originally meant the persistent attack on a person by evil spirits from without, and was distinguished from posses-sion*, where an evil entity was thought to enter the stronghold of the vic-tim's mind and operate from within. It was commonly believed that a vir-tuous person could only be obsessed and was immune to possession. St Anthony (d. 356), the desert hermit, was obsessed not possessed by demons. Another difference between the two states is that in obsession the subject retains both his consciousness and intelligence, whereas in possession the operating intelligence and consciousness are not those of the person him-self but of the invading alien entity. The term obsession is also loosely applied to possession itself, as in the possession of a medium by an evil spirit, tending to the displacement of the medium's normal personality even out of the trance state.

Strictly, obsession is a morbid psychological condition in which an idea persists in a person's mind, without apparent reason, as a consequence of which he is impelled to perform, even against his will or better judgment, certain actions prompted by it, which actions if not performed would leave him with a feeling of guilt, anxiety* and frustration. It covers many kinds of compulsive behaviour.

Obsessional tendencies are inherent in every individual, and nearly every-one has had a passing obsession of some kind or other in his life. But only when it becomes a dominating influence, exercising an irresistible control over his actions and feelings, can it be termed a true obsession. Obsessions often give rise to feelings of persecution, delusions of grandeur, phobias and fears of various kinds. Some subjects think they have committed a heinous crime and deserve to be punished. In cases of guilt-complex this may rise to a pitch where a person will try to inflict the punishment on himself. There is no idea, no torturing fancy, which may not be capable of assuming compul-sive force in the mind.

Obsession attacks people of both sexes and all ages and in all walks of life. Statesmen, bricklayers, engineers, doctors, butchers, priests, psychiatrists, truck-drivers, scientists, all swell the ranks of those treated for obsessive delusions. Some, like Dr Samuel Johnson (d. 1784), must count railings, pillars and posts on the street; others must count steps, or stride over the lines separating the paving stones as they walk. Some fear contamination and must wash their hands all the time. In its minor manifestation people feel the urge to open a letter they have just sealed to make sure that it is there and not a blank sheet or a rough draft; to confirm that the gas has been turned off, or the garage door is locked; or wake up at midnight and look under the bed to satisfy themselves that no one is hiding there. Some are worried to death at the thought that they have made some calamitous mistake in their professional work, or have forgotten something of great importance in their daily round or have committed a social *faux pas* of some kind. Some feel an irresistible urge to use profane language in church, or at funerals or public meetings.

There have been people totally obsessed with the idea of trying to solve absurd metaphysical problems and riddles, and unable to desist because they feel that some cosmic destiny is involved in it. Some again believe that germs abound everywhere, especially in furniture, and live for years in a completely empty room and sleep on the floor. Others keep minute accounts of everything they buy; or meticulously enter in dozens of ledgers the current value of thousands of items of not the remotest concern to them.

Obsessional acts have a strange, stilted, ritualistic quality, and often appear to the victim to be directed from outside. Martinets and disciplinarians are plagued with the urge for stability and order almost as if they were not motivated by their own volition. The table must be set in a special way, the bed made in a certain manner, times must be observed to the minute. The order of things under their control seems to take on a symbolic significance. Any deviation from an established procedure becomes a source of great discomfort, psychic disturbance and anxiety. They have an uneasy feeling that the welfare of the state, indeed of the world, will be affected by any alteration in the rigid routine of their own lives and that of their immediate circle.

Sigmund Freud (d. 1939) discerned an anal fixation in the obsessional character. Such a person tends to be perfectionist, routine-minded, obstinate, parsimonious, mean and pedantic. It represents a rebellious reaction connected with bowel-training in infancy, that makes the adult anxious about 'losing control'. He is inclined to be constipated*, and fears sexual activity since it involves the loss of semen and the surrender of the self.

Occultists sometimes see in obsession the influence of some prevailing thought-form, with which the psyche of the victim has become enmeshed and through which it is permanently influenced.

Certain kinds of mental disorder in which a person's obsession is confined to a single idea, are treated as forms of monomania*, which may amount to schizophrenia*.

Books

Campbell, C. M., *Destiny and Disease in Mental Disorders*, W. W. Norton, New York, 1935.
Carson, C. H., *Obsession*, London, 1933.
Freud, Sigmund, *Obsessive Acts and Religious Practices*, Hogarth Press, London, 1959.
Janet, P., *Les Obsessions et la psychasthénie*, Alcan, Paris, 1903.
Linton, Ralph, *Culture and Mental Disorders*, Thomas, Springfield, Illinois, 1956.
Oesterreich, T. K., *Possession, Demoniacal and Others*, Kegan Paul, London, 1930.
Peebles, Dr, *Spirit Obsession*, London, 1925.
Sargant, William, *The Mind Possessed*, Heinemann, London, 1973.
Zilboorg, G. and Henry, G. W., *A History of Medical Psychology*, Allen & Unwin, London, 1941.

OCCUPATIONAL THERAPY

As its name implies, occupational therapy is healing through work. It is a form of paramedical treatment, supplementary to regular medical and nursing care, and more specifically to physiotherapy*. Whereas physiotherapy* is concerned with restoring the primary muscular and nerve patterns of a handicapped person, occupational therapy is concerned with the uses to which the patient puts them.

The value of work has been recognized from very early times. Having a craft of some kind and being able to do something with one's hands, was regarded as both useful and meritorious. The ritual disciplines of the priesthood, the soldierly activities of the warrior, the labours of the hunter, the farmer and the carpenter, were not only necessary for their livelihood but essential for their wellbeing. The Jews of the Middle Ages, even those who were wealthy and of good family, were always taught some kind of manual work, as a supplement to any other intellectual or financial skills they might have. The great philosopher Baruch Spinoza (d. 1677), after his excommunication from the synagogue, earned his living polishing lenses, a skill he had acquired in his boyhood.

It was also early realized that keeping busy and occupied was an essential factor in the cure of mental patients. Philippe Pinel (d. 1826), when he struck off the chains of the insane and provided them with various occupations, complained that among his patients were members of the nobility who disdained to work and were consequently very difficult to cure.

The idea of occupational therapy was first systematically propounded by Johann Spurzheim (d. 1832), one of the founders of phrenology. It was further developed by George Combe (d. 1858), philosopher, lawyer and phrenologist of Edinburgh. Richard Bucke (d. 1902), one of the pioneers of Canadian psychiatry, insisted on making his patients work as part of their cure. Idleness is the bane of institutions like asylums, jails and old people's homes. Those who retire without having a hobby of some kind soon fall a prey to mental or physical illness. It has been found that when patients are provided with employment the need for sedative drugs is reduced.

Previously many asylums and hospitals had large farms and workshops where a simple kind of occupational therapy could be tried. Men and women worked in workshops, laundries and kitchens. But trade unions objected to this kind of 'exploitation' of patients, and to their doing work that rightly belonged to working men. Many farms, market gardens and hospital workshops had to be closed down, and pottery, basket-weaving and other schoolchild hobbies imposed on patients instead.

The aim of occupational therapy is restorative and rehabilitative. It creates self-confidence, restores self-respect, helps people to attain maximum recovery and independence. Treatment involves both rehabilitation and resettlement. Severely handicapped patients are re-educated for the activities of daily life (ADL), including self-care and work skills.

As a method of purposeful and active treatment it covers a wide field, providing opportunities for various skills, motor and sensory. Improvement is sought in body movement, co-ordination, posture, balance, speed, mobility

198

and effort. Also sight, touch, hearing, concentration, memory, judgment and initiative are improved.

The various kinds of occupation deemed suitable for patients might be roughly classified as follows. *Outdoor*: gardening, farming, agriculture, horticulture, floriculture. *Industrial*: assembly-work, woodwork, simple industrial skills. *Domestic*: cookery, housewifery, dress-making, laundry-work. *Creative*: pottery, puppetry, model-making, basket-work, crafts. *Commercial*: typing, book-keeping, filing. *Recreational*: archery, old-time dancing.

Most forms of occupational therapy concentrate on physical movement, or the co-ordination of hand and brain. But there are others that emphasize the mental rehabilitation or development of patients. Such educational therapy, as it is sometimes called (and often classed as a form of psychotherapy*), concentrates more on the intellectual side and includes subjects like language, mathematics and history. Similarly speech therapy is concerned with the patient's ability to interpret what he feels, sees and hears, and to associate these with the spoken and written word. The speech therapist relies on the physiotherapist to improve those neuromuscular reflexes which affect speech, e.g. breathing and mouth movements. The speech therapist takes up from there. Bibliotherapy includes reading, especially books of high literary quality and poetry. Related branches include drama (*see* psychodrama), music therapy*, and art therapy*.

Books

Fidler, G. S. and J. W., *Occupational Therapy: A Communication Process in Psychiatry*, Collier-Macmillan, London, 1963.

Gardiner, M. D., *The Principles of Exercise Therapy*, Bell, London, 1963.

Greifer, Eli, *Principles of Poetry Therapy*, Poetry Therapy Center, New York, 1963.

James, Eileen, *Realistic Remedies: Occupational Therapy*, Educational Explorers, Reading, 1973.

Jones, M. S., *An Approach to Occupational Therapy*, 2nd edn, Butterworth, London, 1964.

Macdonald, E. M. (ed.), *Occupational Therapy in Rehabilitation*, Ballière, Tindall & Cassell, London, 1964.

Mountford, Stella, *Introduction to Occupational Therapy*, Livingstone, Edinburgh, 1971.

West, W. L. (ed.), *Occupational Therapy for the Multiply Handicapped Child*, University of Illinois, 1971.

Willard, H. S. and Spackman, C. S., *Occupational Therapy*, Pitman, London, 1963.

OPPOSITES

Opposites represent the two contrary poles of a dynamic whole. They exist in all situations, for opposites are found in religion, philosophy, science, nature and the human body. Together they give coherence, vitality and, indeed, existence to all creation.

In metaphysical medicine they are the participating agents in several important concepts, which can be better understood because of them. Sometimes, though not necessarily, they imply an exclusive and hostile antagonism, sometimes a reconciling and integrative synthesis, depending on the context in which they are considered and the condition to which they apply. The basic opposites in the subject are listed below:

Eros (love)	Thanatos (death)
life	death
nature (heredity, instinct)	nurture (environment, training)
masculine	feminine
sexuality	anxiety*
pleasure	pain*
fecundity	sterility (*see* infertility)
mind	body
asoma (non-physical body)	soma (physical body)
psyche	soma
spiritual body	astral body
astral body	etheric body
psychology	biology
functional	structural
dominance	submission
anal sexuality	oral sexuality
in vivo (in life)	*in vitro* (in glass, i.e. in the laboratory)
homoeopathy*	allopathy*
herbalism*	chemotherapy
pyretotherapy	cryotherapy (*see* thermosomatics)
behaviour* analysis	depth analysis (*see* psychodiagnostics)
physician	surgeon
medicine	surgery
acute (sudden and of short duration)	chronic (of long duration)
crisis (sudden turning-point of disease symptoms)	lysis (gradual disappearance of disease symptoms)
dyscolic (unable to endure pain)	eucolic (able to endure pain)
dyspeptic (tending to indigestion)	eupeptic (having a good digestion)
dysgenic*	eugenic*
dyscrasis (bad mixture)	eucrasis (proper mixture) (referring to the mixture of the four humours)
fever*	colds
malaria	syphilis*
leprosy*	syphilis
leprosy	haemorrhoids
leprosy	plague (*see* epidemics)
scurvy	plague
sneeze	hiccup
belch	flatus
gout	palsy
tuberculosis*	typhoid
diabetes	hypoglycaemia

thyrotoxicosis (hyperthyroid-ism)	myxoedema (hypothyroidism) (*see* hormone therapy)
introvert	extravert
bilious; melancholic (introvert)	sanguine; phlegmatic (extravert) (in humoralism)
phosphoric; fluoric (introvert)	sulphuric; carbonic (extravert) (in homoeopathy)
shame (personal)	guilt (social)
phobia	philia (*see* monomania)
neurosis*	psychosis (*see* mental illness)
psychopathy*	psychosis
dysthymia (obsessional anxiety)	cyclothymia*
depression	mania*
hypothymia	hyperthymia
manic depression	dementia praecox
schizophrenia*	cyclothymia
schizophrenia (an introvert ailment, male)	hysteria (an extravert ailment, female)
schizophrenia	epilepsy
catatonia (passive form of schizophrenia)	paranoia (active form)
schizophrenia	cancer and virus infections
hypochondria (a male disease)	hysteria* (a female disorder)
persecution complex	delusions of grandeur
martyromania	megalomania
melancholia*	epilepsy*
myopia, short sight (introvert)	hypermetropia, long sight (extravert)
buttock-oriented male (intro-vert)	breast-oriented male (extravert)
central nervous system (con-trolled by the will)	autonomic nervous system (self-controlled)
sympathetic nervous system (emergency system)	parasympathetic nervous system (rest-ing system)
adrenergic (sympathetic)	cholinergic (parasympathetic)
catecholamines	acetylcholine (neurohormones)
adrenergic (MAOI)	antiadrenergic (MAO)
cholinergic	anticholinergic (cholinesterase)
anticholinesterase	cholinesterase
sympathico-mimetic	sympathico-lytic
parasympathico-mimetic	parasympathico-lytic
adrenals	pituitary
pineal	pituitary
somatotropic hormone (STH)	ACTH
anterior lobe of pituitary (masculine)	posterior lobe of pituitary (feminine)
adrenalin (releases blood sugar)	insulin (lowers blood sugar)
glucagon (increases blood sugar)	insulin (*see* hormone therapy)
hormones	enzymes

201

antigen (foreign substance)	antibody (defensive substance) (*see* organotherapy)
serum	antiserum
toxin (poison)	antitoxin (antidote)
aphrodisiac*	anaphrodisiac*
potassium	sodium (*see* stress)
glucose	salt
acid	base
acid	alkali
amphetamines (CNS stimulants)	barbiturates (CNS depressants)
tranquillizers	stimulants
chlorpromazine	LSD
euhypnic	dyshypnic
psycholeptic	psycholytic
psychoanaleptic	psychodysleptic
psychotomimetic	antipsychotomimetic

Books

See under hormone therapy, psychodiagnostics, *and* drug therapy

ORGANOTHERAPY

Organotherapy, or opotherapy, prescribes animal organs, extracts and juices in its treatment of disease. It has its roots in the ancient past, arising from the doctrine of analogy, which made the primitive believe, for instance, that eating the heart of a brave warrior would make him brave. Advocates of meat-eating, as opposed to vegetarianism, point to the greater food value of flesh. Earlier variants of organotherapy are found in scatotherapy*, where urine, dung, sweat, blood, semen and other bodily substances were thought to have therapeutic value; and borboric therapy*, which rests on the alleged healing properties of bones, claws, feathers, dirt and moulds.

In more recent times there have been various forms of organotherapy based on the superior value of biological, as opposed to chemical, methods of treatment. For example, there was the autohaemic therapy of Dr Loyal Rogers (*c.* 1916) of Chicago, who made medicines by 'attenuating, haemoliz-ing, incubating, and potentizing' a few drops of the patient's own blood. Dr Charles Duncan (*c.* 1918) introduced autotherapy, in which the diseased parts of the patient were used to cure him. Thus, boils were healed by giving the patient an extract of his own boil. What is called haemotherapy also uses blood for healing, or for 'purifying and strengthening the blood'.

It has been pointed out that modern blood transfusion is in effect a more scientific version of the ancient superstition. Blood itself has properties of youth and age, hence the kind of blood used in all these therapies is impor-tant. The experiments of the French biologist Alexis Carrel (d. 1944) sugges-ted that only young serum kept his famous chicken-heart tissue culture alive for over thirty years, and that when old serum was used the tissues died.

Modern research in what is called plasmapheresis (Gk. *aphairesis*, 'withdrawal'), in which large quantities of blood are drawn from an animal, the toxins removed and the blood restored, seems to indicate that blood tends to store certain impurities, and that a change of blood might in some cases be beneficial. Some substances in the blood, like collagen (a fibrous protein), do lead to decline in vigour, and cause ageing.

Most rejuvenation* therapies use the glandular extracts of men and of animals. Organotherapy also forms the basis of preventive medicine, as in immunization, vaccination and inoculation. Immunization is the process by which the body makes itself insusceptible to various foreign substances and bacterial poisons. Briefly, an antigen is a substance that is foreign to the body's own substance; to defend itself against the invading antigen, the physical organism has to produce an antibody (anti-foreign body). Serotherapy, or serum therapy, is based on the acquired immunity of serum, the liquid part of the blood (not to be confused with plasma, containing serum plus clotting elements), which, when it has acquired such immunity to a particular infection is called an antiserum, and contains antibodies against that infection. Again, toxins which are the poisonous substances released by disease-causing bacteria, are neutralized or destroyed by antitoxins formed naturally in the body.

A number of modern remedies are obtained from animal organs. Thus, from the liver we get the drug heparin, used to prevent the coagulation of blood. Liver extract is prescribed in pernicious anaemia. The products of various glands (many now synthesized) are used for diabetes, cancer, infertility, high blood pressure and other diseases. Many of these substances are the products of the animal's internal secretion glands or the cells of the nervous system (*see* hormone therapy).

Books

Cobb, I. G., *The Glands of Destiny*, Heinemann, London, 1927.
Gardner, Martin, *Fads and Fallacies in the Name of Science*, Dover, New York, 1957.
Gordon, B. L., *Medicine Throughout Antiquity*, Philadelphia, 1949.
McGrady, Patrick, *The Youth Doctors*, Arthur Barker, London, 1969.
Parish, H. J., *A History of Immunization*, Edinburgh, 1960.

OSTEOPRACTIC

A term recently coined to cover two methods of healing, both based on the earlier skill of 'bone-setting'. Osteopractic is based on the notion that all remedies necessary to health exist in the human body, but the body cannot function at its peak of efficiency unless the structure is sound. Illness results from structural or mechanical defects, which are mainly osseous, that is, concerned with the bony framework of the body. All disease stems from defects in the normal articulation of the bony framework, from strains and stresses. When bones, joints or ligaments get out of position, either through sudden dislocation or long misuse ('postural abuse'), manipulative surgery is needed, in order to adjust the body so that the natural remedial agents can muster their forces and effect a cure. Detailed charts are drawn up showing the connection between the bones and the various organs which help the practitioner to localize the trouble.

The Edwin Smith Papyrus (*c.* 1600 BC) of ancient Egypt prescribes muscular, osseous and spinal adjustment for sprains and dislocation of the back. Hippocrates (d. 359 BC), the Greek physician, was also well aware of the relationship of the spine with bodily health and advised, 'Look well to the spine for the cause of disease.'

One form of osteopractic known as *osteopathy* was founded by Andrew Taylor Still (b. 1828), a country doctor of Virginia, who in 1874 formulated the Rule of the Artery, which stated that the beginning of all disease was traceable to the malfunctioning of an artery, due to pressure upon it. The pressure had to be discovered and adjusted, and nature would do the rest. His motto was, 'Find it, fix it, and leave it alone.' He held that blood, carrying the vital energy through the body, must circulate without impediment. If prevented for any reason from flowing freely it would become sluggish and sour, and illness would result. Though he was not very clear how this happened and could not explain the process, he wrote, 'It matters not what you call it: here is your mystery.'

The second form of osteopractic, called *chiropractic*, was founded by an unqualified Iowa practitioner from Canada named Daniel David Palmer (*c.* 1890), who established the Rule of the Nerve. He and his followers laid greater emphasis on displacements and 'subluxations' (partial dislocations) of the spinal vertebrae, or of the intervertebral disc of cartilage later known as the 'slipped disc', which press on the nerves, which in turn fail to transmit to the bodily organs the necessary impulse for their proper functioning. The chiropractor, by skilful manipulative adjustments, corrects the fault and permits the nerves to function freely. Another related technique, which is approved by orthodoxy, is physiotherapy*, dealing with the softer tissues and muscles, rather than with the bones.

It is to be noted that in all kinds of osteopractic teaching, the student can be helped only to a limited extent. The skilled practitioner depends on the degree of rapport he is able to establish with the patient, on his intuitive understanding of the body as a functioning organism, and on his flair for manipulating without conscious control. The best practitioners seem to let their hands work out the pressures on their own.

Books

Chaitow, Leon, *Osteopathy: Head-to-Foot Health Through Manipulation,* Thorson, London, 1974.
Dintenfass, Julius, *Chiropractic: a Modern Way to Health,* Pyramid, New York, 1966.
Downing, A. H., *Osteopathic Principles in Disease,* San Francisco, 1939.
Hoag, B., *Theory and Practice in Osteopathic Medicine,* McGraw-Hill, London, 1969.
McClusky, T., *Your Health and Chiropractic,* New York, 1962.
Puttick, R. W., *Osteopathy,* London, 1956.
Schofield, Arthur, *Chiropractic,* Thorson, London, 1973.
Stoddard, A., *Manual of Osteopathic Techniques,* Heinemann, London, 1959.
Weiant, C. W. *et al.,Medicine and Chiropractic,* New York, 1959.

P

PAIN

A sensation quite distinct from that communicated by the sense of touch. It possesses mysterious qualities all its own. A local anaesthetic will not abolish the sense of touch, so that a patient may be fully aware of the part of his body being operated upon, although he feels no pain.

What actually causes the feeling of pain is not clear, and cannot always be attributed to physical causes, like injury or inflammation. One theory is that it may be due to a disturbance of electrical tension or chemical imbalance in the affected cells. Speusippus (d. 330 BC), successor of Plato in the Academy, said that pain and pleasure were opposite evils. Indeed, both are rooted in the etheric body, according to occult theory. Ultimately then, pain, like pleasure, may best be described not only in neurological and physiological terms, but also in etheric terms. Pain originates in the etheric system, which is the seat of sensation and brain consciousness. It is what one has to suffer for the privilege of consciousness, for we can only feel pain when we are conscious.

The gradations of pain are also difficult to determine, and methods of estimating its intensity remain unsatisfactory, largely because of the difficulty of establishing a quantifiable norm. But it is generally agreed that the range of possible pain experience extends roughly between a mild headache and third-degree burns.

The ability to endure pain depends on the so-called pain threshold, and varies greatly with different people. It seems to be linked with race, age, sex, general health and even the time of day and season of the year. Different nationalities seem to have different thresholds. The Swedes and Irish are apparently less sensitive to pain than the French and Italians. In general, women tolerate pain much better than men, just as they seem to possess some special factor that enables them to withstand the stresses of life better than men in the long run. The introverted, the neurotic and the anxious feel pain to a greater degree than others. Excitement, such as arises at the height of a game or battle, raises the pain threshold so that people can stand more pain without discomfort, sometimes without even being aware that they have been hurt. Good pain-endurers are called eucolic, and those who cannot endure it, dyscolic.

Analgesic drugs, which deaden pain without loss of consciousness, such as aspirin, barbiturates, alcohol, work by raising the pain threshold. They do not stop the pain at source, but by gradually dulling the nerve impulses, increase the level of pain the nervous system can tolerate before it begins to register the sensation of hurt.

Certain parts of the body normally register lessened pain reactions, or even none at all. The interior of the brain feels no pain, so that surgeons can carry out major brain operations with only a local anaesthetic. The inner lining of the mouth opposite the second molar tooth is also insensitive, which makes it possible for the wonder-worker to pass a needle through the cheek at this point without undue discomfort. The vagina is comparatively insensitive to pain or pleasure. Sensation is also lost when certain diseases are present, like leprosy*.

Because of the intricate interweaving of the nervous system, or the ramifications of the subtle arteries, a pain stimulus in one part of the body may sometimes be felt somewhere else. This is known as referred pain. Gallstones and liver disease may cause pain near the shoulder-blades; the pain of an inflamed appendix often makes itself felt just below the breast bone. There have been cases of pneumonia patients being operated on for appendicitis because of the strongly placed pain experienced not in the chest, but in the abdomen. Headache and stomach-ache are the commonest of referred pains.

Another peculiarity is that pain often continues to be felt in a limb that has been amputated. This pain in a phantom limb is explained in terms of the nerve communications network that is left unimpaired and continues to function even after the organ to which it relates has been removed. It can also be explained as a form of paraesthesia* or displacement of sensory perception.

Pain has often served as a spiritual aid, and has been sought by ascetics, mystics and martyrs as a mode of understanding the deeper significance of life. It tends to bring on certain xenophrenic* states. The minor variants, as manifested in algolagnia (sadism and masochism) not only arouse sexual desire, but sometimes provide a mild feeling of transcendence. It is known that torture, mutilation, and other forms of mortification of the flesh cause large quantities of histamine and adrenalin to be released into the blood stream, which brings about changes of consciousness.

As a phenomenon of the etheric body pain has certain occult connotations. And it has moral and religious overtones as well. Flagellation, long a therapeutic fashion in Europe, was also recommended by the church as a form of spiritual discipline. The word pain comes from the Latin *poena*, 'punishment', based on the notion that we suffer pain because we deserve it. It is a well-established psychological fact that pain is often self-inflicted as a means of lightening the burdened mind and easing the conscience. Guilt feelings lie behind many illnesses, and patients sometimes welcome pain.

There are also those who feel that existence without pain and suffering is unnatural, and are actually comforted by the periodical onset of pain. Dr Thomas Arnold (d. 1842), headmaster of Rugby, as he lay on his death-bed, racked with the excruciating pain of angina pectoris, thanked God for giving him pain, since he had suffered so little pain in his life. Some, indeed, believe that though men are often drawn to seek pleasure, everyone has a secret preference for what is painful and unpleasant (de Rougemont, 1956, p. 62).

Books

Bakan, David, *Disease, Pain and Sacrifice*, Beacon Press, Chicago, 1968.
Brena, Steven, *Pain and Religion*, C. C. Thomas, Springfield, Illinois, 1972.
Buytendijk, F. J. J., *Pain: Its Modes and Functions*, University of Chicago Press, 1962.
Crue, Benjamin, *Pain and Suffering*, C. C. Thomas, Springfield, Illinois, 1970.
Keele, Kenneth, *Anatomies of Pain*, Oxford University Press, 1957.
Lewis, C. S., *The Problem of Pain*, London, 1940.
Melzack, Ronald, *The Puzzle of Pain*, Penguin Books, Harmondsworth, 1973.
Merskey, H. and Spear, F. G., *Pain: Psychological and Psychiatric Aspects*, London, 1967.
Rougemont, Denis de, *Passion and Society*, rev. edn, Faber & Faber, London, 1956.
Szasz, Thomas, *Pain and Pleasure: a Study of Bodily Feeling*, Basic Books, New York, 1957.

PAIN THERAPY

The infliction of pain in order to cure disease, has had a wide application in the past. It was regarded both as physically therapeutic and mentally cathartic. The methods employed were usually variations of cutting, burning and stinging. Thus scarification, or scarring with red hot irons, or gashing with a knife, was commonly practised in primitive societies with, as a rule, the idea of improving muscular strength and virility. Vesication or raising blisters by beating with nettles, or other blistering herbs, or using hot metal, was a standard remedy for lumbago, neuralgia, rheumatism and sciatica.

In cauterization (Gk. *kautĕr*, a hot iron) burning metal was held to the flesh to sear boils and tumours. Sometimes the head was shaved and the hot iron applied direct to the scalp to cure epilepsy*. Hippocrates (d. 359 BC) said: 'What cannot be cured by medicines may be cured by the knife. What the knife cannot cure may be cured by cautery. What cannot be cured by cautery is incurable.' Till the beginning of the last century it was accepted medical practice to apply hot instruments to a wound or incision in order to seal the ends of open blood vessels.

According to the Roman physician Celsus (fl. AD 50), four symptoms accompanied inflammation, namely: calor (heat), rubor (redness), tumor (swelling) and dolor (pain). To this Galen (d. AD 201) added the dictum: 'No wound can heal unless an evil-smelling laudable pus appears.' These axioms gave rise to a spate of often barbarous remedies in which the four symptoms of Celsus, and the 'laudable pus' of Galen, were induced artificially in order to effect a cure, and to create, as it were, a focus from which the bad 'humours' could be discharged.

In setonation (Lat. *saeta*, a bristle) a thin string made of several strands of twisted horsehair, silk or linen, was passed through a fold of skin by means of a large needle and left there for several months until it festered. It could, for example, be threaded through the calf for a wounded knee, or through the neck for eye trouble. Setoning went out of fashion about a hundred years ago.

Another standard method was to relieve the symptoms in one part of the body by producing a counterirritation in another part, usually at a site on the opposite half of the body. Thus, in order to heal a tumour on the right shoulder, the flesh of the left shoulder or arm was cut and irritants applied, or an artificial ulcer (fontanelle) induced there, in order to divert the body's preoccupation with the original tumour.

Flagellation, self-inflicted or administered by others, with nettles, twigs, whips or chains, was among the therapeutic ordeals of many communities especially in the Middle Ages. It was sometimes carried to extreme lengths and involved protracted pain, deep laceration, and even mutilation of the body. This was referred to as basanotherapy (Gk. *basanos*, 'torture') and was common among many monastic sects. It is a remarkable fact that many ascetics who inflict the most terrible tortures on themselves seldom suffer from commonplace ailments, do not succumb to any prevailing epidemics, survive as if by a miracle from the sores and infections that beset them, and live to a ripe old age.

Students of pain therapy have observed that external pressures strengthen resistance to pain, and access to relief resources accelerates susceptibility to pain. We break down quicker when we get aid or when aid is known to be available. Under the most terrible of all régimes, the German concentration camps, suicide and attempted suicide were rare; symptoms of phobia in phobia-afflicted patients either completely vanished, or improved to such an extent that patients could work. In spite of injury, starvation and exhaustion, and extremities of suffering in circumstances that would have killed them in the normal course, thousands of men, women and children survived. Almost immediately after liberation, the symptoms of illness and pain that had been suppressed for years, recurred with remarkable rapidity.

Pain therapy in various forms has been practised for centuries in asylums* for the insane, usually in the form of shock therapy. This involves subjecting the patient to conditions that cause a sudden and extreme physical and nervous crisis. It could be that shock stimulates the pituitary and adrenal glands, and liberates histamines and other neurohormones, and thus in an indirect way does have some therapeutic value.

Among the more recent forms of shock therapy is insulin coma therapy (ICT), or insulin shock therapy, for the cure of schizophrenia*, introduced in 1933 by the Viennese physician Manfred Sakel (d. 1957). Here the patient is first given large doses of insulin to reduce the amount of sugar in the blood and produce hypoglycaemia (low blood sugar). This results in mental confusion and excitement, following which the patient jerks and twitches for an hour or so, before passing into an insulin coma. Then sugar is administered and he wakes up feeling better. This method is now largely discredited.

There are several other forms of shock treatment known as convulsant (or convulsive) therapy, based on the old idea of the intrinsic antagonism between epilepsy and schizophrenia; to treat schizophrenia, it was thought desirable to induce epilepsy artificially. In 1935 Ladislos Jos Meduna (d. 1964) of Budapest induced convulsions by intravenous injections of a camphor derivative, cardiazol (known as metrazol in the USA), a crude and frightening treatment which produces a horrifying fit, after which the patient becomes normal for a time.

In 1938 Ugo Cerletti (d. 1963) of Milan replaced cardiazol after he developed electroconvulsant therapy (ECT), also called electric shock (electroshock) treatment (EST). It is said that Cerletti got the idea when he noticed, during a visit to one of the abattoirs in Rome, that in those pigs that did not immediately die of electrocution, there were marked changes in behaviour. ECT is commonly employed in cases of severe mental depression*, and acute schizophrenic catatonia. The patient is laid on a couch and given anaesthetics and muscle relaxants; electrodes (metal plates) are placed on his temples, and a powerful current sent through the brain. The ensuing shock sends him into a convulsive fit resembling epilepsy. The muscle relaxants help to reduce the bodily spasms. The beneficial effects of the shock last for some time, but the treatment often results in loss of memory which may continue for several weeks.

Critics of the 'shock mills' feel that the long-term effects of altering the chemical and electrical balance of the brain could lead to irreversible brain and personality damage to the patient.

Books

Kalinowsky, L. and Hippius, H., *Pharmacological Convulsive and Other Somatic Treatments in Psychiatry*, Grune & Stratton, New York, 1969.

Merskey, H. and Spear, F. G., *Pain: Psychological and Psychiatric Aspects*, London, 1967.

Zilboorg, G. and Henry, G. W., *A History of Medical Psychology*, Allen & Unwin, London, 1941.

PARAESTHESIA

A generic term applied to all derangements of sense perception, where sensations are misinterpreted, misplaced, or abnormally felt or not felt at all. It includes: hyperaesthesia, a heightening of the sensory faculties; anaesthesia, or insensitivity to pain; synaesthesia, the mixing up or transposition of the senses; allaesthesia, the experience of sensation at a point other than the point of stimulation; polyaesthesia, or the multiplication of the senses, where a stimulus applied to one part of the body is felt in other parts as well; allocheiria, the experience of a sensation in a part of the body symmetrically opposite to the point of stimulation, as when a pinch on the right hand is felt on the left; pseudaesthesia or false feeling, arising without any stimulation whatsoever, such as the pain felt in an amputated limb. A few of these abnormalities are further considered below.

Hyperaesthesia is the condition of abnormal sensitivity often due to an unusually low threshold of sensation, resulting in an extraordinary extension of the physical senses. It usually refers to the hyperacuity of one or more of the bodily senses.

In tactile hyperaesthesia a person can read a page of print (not raised letters or braille) by merely touching the lines with his fingers. In olfactory hyperacuity he can smell a glove and then, animal-like, 'smell out' its owner in a roomful of people. In auditory hyperacuity a person in one room can hear something whispered in another room.

By visual hyperacuity the Australian Aborigine tracker will follow trail marks quite imperceptible to ordinary eyes. Visual acuity also enables a person to read print in the dark. Some people have the condition called nyctalopia, 'day blindness', and can see clearly in the dark and less clearly in the day. The French philosopher Henri Bergson (d. 1941), in the course of an experiment with a man reputed to have telepathic powers, found that while he was reading a book, the man was reading the reflection in the cornea of Bergson's eyes.

Sexologists speak of sexual hyperaesthesia, referring to an abnormal or insatiable sexual desire.

Psychics also speak of the paroptic sense (Gk. *para*, 'beyond'; *optikos*, 'sight'), the paranormal faculty of seeing without the use of the physical sight, in which the vision of the etheric or astral double presumably comes into operation.

Anaesthesia is partial or total insensibility to bodily feeling. When produced by anaesthetics, it plays a major role in surgery, dentistry and childbirth. The discovery of modern anaesthetics, the most important single advance in the history of surgery, is little more than a century old. The earlier methods of inducing insensibility included: giving the patient a few sharp taps on the head with a leather-covered mallet until he became unconscious, the process being repeated if he showed signs of coming round; dosing the patient with opium, hashish or wine; placing a 'soporific sponge', a sponge dipped in a mixture of soporific herbs, firmly over the patient's nose; freezing the area to be operated upon with ice or snow; applying pressure to the carotid artery, used by Ambroise Paré (d. 1590), not always with success; 'mesmerizing' the patient, used by the followers of Franz Mesmer (d. 1815), with even less success.

The conditions under which patients were operated on in earlier days are almost beyond belief. They were tied with ropes or held down by strong assistants. Amputations were performed while the patient was conscious. Many died during or immediately after the operations from the rough handling, pain, loss of blood, weakness, shock or heart failure, and of those who survived many more died of infection. Among the primary requirements of a surgeon were 'a cast-iron stomach and nerves of steel', mainly to withstand the screams of the victim.

To a limited extent anaesthesia can also be achieved by training, or occur spontaneously. Thus, the fire-walkers of Fiji and other places seem to be immune for short periods to the heat of a blazing fire-pit. The Isawa dervishes of north Africa hold red-hot pieces of iron in the hands, place live coals on their tongue, and tear thorny cacti with the teeth, all with complete immunity. In the past the bokte wizards of Tartary and the Pawnee medicine-men of Nebraska would inflict the most ghastly wounds on themselves which would heal within a few minutes.

In 1660 during an epidemic of 'possession' at the Ursuline convent of Auxonne, the nuns felt no pain when long needles were thrust under their finger-nails. The Convulsionaries of Paris (*c.* 1730) and the Fareinists of Lyons (*c.* 1775) allowed themselves to be beaten with iron rods and pierced with iron spikes without feeling pain or suffering injury. These astonishing phenomena were witnessed and authenticated by sceptical, even hostile, witnesses, among them the philosopher David Hume.

In the same way modern Egyptian fakirs have allowed themselves to be skewered and gashed with knives until the blood flowed freely, and have then stopped the flow at will. European wonder-workers have thrust their hands into an open hearth long enough to toast a slice of bread, without harm, and have allowed themselves to be used as human pincushions, with stilettos thrust into their bodies.

One contemporary writer describes how in a kind of trance-like state he found himself impervious to injury or pain, and in the presence of a dozen witnesses was able to extinguish glowing cigarette tips (temperature 1,380°F) by grinding them out against the sensitive areas of his body, including the cheeks and eyelids. There were no blisters and no after-effects (Pearce, 1973, p. 4).

All these facts, as well as the almost miraculous elimination of pain achieved by acupuncture*, and during so-called 'psychic surgery'*, have caused a revision of our concepts of pain* and anaesthesia.

Synaesthesia, a wrongly localized sensation, is commonly spoken of as the transposition of the senses. Here the functions of the separate senses seem to fuse, get blurred and mixed up, so that the stimulus appropriate to one sense organ is received by another, or a stimulus provoked at one point is sensed at a different point.

Thus, in colour hearing, colours will produce sound impressions, and music may be seen visually as well as heard. Sight is especially subject to synaesthesia.

Reading with the finger-tips is a rare but now well-established phenomenon. Researchers believe that the skin does have a 'sight potential', and where this is well developed we have the faculty of eyeless sight, or skinsight. In 1963 a team of Russian scientists at the Soviet Institute of Biophysics in Moscow investigated the skinsight of a 22-year-old housewife from the Urals, Rosa Kuleshova, who 'saw' with her fingers. She could also read, though less accurately, with her toes and tongue. These experiments were very thoroughly carried out, with maximum precautions, to exclude any possibility of telepathy, unconscious prompting and risk of fraud.

Experts suggest that the phenomena may be due to certain microscopic nerve endings, primitive ocelli, photosensitive cells, scattered all over the skin surface, of which one set, the eye-spots, evolved through the ages into the more complex mechanism of the eye. Other areas of the skin still retain vestiges of this endowment and for some reason become activated in cases of hysteria* or other nervous conditions. In some cases of synaesthesia, sight seems to be centred in the epigastrium, and if a person is blindfolded he can 'see' objects presented to the pit of his stomach.

Numerous theories have been put forward to explain paraesthesia. Thus, it is said that organic disease, nervous disorders, spinal injury, damage to the sensory nerves and damage or pressure on certain nerve centres can result in sensory confusion leading to paraesthetic experience. Surgical manipulation of the nerves can also bring about synaesthesia. Thus, if a nerve fibre from the tongue is connected to a nerve fibre leading from the ear to the brain, vinegar can be experienced as a loud explosion.

PATIENT

Again, there is an affliction of the nervous system that can account for some forms of anaesthesia. In this rare disease, known as syringomyelia, the patient retains his sense of touch but is immune to heat, cold or pain, and is therefore in constant danger of harming himself without being aware of it.

Some drugs like the hallucinogens, also some intoxicants and anaesthetics, cause anomalous reactions in the sense organs. Various other factors such as shock, hysteria*, epilepsy*, 'possession'*, hypnotic suggestion, torture, stress*, injury, migraine*, trance or other xenophrenic* states, might precipitate a paraesthetic experience. The faculty may be developed through practice and occult training. Occultists believe that some cases of paraesthesia may occur as a result of partial discoincidence in the plexal areas between the physical body and its etheric double.

Books

Cannon, Alexander, *The Power Within*, Rider, London, 1950.
Farigoule, L., *Eyeless Sight: a Study of Extra-Retinal Vision and the Paroptic Sense*, London, 1924.
MacQuitty, Betty, *The Battle for Oblivion: The Discovery of Anaesthesia*, Harrap, London, 1969.
Ostrander, S. and Schroeder, L., *PSI: Psychic Discoveries Behind the Iron Curtain*, Sphere Books, London, 1970.
Pearce, Joseph, *The Crack in the Cosmic Egg*, Lyrebird Press, London, 1973.
Rawcliffe, D. H., *Illusions and Delusions of the Supernatural and Occult*, Dover, New York, 1959.
Sudre, René, *Treatise on Parapsychology*, Allen & Unwin, London, 1960.
Weil, Andrew, *The Natural Mind*, Jonathan Cape, London, 1973.
Williams, Guy, *The Age of Agony*, Constable, London, 1975.

PATIENT

Under the Hippocratic oath the physician's chief concern is for the welfare of his patients. The doctor swears: 'I will keep them from harm . . . my visit to them shall be for the benefit of the sick.' A sympathetic understanding of the patient's predicament is basic to the medical code in all parts of the civilized world. 'May I never see in the patient anything but a fellow creature in pain', said Maimonides (d. 1204), Jewish physician and philosopher.

Sickness is viewed as an affliction and the patient as the victim of biological circumstances who cannot be held accountable for becoming ill. He is excused from his normal social role, and allowed to retreat from his responsibilities and from the daily struggle. He belongs to a special category, and is in a position of special relationship with his doctor, to whom he entrusts his health and physical welfare. He is an individual, sick and in pain, who comes in good faith to his doctor hoping to be cured.

It has been pointed out that socialized medicine has somewhat altered the status of the patient. Men become demoralized by easy access to welfare concern for every trivial ailment, and doctors react by becoming insensitive to their complaints. Many patients visit their doctors to replenish their stock of sleeping pills or tranquillizers, or to obtain the necessary certificate to enable them to take a break from their work without loss of face or income. This tends to foster not only dependence, but malingering. Furthermore, medical assistance is prodigally misspent by disbursing it free to everyone, and so squandering it on the affluent.

It has been found that a form of Parkinson's law has suddenly come into operation in this area, too. The more doctors you have, the more patients mysteriously appear who need their services. The more hospitals you have, the more people seem to get sick to fill them. Some hospitals maintain waiting-lists on principle, using them as a means of rationing resources. It is a mistake to believe that the nation's health improves as the national health bill rises.

On the other side, in the overall sphere of sociopsychosis*, the patient might be said to symbolize a widening range of dichotomies of the us-and-them type in the social and political scene, since most people in our society today are under surveillance of some kind, whether for scientific, social or political reasons. There is a lay world and the orthodox world; the world of the bureaucrat and that of his victim; of the expert and the ignoramus; of the doctor and the patient.

The patient has become a set of mechanical parts, and medical progress seems to be gauged by the endless subdivision of the parts into smaller units, each nut-and-bolt specialist concerned only with his little area, more and more out of touch with the individual who is his patient. It has been said that the patient does not know what he has, but he does know how he feels; the doctor knows what the patient has, but does not know how he feels. Few doctors today bother, or have the time, to understand their patients as persons who need both technical assistance and pastoral care.

Quite often the patient is not a subject to be cured, but a depersonalized object in a research project. He has been converted from a man into a thing, from a human being into a case, from an individual into a number. Healing is a matter of continuous assault on the patient in the name of treatment, but often for purposes of research. He becomes a victim of molecular biology*, artificial generation*, transplantation and other ventures in experimental medicine.

Dr C. A. H. Watts relates how as a medical student he was asked by a very eminent surgeon to name the most important person in the operating theatre. He mentioned the surgeon, then the theatre sister, and finally the anaesthetist, but each time was told that he was wrong. The fact that the patient was the most important person in the theatre had never crossed his mind.

Those who have made a study of the doctor—patient relationship have reason to believe that nowadays the view that stresses the importance of the patient as a person, is fast becoming old-fashioned. The patient is merely an incident in the medical process. He is a counter in an elaborate scheme, and his individual care is not the primary objective of medical concern. In bulk he receives technological treatment, and becomes part of a medical statistic. Except in the case of a bungling surgeon or grossly careless nursing, the patient will pull through, and if he does not the process continues. The doctor can still say, without any humorous or snide overtones: 'The patient died, but the treatment was a success.'

PHYSIOTHERAPY

Books

Balint, Michael, *The Doctor, His Patient, and the Illness*, 2nd edn, Pitmans, London, 1968.
Cartwright, Ann, *Patients and Their Doctors*, Routledge & Kegan Paul, London, 1967.
Entralgo, P. L., *Doctor and Patient*, World University Library, London, 1969.
Fox, René, *Experiment Perilous: Physicians and Patients Facing the Unknown*, Free Press, Chicago, 1959.
Greenblatt, M. *et al.*, *The Patient and the Mental Hospital*, Free Press, Chicago, 1957.
Hodson, Mark, *Doctors and Patients*, Hodder & Stoughton, London, 1967.
Platt, Lord, *Doctor and Patient*, Nuffield Trust, London, 1963.
Ramsay, P., *The Patient as Person*, Yale University Press, 1970.
Regan, L. J., *Doctor and Patient and the Law*, 3rd edn, Mosby, London, 1956.
Robinson, David, *The Process of Becoming Ill*, Routledge & Kegan Paul, London, 1971.
Steinzor, B., *The Healing Partnership: the Patient as Colleague in Psychotherapy*, Harper & Row, New York, 1967.
Watts, C. A. H., *Depression: the Blue Plague*, Priory Press, London, 1973.

PHYSIOTHERAPY

Physiotherapy treats bodily ailments by manipulation and adjustment of the physical structure. In its earliest form, as exercise and massage, it remains an essential routine in the training of athletes and others who are in good health and wish to remain strong and fit. A variant, called kinesiotherapy*, concentrates largely on posture and movement. In its more unorthodox form physiotherapy is known as osteopractic*, which is concerned with the skeletal structure and the adjustment of nerves, muscles and bones, that have been displaced.

Physiotherapy proper concerns itself principally with the revival of function in bones, joints, tendons and ligaments, with muscle strength and nerve activity, as well as general patterns of movement, breathing, speech, and so on. It applies external aids like heat, sunlight, hot springs, and also various kinds of electrotherapy*, like diathermy, which heals by creating warmth in the deeper layers of the body tissues. Physiotherapy is closely connected with occupational therapy*, which takes up where physiotherapy leaves off, and goes on to rather more purposeful and generalized activity.

Physiotherapy also covers orthopaedics, or orthopaedic surgery, which deals primarily with troubles resulting from fractures, burns, muscle strain, stroke and nerve injury. Great strides have been made in correcting bone deformities arising from disease or injury, especially in childhood.

An important branch of physiotherapy is prosthetics, the replacement or supplementation of broken or damaged parts of the body by artificial ones, including functional training and rehabilitation. It is to be distinguished from transplantation, which replaces internal organs, usually by natural organs. The prosthesis or artificial organ is commonly an arm or leg, but may include such things as false teeth and glass eyes.

Generally the replacement of damaged or missing soft tissues like the nose and eyes, as well as skin grafting, is the province of plastic surgery, which, though done for cosmetic purposes, has great psychological value, removing feelings of deficiency and deformity. Today plastic surgery is performed for face lifts, thigh lifts, arm lifts, abdominal lifts, hair transplants, removal of wrinkles, frown lines, baggy eyelids, reduction of oversized breasts, enlargement of small ones, reconstruction of nose, ears and chin. Operations on the sexual organs have been successful on women only; for while the opening of the vagina can be narrowed, it is not possible to replace a damaged penis by a substitute that works.

The art of making and fitting replacement parts was known to many ancient peoples. In Europe it was first developed by Ambroise Paré (d. 1590), but the most celebrated exponent before the present century was the Italian surgeon Gaspare Tagliacozza (d. 1599) about whom many extravagant tales were told. He specialized in noses, and took the spare parts from slaves, but the part survived, it was said, only so long as the slave was alive, and then dropped off.

Books

Cash, J. E., *Textbook of Medical Conditions for Physiotherapy*, Faber & Faber, London, 1971.

Gardiner, G. M. D., *Physiotherapy*, Hale, London, 1964.

Grant, W. R., *Principles of Rehabilitation*, Livingstone, Edinburgh, 1963.

Hirschberg, G. G. *et al.*, *Rehabilitation: a Manual for the Care of the Disabled and Elderly*, Lippincott, Philadelphia, 1964.

Krusen, F. H., *Concepts in Rehabilitation of the Handicapped*, Saunders, Philadelphia, 1964.

PHYTOTHERAPY

Phytotherapy (Gk. *phyton*, 'plant'), also called botanotherapy or vegetotherapy, makes use of plants and trees for therapeutic purposes. Exponents maintain that plants provide all the food required by man for his health and wellbeing, as well as all the ingredients necessary for the prevention and cure of every ailment. Plants respond to love and care, and convey their vitality through fruit, flowers and scents.

Phytotherapy includes herbalism*, which makes use of the roots, leaves, seeds and stems of plants and herbs in various ways. It also includes floritherapy*, or healing with flowers; and aromatherapy*, which employs scents, aromatic herbs and spices. Because plants transmute the elements in the soil that we ourselves are unable to use, they provide us with important minerals and metals that make for health and vitality. Plants and plant products are the source of almost every important drug used in ancient and modern medicine. They are sedative, hallucinogenic, excitant, purgative, narcotic, aphrodisiac. Even those that are poisonous have their uses when taken in the correct dosage.

Fruits, with their smell, flavour, colour, taste, pulp, combine to form a health meal that is unequalled by any cooked food. Nuts form a natural capsule providing a source of energy better than any tonic. Plant essences and perfumes provide an important ingredient in all incenses, which directly affect the psyche, and thus the body.

PLACEBO

Trees spread their branching antennae heavenwards, and draw down beneficent electrical influences. They send their roots downwards, imbibing
magnetic energy from the vital tissues of Mother Earth. They radiate strength,
and pleasant psychic vibrations; their presence is healing and invigorating. The
Iron Chancellor, Otto von Bismarck (d. 1898), when fatigued from the stress
of his responsibilities of state, took the advice of his personal physicians, and
used to sit against a tree, or put his arms around it for ten or fifteen minutes
at a time to restore his energies.

According to plant lore, close association with trees can change mood and
even character. For example, the poplar breeds contemplation; the beech
gives assurance; the chestnut, restraint; the elm, understanding; the willow,
patience; the ash, piety; the elder, temperance; the birch, chastity; the oak, a
man's tree, gives courage, resolution and endurance.

Books

Brown, Beth, *ESP with Plants and Animals*, Essandess, New York, 1972.
Dodge, Bertha, *Plants that Changed the World*, Dent, London, 1963.
Palaiseul, Jean, *Grandmother's Secrets: Her Green Guide to Health from Plants*, Barrie
& Jenkins, London, 1973.
Quinn, V., *Roots: their Place in Life and Legend*, Philadelphia, 1938.
Tompkins, P. and Bird, C., *The Secret Life of Plants*, Allen Lane, London, 1974.

PLACEBO

Placebo (Lat. 'I shall please') originally referred to a 'medicine' with hardly
any curative value, given to a patient to keep him contented. It has been
known for ages that a large proportion of patients react favourably to any
medication prescribed for them, even if what is prescribed has no curative
value at all. Thus, a peasant whose temperature was being taken and believing that it was part of the cure, said he was feeling better as soon as the
thermometer was removed from his mouth. The success of the quack can to a
great extent be accounted for in terms of the suggestion implanted by him
in the mind of the patient for his sugar pills and make-believe remedies.

Most patients want something in addition to the bedside manner and
general advice. They insist on visible and tangible treatment. They like to go
through the ritual procedures of taking a drug, or to have some form of
treatment administered to them. Doctors too feel they are doing something
beneficial and positive in this way, and so resort to prescribing a placebo, a
harmless and chemically inert medication.

In 1933 two London cardiologists, William Evans and C. Hoyle, treating
a group of patients suffering from angina, gave them pills made from bicar-
bonate of soda. The patients assumed that the pills would ease their condition, and over a third reported that the pain had been satisfactorily eased.
Later experiments conducted on a wider scientific basis confirmed that the
healing power of faith and confident expectation was of the greatest importance in the cure of disease, and that the chemical composition of a drug was
not the only determining factor in a patient's reaction to it.

216

Subsequent experiments went even further. A woman suffering from recurrent attacks of nausea and sickness was given an emetic (that would induce nausea and so aggravate the condition), but was told that it would stop her from feeling sick. Her body reacted accordingly. In spite of the presence of the emetic in her system, her mind responded to the suggestion and her nausea abated.

Such research is essential in order to determine the efficacy and side-effects of new drugs, and experiments on placebo medication are often carried out without either the doctor or the patient knowing what the medicine contains, and whether it is a potent drug or a simple placebo. These 'double blind' studies as they are called, enable useful information to be obtained regarding the value of a drug.

Subjects who react to a placebo as to a chemically active drug, are called placebo-reactors, and such people are sometimes regarded as suggestible, gullible, passive and neurotic. But this correlation is denied by other observers, who say that placebo reaction depends not on the individual, but on circumstances, such as: the nature of the illness, the place where medication is being carried out (hospital or home), the sophistication of equipment, the treatment by nurses, the personality of the doctor. Placebo experiments have shown that there are many complex reactions between the patient and the doctor which play an important part in the patient's improvement.

Books

Beecher, H. K., 'Surgery as Placebo: A Quantitative Study of Bias', *Journal of the American Medical Association*, 176, 1961, 1102-7.
Claridge, Gordon, *Drugs and Human Behaviour*, London, 1970.
Frank, J. D., *Persuasion and Healing*, London, 1961.
Kissel, P. and Barrucand, D., *Placebos et effet placebo en médecine*, Paris, 1964.
Tuckey, C. L., *Treatment by Hypnotism and Suggestion*, London, 1913.

PNEUMOPATHY

Pneumopathy (Gk. *pneuma*, 'breath'), or breath therapy, is also known as *aerotherapy* (Gk. *aēr*, 'air'), though the latter is more strictly limited to breathing exercises in the fresh air. Pneumopathy entails a knowledge of the breathing processes, including inhalation, retention, exhalation, retention; control of the breathing rate; the depth of breathing. It is well established in physiology that all these elements of the respiratory process have a profound effect on mind and body.

Above all, pneumopathy is based on the old hermetic belief that there are various life-giving currents and noxious toxins in the 'pneumosphere', and the skill of the physician lies in prescribing the most suitable kind of air required for a particular ailment, and in advising the avoidance of certain kinds of smells for the prevention of disease.

Indeed, scents and odours affect all living things in strange ways that cannot be scientifically explained. They can exalt the consciousness, or stir the unconscious into activity. Long-forgotten incidents and events of one's childhood or youth can be instantly recalled by a smell. Every smell has a special potency and a particular effect. What is called 'olfactory intoxication' touches the mental, psychic and spiritual centres in man.

Every odour, agreeable or otherwise, has its own properties, which when inhaled into the lungs can cause both physiological and psychological changes, affecting the blood circulation, the heart rate and the higher brain centres, stimulating the glands and thus setting up strong emotional responses that heal or hurt. Pneumopathy endeavours to select the right smell for the right malady, and relieve it by inducing the right mood. Flowers and fruit, perfumes and incense, which are the province of floritherapy* and aromatherapy*, form part of the pneumopathic repertory.

Artificially blended perfumes, even from natural substances, have to be prescribed with care, for they can be overpowering. Most of them are too strong for children, for the aged, for the sick. Some can create sickness. Exotic perfumes with strong animal ingredients work direct on the etheric body and arouse the lower instincts. Thus, women who try to attract men by means of strong perfumes often find that the passions they arouse have been ephemeral.

The smell of earth, a powerful rejuvenant, was recommended for numerous ills. Francis Bacon (d. 1626) held that the smell of earth, newly turned up with a spade, was a great tonic, and that women would do themselves much good by weeding, especially in spring when the land exhaled its most vitalizing breath. The pure air in the vicinity of mountains and seas, now known to contain a high degree of health-giving ozone, is still supposed to be very beneficial for body and mind.

In the same way certain seasons bring their own 'airs' with them, sometimes invigorating, sometimes laden with noxious vapours. In the Middle Ages it was thought that virulent epidemics like the Black Death were the result of pestilential winds borne across the land, which contaminated all the countries over which they passed. Many curious methods were devised to filter this air and make it fit to breathe. Some people wore a prophylactic mask with a parrot-like beak stuffed with medicinal spices. Some wore perfumed objects around their necks or held them to their nostrils. Animals were brought into the house to absorb the ill winds. Often a herd of bulls, cows, sheep or goats would be driven through the town to inhale the noxious air and breathe out the purifying vapours from their own lungs.

This latter deep-rooted belief in the therapeutic value of cattle exhalations was widespread in many parts of the globe. In Eastern countries and even in Europe it was long held that the breath of cattle and the warm vapours exuding from their bodies had a curative effect on chest complaints. The breath of cows particularly, was a specific for consumption, and it was good to sleep over a shed where the animals were kept. The Russian mystic George Ivanovich Gurdjieff (d. 1949) enthusiastically advocated this. One of his disciples, the talented writer Katherine Mansfield, ill with tuberculosis, was persuaded to sleep in a cowshed, and it was in the cowshed that she died in 1923, without being cured.

Bodily and organic smells were also considered to be curative. The hermetic philosopher and alchemist known as Artephius (d. 1150) attributed his phenomenal longevity to the fact that he would distil a spirit from the blood of young men and inhale it. In Iraq they said that a child suffering from the ill-effects of *rīha*, or mal-odour, could be cured if held over a pit into which the blood of a slaughtered beast was drained off; the worse the smell, the better for the child. In many parts of Europe there was a notion that a girl suffering from anaemia and listlessness could be restored to health and made beautiful if she inhaled the smell of a handkerchief into which a healthy man had ejaculated his semen.

Altogether, the inhalation of unpleasant smells was thought to have excellent tonic properties, and belief in the beneficial odours of lavatories, tanneries, cesspools and decaying animal and vegetable matter, including scatological substances, was widely current all over the world. Pestilential fumes could be counteracted by inhaling even more nauseous smells, so that the most disgusting things were smelled, or else were burned and the fumes inhaled. Some recommended standing over a latrine and breathing in the stench arising from human excreta, based on the alleged statement by Paracelsus (d. 1541) that in times of plague all excrement, especially human, was healthy. Some used to break wind into a bottle, and this 'bottled air', or 'fart bottle', was unstoppered and sniffed as required. Bad breath from the mouth or stomach could be cured by standing over a privy with the mouth open and taking in deep breaths, 'the greater stink of the privy drawing unto it, and carrying away the less', said Sir Kenelm Digby (d. 1665). Until the 1930s there was a superstition in Norfolk that whooping cough could be cured by holding the child head downwards in the privy.

Early pneumopathic concepts led to modern developments in inhalation therapy and anaesthesia. Gases like nitrous oxide; chloroform and ether are used in surgery, and some of them can produce xenophrenic* states and bring on ecstatic experiences, and thus occasionally lead to addiction. When Joseph Priestley (d. 1804) first discovered oxygen, he wrote about it as follows: 'This pure air may become a fashionable article of luxury, though hitherto only two mice and myself have had the privilege of breathing it.' Priestley also discovered nitrous oxide.

Doctors soon became interested, and 'pneumatic medicine' became very popular in the treatment of respiratory diseases and even scurvy and cancer. Thomas Beddoes (d. 1808) opened a Pneumatic Institute at Clifton, which offered cures by inhalation of various gases. His assistant Humphry Davy (d. 1829), while experimenting with nitrous oxide, happened to inhale some himself, and noted the lightness and relaxation he experienced. It was so agreeable that he broke out laughing, and this happy quality gave it the name of laughing gas. Davy made silk bags to hold the gas and tried it out on friends. The poet Samuel Taylor Coleridge (d. 1834) volunteered, and wrote, 'I experienced the most voluptuous sensations and had the most entrancing visions.' Some young ladies who tried it declared, 'Mr Davy's silk bags hold the key to paradise.' But doctors were quick to realize the dangers of administering nitrous oxide; its indiscriminate use was made illegal in England, and Dr Beddoes had to convert his institute into a hospital.

Chemical gases form an important branch of pneumopathic research.

Poison gas and nerve gas have been used in recent warfare with terrifying results, and it is well known that industrial gases cause great harm to factory workers. Petroleum vapours are known to produce sensations not unlike those produced by drugs, including palpitation, dizziness and hallucinations. Juveniles sometimes take to inhaling petrol fumes for 'kicks'. In 1968 it was reported that certain north Australian tribes were damaging drums of high octane fuel in remote airfields to inhale the fumes, and this became quite a problem with the authorities.

Those who constantly handle gases in hospitals can also become addicted. Nurses and anaesthetists take to sniffing ether bottles or opening cylinders of nitrous oxide to satisfy their craving. Similarly workers who deal with dry-cleaning fluids, paint-thinners, liquid shoe-polish, cellulose paints, glue and other such commercial and domestic solvents, also run the danger of addiction. The addictive inhalation of glue, known as 'glue-sniffing', is not uncommon. Still another discovery is that a kind of euphoria can be achieved by inhaling certain aerosol sprays, deodorants and propellants, but these can have a fatal outcome.

The pressure under which gases are inhaled assumes great significance in certain professions. Deep-sea divers run the risk of nitrogen narcosis from breathing air under pressure. The degree of tolerance to hyperbaric nitrogen (nitrogen under pressure) varies with individual divers. Popularly known as 'the narks', its symptoms include light-headedness, garrulity, rashness, euphoria, intoxication and often a feeling of beatitude. In the same way oxygen under pressure (hyperbaric oxygen) is used in treating many critical conditions, such as carbon-monoxide poisoning, coal-gas poisoning and brain damage. There is, however, a risk of blindness when used on babies. In carbon-dioxide therapy, which is used to produce emotional abreactions and alleviate anxiety, carbon-dioxide gas is administered till the patient is unconscious.

Books

Bedichek, Roy, *The Sense of Smell*, Michael Joseph, London, 1960.
Bloch, Iwan, *Odoratus Sexualis,* Panurge Press, New York, 1934.
Cousteau, J. Y., *The Silent World*, Hamish Hamilton, London, 1953.
Duncum, B. M., *The Development of Inhalation Anaesthesia*, London, 1947.
Miller, Albert H., *Thomas Beddoes, Pioneer in Inhalation Therapy*, New York, 1932.
Nohl, Johannes, *The Black Death*, Ballantine, New York, 1960.
Pauwels, Louis, *Gurdjieff*, Douglas, Isle of Man, 1964.
Ramsay, Sir W., *The Gases of the Atmosphere*, London, 1896.
Wellman, M., *Die pneumatische Schule bis auf Archigenes*, Berlin, 1895.

POSSESSION

The apparent invasion and taking over of an individual's mind and body by a non-human or demonic entity, causing raving and convulsions. It is to be distinguished from mediumistic trance, when the spirit of a dead person makes temporary use of the medium's physical apparatus in order to communicate with the living. Some authorities even distinguish between demon possession and the possession of shaman priests by ancestral spirits, or of voodoo practitioners by the *loa* or cult deity, since such possession, like mediumship, is voluntary, does not interfere with normal life or lead to disintegration of the personality. Possession is further to be distinguished from obsession*, in which the victim's mind remains his own. Obsession is a psychological concept, possession a demonological one. In true possession, the victim's mind is displaced altogether; the occupying spirit is evil or earth-bound; it could be that of a criminal, suicide, a sorcerer or an actual demonic entity.

Belief in diabolical possession is very old. Egyptian, Greek and Roman literature teems with instances of people being possessed. The Bible records that Saul was 'troubled with an evil spirit', and Talmudic writings confirm that the ancient Jews accepted possession as a fact. The several cases recorded in the New Testament are all cured by Christ commanding the residing demon to depart. Medieval writings are similarly filled with instances of persons being possessed by devils. The victim was referred to as an energumen (Gk. *ergon*, 'work'), because the devil was thought to work within him.

The nature of the manifestation in any locality is determined by the prevailing customs and traditions, and the religion and beliefs of the place, which accounts for the slight variations in possession cases. But in general, descriptions of the onset, symptoms and aftermath are everywhere the same. Commonly the victim is an adolescent. He is gradually overcome by a feeling of uneasiness and restiveness which he can neither account for nor control. He gets palpitations and has a growing sense of fear. Strange fancies take hold of him which he is unable to shake off. He feels giddy and the ground seems to rock and sway beneath his feet. He has a sensation of constriction in the throat, an oppression in the chest.

After these preliminary skirmishes the actual attack is quite sudden. The victim falls into a fit resembling epilepsy*, and goes through all the phases of convulsions*. He grimaces horribly, sticks out and retracts his tongue rapidly like a snake, grinds his teeth, foams at the mouth, and is gripped with horrible contortions. The plasticity of the body during possession is unbelievable, and the neck, face and limbs are twisted beyond the person's normal capabilities. His eyes roll in all directions, or glare frighteningly at others; often they are unfocused as though he were looking into some other dimension. The mind seems to be seething with dark thoughts.

He raves, snorts, screams hysterically, mouthing obscene, abusive language, or babbling utter gibberish. His laughter is maniacal, his voice quite unrecognizable, deep and gruff. Occasionally beast-like sounds and terrifying groans and roars emanate from his throat. When violent, he has extraordinary strength. A frail, weak boy cannot be held down by three strong men when possessed; he flings them off as though they were infants. He can and frequently does inflict injury on himself without apparently feeling any pain.

He sometimes complains of burning, biting, pinching or other painful sensations in his entrails, head and chest. Often he will tear off his clothes and expose his private parts, masturbate or go through the motions of sexual intercourse. He breaks wind, vomits and defecates without restraint, and what is exuded seems to have a more foetid stench than such products normally have. His breath is stale, acrid and overpowering.

POSSESSION

What was once thought to add strength to the theory that such persons are possessed by a demon, was the fact that in some instances rapping noises are heard, tables, chairs, beds and other items of furniture are moved, and crockery thrown about, as in poltergeist manifestations. Today such phenomena are attributed to bioplasmic activity.

Like other traumatic phenomena, the sight of a possessed person can often lead to a sensitive onlooker becoming 'possessed' and hysterical himself. Cases of mass hysteria* are not uncommon in social and religious history.

On awakening from the attack, the victim continues to be in a dazed condition for some time. There is extreme sensitivity to light, together with a feeling of nausea, drowsiness, dizziness and exhaustion. Seldom is any remembrance brought back of what has taken place. After a pause of a few hours, days or weeks, there may be a recurrence of the attack.

The causes of possession are still not clear. Psychologists regard it as a mental pathology on a par with hysteria*, epilepsy and insanity, and believe that all the manifestations arise from a deeper, unconscious layer of the mind buried in the subego, and perhaps brought to the surface by a physical or mental shock of some kind. Others attribute it to such things as prolonged indulgence in drugs, morbid preoccupation with spiritualism and the occult, the practice of table-tapping or playing with the ouija board.

The traditional methods of driving the demon out have been many and varied. Primitive man was often trepanned to release the demon from his head. In other places the remedies included whipping the unfortunate victim, dowsing him with water, starving him, blowing air up his nostrils, fumigating him, making him smell burnt rags, pulling his hair, administering emetics and enemas. The demon was threatened, entreated, cajoled, abused. Most commonly exorcism* is performed, which is a rite of banishment, with prayers, and invocations of the divine name, accompanied by adjurations to the demon to depart.

Many authorities who have devoted years to the subject still feel that possession is an actual invasion by an alien entity, and that mental patients are often possessed by conscious beings. After thirty years' clinical study, Dr Carl Wickland (c. 1924) of the Psychopathic Institute of Chicago, and member of the American Association for the Advancement of Science, came to the conclusion that many inmates of asylums were not insane, but possessed by spirits who were deluded in some cases by a false belief in reincarnation, which rendered them earth-bound. Shaw Desmond mentions an ex-president of an international congress of alienists who admitted that the specialist in mental illness 'had now seriously to take into account the possibility of possession by spirit entities'. Referring to the massive historical tradition about possession based on concrete evidence, William James (d. 1910), the eminent psychologist, said that the refusal of modern scientific enlightenment to regard possession as a likely hypothesis was a curious example of the power of fashion in scientific matters. He concluded: 'That the demon theory (not necessarily a devil theory) will have its innings again is to my mind absolutely certain.'

Books

Alexander, W. M., *Demonic Possession in the New Testament*, Clark, Edinburgh, 1902.

D'Assier, Adolphe, *Posthumous Humanity*, trans. and annotated by H. S. Olcott, George Redway, London, 1887.

Desmond, Shaw, *Healing, Psychic and Divine*, London, 1956.

Freud, Sigmund, *Collected Papers: a Neurosis of Demoniacal Possession in the 17th century*, Hogarth Press, London, 1924.

Howton, R., *Divine Healing and Demon Possession*, London, 1909.

Lhermitte, J., *Diabolical Possession, True and False*, Burns & Oates, London, 1963.

Nevius, J. L., *Demon Possession and Allied Themes*, 3rd edn, Revell, New York, 1894.

Oesterreich, T. K., *Possession*, Routledge & Kegan Paul, London, 1930.

Peebles, Dr, *Spirit Obsession*, London, 1925.

Prince, Raymond (ed.), *Trance and Possession States*, Bucke Memorial Society, Montreal, 1966.

Raupert, J. Godfrey, *The Dangers of Spiritualism*, London, 1920.

Sargant, William, *The Mind Possessed*, Heinemann, London, 1973.

Sharp, Granville, *The Case of Saul, Showing that his Disorder was real Spiritual Possession*, London, 1807.

Wickland, Carl, *Thirty Years Among the Dead*, Los Angeles, 1924, reprint, Spiritualist Press, London, 1968.

Zilboorg, G. and Henry, G. W., *A History of Medical Psychology*, Allen & Unwin, London, 1941.

PRIMITIVE MEDICINE

Primitive medicine embraces all unorthodox and unscientific procedures of healing, usually with the aid of remedies obtained direct from natural products. It includes: (a) the tribal remedies of simple and undeveloped societies; (b) the ancient medical systems of early developed civilizations, such as Egypt, Mesopotamia and China; (c) the traditional country and folk-medicine practised by rural populations in modern advanced societies.

Most forms of primitive treatment involve the use of plant and animal substances, including herbs, roots, snails, spiders; scatological* substances or the exuviae of men and animals, like faeces, urine, blood, sweat, semen; and borboric* substances like offal, mud, mould. In tribal societies healing methods often call for ritual procedures, like performing some action at a certain time, in a set manner, usually to the accompaniment of incantatory verses of magical import.

A great deal of symbolism is implicit in all primitive medicine. Thus, much emphasis is laid on the relationship between things that are externally alike. In medieval times this was elaborated in the doctrine of signatures, a signature being any distinctive feature or quality that indicates a connection between the remedy and the malady. Herbs, animals and minerals, it was said, 'have marked upon them, as it were in hieroglyphics, the very signature of their virtues'. So, the aspen whose leaves tremble, was good for the palsy; powder made from pulverized red rocks was good for staunching blood; because a lion had a luxurious mane, lion-fat was rubbed into the scalp to prevent baldness.

A natural extension of this principle of inter-relatedness was that of a homoeopathic connection between the cause of a disease and its cure. Variants of this were once commonly accepted in Europe, especially during the sixteenth and seventeenth centuries. It was thought, for example, that there existed an occult rapport between the wound and the weapon that inflicted it. So if a person received an injury in a duel, the wound was washed clean but otherwise left unattended, while a special salve made of many strange ingredients, including bear's fat and moss found growing on a skull, was rubbed on the sword. Francis Bacon (d. 1626) says: 'It is constantly received and avouched (though myself as yet am not fully inclined to believe it) that the anointing of the weapon that maketh the wound will heal the wound itself.' His younger contemporary, Sir Kenelm Digby (d. 1665), brought the salve, or powder of sympathy, as it was then called, to the notice of the recently formed Royal Society of England.

Another curiosity of primitive medical theory is the widespread belief in transferation, 'bearing off', or curing a disease by transferring it to something else. Here, disease is treated like an object which is ceremonially placed upon another person, animal, plant or inanimate thing, and thus transferred to it. Until the seventeenth century in England, a standard household remedy for common ailments, such as a cold or headache, was to place a hair from the head of the sufferer between two pieces of bread, and feed it to a dog while intoning the following verse: 'Good luck hound, may you be sick and I be sound.' Diseases could also be ritually transferred to an egg, onion, potato, block of wood, piece of paper, and the object then burned, buried or sunk in a stream.

Although most orthodox physicians have tended to scorn the methods used by primitive healers as so much superstition, there is today a growing appreciation of the genuine value of some of these methods. Centuries of experience have gone into the evolution of primitive healing, and their cures, both psychological and medicinal, have often been very remarkable.

Throughout the history of medical practice the orthodox forms of healing were confined to the rich. The poor had to depend on the skill of the local 'quack', and were often the better for it. Thomas Sydenham (d. 1689), known as the English Hippocrates, speaking of his own day, said that it would have been better for many wealthy patients if the art of medicine had never been invented, remarking that many poor men owed their lives to their inability to afford conventional treatment. Folk-remedies have had many eminent supporters. Notable was the great John Wesley (d. 1791), whose collection in a book entitled *Primitive Medicine* is still being republished and has found readers all over the world.

Primitive healers applied the earliest psychotherapy*, in the form of suggestion, confession, group therapy*, music therapy*, art therapy* (sand-painting), religious healing and hypnosis*. The kahuna or native hierophants of Polynesia, were famous for their cures through psychological *huna* techniques. The research psychologist Kilton Stewart working among the Senoi tribe of Malaysia and studying the extraordinary use they made of dreams in maintaining the welfare of the community, concluded that the Senoi system of interpersonal relations based on dreams and dream interpretation was 'in the field of psychology perhaps on a level with our attainments in such areas as television and nuclear physics' (Tart, 1969, p. 161).

Surgery of a fairly advanced kind was performed by many ancient peoples. Primitive medicine-men carried out amputations, set broken bones, performed lithotomy (cutting for stone in the bladder), and operated for hernia and varicose veins. Embryotomy in difficult cases of childbirth was performed by skilled women in many tribal communities with little or no risk to the mother. The surgical skill of the Cherokee healer in the treatment of wounds was considerable; so was that of the Fijian. The Indians of Ecuador did Caesarean section, dreaded by Western surgeons until a few decades ago. The Yoruba healer of Nigeria effectively treated cataract by surgical detachment of the lens of the eye.

Trepanning or trepanation was especially widespread. This entails the removal of a piece of the skull by boring or cutting out with a sharp instrument. It is one of the earliest of all surgical operations, and was practised from Scandinavia to North Africa from the time of the polished stone age, with the most primitive tools, and usually for the cure of mental disorders, such as epilepsy*, hysteria* and convulsions*. Such diseases were believed to be due to possession by spirits, so a hole was bored in the skull to provide a door by which the invading spirit might be allowed to escape. The custom survived in remote rural areas till the end of the last century and was quite common. According to Baring-Gould, the native inhabitants of certain parts of the Balkans, 'had recourse to trepanning on the smallest provocation, simply because they had headaches'. Some people were trepanned as many as seven or eight times.

Primitive healers used ingenious anaesthetic methods and were well aware of the value of antiseptics such as hot water, wine-soaked bandages and fumigations. The ancient Egyptian art of bandaging, not only mummies but living patients, has never been equalled. Folk-healers were acquainted with many useful medical aids: massage, bleeding, cauterization, fomentation, poulticing, ligaturing, diet, mud-packs, sweat-baths and heliotherapy.

In time, various bush remedies and old-world folk-remedies were confirmed by modern research. Thus, the 'absurd African superstition' that malaria was caused by the bite of a mosquito was proved right in the early 1900s. Variolation, or inoculation of the skin with the infected discharge from a mild case of smallpox, had been known to the peasants of rural Turkey for centuries. The subsequent experiments of Edward Jenner (d. 1823) were inspired by a local custom among the Gloucestershire dairy maids, who used to immunize themselves by vaccination with cowpox.

The practice of smearing open wounds with mouldy substances, widely followed both among ancient tribal peoples and among the peasantry in Europe, looked like pure superstition until Alexander Fleming (d. 1955) discovered penicillin in one kind of mould. Cowdung, human urine, saliva, cobwebs, have all since been found to possess healing enzymes and other therapeutic properties (*see* borboric therapy).

The value of liver for anaemia was already known to the ancient Chinese. Cod-liver oil is an old Scandinavian folk-remedy for rickets. Sir Thomas Browne (d. 1682), writing about the birds of Norfolk, says: 'Many rooks are killed for their livers in order to cure the rickets.' Today the liver treatment holds good for both anaemia and rickets.

Male fern was an old English rural remedy for tapeworm. In 1763 Edmund Stone wrote a paper based on old wives' remedies on the effectiveness of willow bark in the treatment of ague and malaria. In 1838 salicylic acid was extracted from willow bark, the forerunner of aspirin. The medieval old wives' tales about the virtues of henbane, aconite, hellebore and belladonna, have been proved right. The Birmingham physician William Withering (d. 1799) discovered digitalis after he found women in Shropshire taking a concoction containing foxglove for dropsy.

Hundreds of items from native remedies all over the world have found their way into the modern *materia medica* of Western medicine, as will be evident from the following brief catalogue:

Egypt. The Ebers papyrus (*c.* 1630 BC) describes an eye disease, probably trachoma, which was treated with copper. Trachoma is treated with copper sulphate today. The Egyptians also knew the value of pyrethrum (pellitory or feverfew) for toothache and fever, besides hundreds of other medicinal herbs.

Mesopotamia. The 'juice' of frog was used for eye troubles. It is now confirmed that frog gall has definite value in some eye conditions. The skin of the frog is also known to contain the valuable drug bufagin.

Persia. The ancient Persians were familiar with numerous animal and herbal remedies, many of which were incorporated into the Greek pharmacopoeia. They used camphor for promoting phlegm and sweat, and were the first to employ chenopodium for hookworm, and opium as an anaesthetic.

Greece. The Greeks made an immense contribution to modern medicine. The bulk of their *materia medica* passed to Rome and thence to the rest of Europe. They used hellebore, podophyllum and aloes for constipation*, and squill as a diuretic.

China. A treatise going back 3,000 years mentions chaulmoogra oil, obtained from a Himalayan evergreen, as a remedy for leprosy*. Recently rediscovered, it has been found very effective. The Chinese used ephedrine (*ma-huang*) to relieve fever, cough and lung ailments. They were also aware of the tonic value of rhubarb, and the rejuvenative properties of ginseng. Among the minerals used medicinally were iron, arsenic, mercury and calcium.

India. Rauwolfia, the plant from which the drug reserpine is made today, was an ancient Indian *ayurvedic* remedy for high blood pressure and heart trouble. The Indians also used the berry from which we now obtain the drug picrotoxin, for stimulating respiration.

Arabia. From the Bantus of Africa the Arabs adopted the use of a concoction of *nux vomica* (which contains strychnine) as a tonic, which they introduced into Europe. From Abyssinia they learned the value of caffeine, found in coffee.

West Africa. The drug physostigmine comes from the famous Calabar bean used in Nigeria.

East Africa. The drug strophanthin obtained from an East African plant has a similar action on the heart as digitalis.

West Indies. Guaiacum, also known as *lignum vitae*, 'wood of life', is a native remedy for rheumatism. From here, too, comes castor oil for constipation.

Siberia. Siberian peasants prepared a sedative from the lichen *usnea*, which they steeped in urine. It is now known to be a rich source of barbituric acid, the basic element of the barbiturates.

America. The Iroquois of North America used lobelia to stimulate breathing and ease asthmatic spasms. They also used cascara for constipation. From the Powhatan Indians of Virginia came tobacco. The Aztecs of Mexico used jalap as a purgative. Pregnant Aztec women chewed pieces of wild yam, now known to contain the chemical diosgenin, convertible into the natural female hormone progesterone, which helps to maintain and protect the placenta and embryo during pregnancy. From the Mayas of Central America comes sarsaparilla. From the Incas of Peru we get perubalm, cocaine, cinchona (from which comes quinine). From the Tupi tribe of the Orinoco comes curare juice, extracted from the sacha plant, for the cure of snake-bite. Also ipecacuanha, from which comes emetine; capaiba, a balsam; and tolubalm, for coughs and catarrh.

Books

Baring-Gould, S., *Strange Survivals*, London, 1892.
Black, William George, *Folk Medicine: a Chapter in the History of Culture*, Folk-Lore Society, London, 1883.
Brockbank, William, *Ancient Therapeutic Arts*, Heinemann, London, 1954.
Hoernle, A. F. R., *Studies in the Medicine of Ancient India*, Oxford, 1907.
Hughes, H. B., *Trepanation*, Foundation for Independent Thinking, Amsterdam, 1971.
Jarvis, D. C., *Folk Medicine*, Pan Books, London, 1961.
Jünling, Johannes, *Die Tiere in der deutschen Volksmedizin alter und neuer Zeit*, Berlin, n.d.
Kennell, Frances, *Folk Medicine: Fact and Fiction*, Marshall Cavendish, London, 1976.
Lawrence, R. M., *Primitive Psychotherapy and Quackery*, Constable, London, 1910.
Leslie, C. (ed.), *Asian Medical Systems*, California University Press, 1977.
Maclean, Una, *Magical Medicine*, Allan Lane/The Penguin Press, London, 1971.
Sigerist, Henry E., *A History of Medicine: Primitive and Archaic Medicine*, Oxford University Press, 1967.
Tart, Charles (ed.), *Altered States of Consciousness*, Wiley, New York, 1969.
Wassen, S. H., *Some General Viewpoints in the Study of Native Drugs of the West Indies and South America*, Ethnos, New York, 1964.
Williams, J. J., *Voodoos and Obeahs: Phases of West Indian Witchcraft*, Dial Press, New York, 1932.

PSYCHIATRY

As a form of mental treatment, psychiatry is to be distinguished from psychotherapy*. Broadly, psychotherapy is a branch of psychology, and psychiatry a branch of medicine. Psychotherapeutic practice consists mainly in verbal treatment, psychiatry includes other, more drastic forms of cure. Psychotherapy can be undertaken in the therapist's consulting room, psychiatry may require treatment in hospital. In contrast to psychotherapy, which regards psychopathology as a mental condition, psychiatry regards it as physical, and treatment is oriented accordingly.

It is in respect of its methods that psychiatry has come in for increasing censure. It has been labelled a modern superstition, on a par with astrology and alchemy. A strong case had been made for treating psychiatry not as a medical speciality, but as one of the social sciences, and not a very advanced science either. The great French physician Philippe Pinel (d. 1826), who reformed the bedlams of his day, took the inmates out of their dungeons and gave them sunny rooms and sympathetic understanding. Modern psychiatrists, say the critics, have sent them back to the dungeons of their own disturbed minds and subjected them to persecution and degradation. Modern treatment includes surgical operations on the brain, shock therapy and other forms of more or less viciously punitive treatment in asylums*.

Some of these methods are being placed in serious doubt, though all of them have in their time been fashionable, and tried out by responsible psychiatrists, in spite of public disquiet and the unheard cries of the victims. Today brain surgeons implant electrodes in the core of the brain of schizophrenic patients to relieve physical and emotional pain. ESB (electrical stimulation of the· brain) can now be administered transdermally, and psychiatrists are looking forward to an 'electro-chemical psycho-civilization' of brainwashed and mind-bent men and women who can be regulated to the last mood and thought by remote control.

Psychiatrists, it has been said, have produced a library of theses full of learned jargon, concerning their secret lore, but those who study their tomes are as confused and uncertain about the treatment of the mentally ill, as the benighted medicasters who lived before Pinel. Psychiatrists themselves don't always understand one another's publications, since much of their content is 'simply indigestible' (Foudraine, 1974, p. xii).

More than half of all the hospital beds in the USA and Europe are occupied by patients with mental illness. The number of cures is abysmally low, and in fact no greater than at the height of eighteenth-century quackery. This, say the critics, is a sad reflection on the value of the expensive equipment, the competence of the highly paid specialists and the usefulness of the countless products lucratively manufactured by the drug companies. Nor is the recommendation in favour of psychiatric treatment improved by the fact that 'the rates of suicide, alcoholism, divorce, and disturbed offspring, are higher in psychiatry than in any other profession' (Rogow, 1971, p. 30).

Yet, psychiatrists are called in to intervene and decide about the responsibility of teenage delinquents, the culpability of gangsters, marriage guidance, the rearing of children, unemployment and hooliganism, and to make judgments on job suitability, disciplinary action and criminal behaviour. Psychiatry today has invaded hospitals, schools and colleges, the law-courts, the government, the army and industry. Psychiatry, they conclude, is not a healing method, but big business.

Books

Alexander, F. G. and Selesnick, S. T., *The History of Psychiatry: an Evaluation of Psychiatric Thought and Practice from Prehistoric Times to the Present*, Harper & Row, New York, 1966.

Barnett, Michael, *People Not Psychiatry*, Allen & Unwin, London, 1973.

Boyers, Robert and Orvill, Robert (eds), *R. D. Laing and Anti-Psychiatry*, Harper & Row, New York, 1971.

Clare, Anthony, *Psychiatry in Dissent*, Tavistock Publications, London, 1976.
Cooper, David, *Psychiatry and Anti-Psychiatry*, Barnes & Noble, New York, 1967.
Foudraine, Jan, *Not Made of Wood*, Quartet Books, London, 1974.
Laing, R. D., *The Divided Self*, Pantheon, New York, 1969.
Martin, D. V., *Adventure in Psychiatry*, Cassirer, Oxford, 1962.
Rogow, Arnold A., *The Psychiatrists*, Allen & Unwin, London, 1971.
Szasz, Thomas S., *The Manufacture of Madness*, Routledge & Kegan Paul, London, 1971.
Wright, F. L., *Out of Sight, Out of Mind*, National Mental Health Foundation, Philadelphia, 1957.

PSYCHIC SURGERY

Psychic surgery is performed by unprofessional men through the intermediary of spiritual guides, using methods contrary to common surgical practice. It is practised today mostly in Brazil and the Philippines, in regions where the cult of Christian Spiritism is prevalent. The majority of the healers work without remuneration.

The best known of the Brazilian healers was José Pedro de Freitas (d. 1971), nicknamed Arigo (yokel), an illiterate farmer who treated over 2 million people in his humble clinic in Congonhas do Campo in the State of Minas Gerais. He was twice jailed for practising without a licence. Arigo was especially noted for his amazing ability to diagnose the most obscure physical ailment without any external aid, and prescribe for it, writing out the prescriptions with great rapidity in Portuguese and German, some requiring as many as 15 different drugs, and giving the correct quantities. Among others who investigated him was a team of 6 doctors and 8 scientists who watched him at work in 1968, as 1000 patients filed past. Without touching them, and taking only a few seconds for each, he diagnosed and wrote out prescriptions, which were found to be 'phenomenally accurate'.

Arigo also frequently performed painless surgery without anaesthetics or any antiseptic precautions, in a room thronged with patients and mobs of children. In one case he ripped open a man's stomach with his finger, removed a cancerous tumour and patched the abdomen while the patient himself remained awake and smiling. Arigo claimed to be guided by the spirit of Dr Adolf Fritz, a German surgeon of the First World War, and used the crudest implements, an ordinary kitchen knife, nail scissors and a pair of tweezers, all of which he kept in a rusty tin can. He was subjected to intensive investigation by the highest members of the Brazilian medical profession who unanimously declared the phenomena astounding and miraculous. Many of his operations were photographed and filmed.

In the Philippines, about 100 miles north of Manila, a group of more than a dozen Filipino mediums, men and women, also practise psychic surgery. Best known among them is Tony Agpaoa, whose operations, like those of Arigo, have been filmed, photographed and closely investigated by scientific organizations like the American Belk Foundation. Agpaoa usually makes a quick slicing movement with his finger on the patient's body, often not even touching it, and an incision appears, without much bleeding. With his bare hands, he then delves into the opening, manipulates it in a haphazard manner, sometimes not even looking at what he is doing. Tissue and other substances seem to grow out of the body, or materialize out of nothing. Existing cancerous growths seem to dematerialize; they just cease to exist and there is no trace of the original lump or tumour. After the operation he closes the opening with a movement of his hand.

Agpaoa, like other psychic surgeons in the group, belongs to the Christian Spiritist sect, and prepares himself and his patients by long prayers.

Lyall Watson who witnessed another of these healers performing, and watched every movement closely, reports that the healer rubbed and kneaded the abdomen of a patient until first blood and then an aperture appeared so that her intestines were visible. He inserted his hand into the gap and continued the moulding, and then suddenly extracted a mass of tissue as big as a tennis ball. After he withdrew his hand an assistant wiped the area with a piece of cloth. There was no trace of any wound, or mark of any kind. The whole operation took about five minutes.

In March 1973 a team of 9 scientists, including doctors, psychiatrists and physicists, from the USA, UK, Germany, Switzerland and Japan, taking 50 of their own patients with them, observed more than 10 healers in action. They left convinced of the existence of several types of 'psycho-energetic phenomena', including the materialization and dematerialization of human blood, tissue and organs.

A remarkable feature of some of these healings is that the incisions appear often while the surgeon is several inches away from the patient. Sleight-of-hand, fake and hypnosis* have been effectively ruled out, but no satisfactory explanation has yet been forthcoming.

Books

Andreas, P. and Adams, G., *Between Heaven and Earth*, Harrap, London, 1967.
Clare, Anthony, *Psychiatry in Dissent*, Tavistock, London, 1976.
Dooley, A., *Every Wall a Door*, Abelard-Schuman, London, 1973.
Fuller, John G., *Arigo: Surgeon of the Rusty Knife*, Crowell, New York, 1974.
Gray, I., *From Materialization to Healing*, Regency Press, London, 1972.
Motoyama, Hiroshi, *Psychic Surgery in the Philippines*, Institute of Religious Psychology, Tokyo, 1972.
St Clair, David, *Drum and Candle*, Macdonald, London, 1971.
Sherman, Harold, *Wonder Healers of the Philippines*, Psychic Press, London, 1967.
Tabori, Paul and Raphael, Phyllis, *Beyond the Senses*, Souvenir Press, London, 1971.
Valentine, T., *Psychic Surgery*, Henry Regnery, Chicago, 1973.
Watson, Lyall, *The Romeo Error*, Hodder & Stoughton, London, 1974.

PSYCHIC VAMPIRISM

The drawing and absorbing of physical, nervous and psychic energy by one person from another. Even where the actual vampirism of folklore may be doubted, there is evidence to show that psychic vampirism is possible, and does occur. Psychic vampires regenerate and recharge their own depleted energies by association with others. The vitality of those with whom they come in contact flows to them. Such vampires are like sponges and are often quite unconscious of their ability to draw strength from others. Some, of course, do it consciously. They feed, as it were, on the biomagnetic* radiation, aura or bioflux of their victims. Occultists say it is possible for the victim, if he tries, to recognize those who thus draw on him, and such victims are advised to avoid the company of those people.

Natural healers usually have a superabundance of vital power which flows easily from them when they function. Most so-called miraculous cures are explained as being the result of the patient unconsciously tapping vigour projected from the tissues of the healer. The touch-healer James Leverett (c. 1637) used to say that he could feel the strength going out of his body every time he performed a cure, and had to take to his bed after a heavy day's stroking.

Sometimes patients naturally tend to draw, albeit unwittingly, on those who are present, and are sustained thereby. The German clairvoyante Frederica Hauffe (d. 1829) used to receive 'nourishment' from the vital energy of her unsuspecting visitors, and many of her friends confessed that they felt weakened after spending some time in her company. A related form of the same phenomenon occurs in the séance room, when the spirit-control or medium draws energy from sitters for their kinetic effects and materializations.

Such vampirism is always going on, the strong vampirizing on the weak, the weak on the strong, the young on the old, the old on the young. The Hermetic philosopher Artephius (c. 1150) used to replenish his energies by engulfing with his etheric body the etheric bodies of young men and draining their psychic vitality. Black magicians are still believed to be able to do this in order to replenish their strength.

Bodily or close contact with young virgins of either sex, especially sleeping with them without sexual intercourse, was once a popular method of rejuvenating the body. But here there is always the danger that the young person might actually vampirize on the emanations of the older one. It was further believed that teachers lived long because they continually took in the virginal atmosphere of their charges. But this, too, is very doubtful. If they do live long, it is perhaps because of the unharassing nature of their occupation and the constant activity of their minds. The magnetic qualities of the young can be very strong and they can absorb more powerfully from older people than the latter can from them. Adults who habitually associate with adolescents often find their vitality is slowly being drained and they are easily fatigued.

Psychic vampirism is often associated with sexual activity. The female normally absorbs vital energy from her husband as a result of invagination, but the male too feeds on her psychic emanations, especially during orgasm. Acclivity techniques are concerned with the deliberate absorption of female sex energy.

Books

See under shunamism

PSYCHODIAGNOSTICS

A form of depth psychology which attempts to probe the unconscious mind and hidden motivations of an individual to discover what lies beneath and within. It is a useful tool in determining personality traits, strength and weakness, predispositions, prejudices, tendencies, secret wishes and aspirations, hates and loves, likes and dislikes. It is valuable in many areas such as vocational guidance, job suitability and marriage compatibility, as well as for the prognosis or prediction of likely future states.

To start with, the outward appearance of the individual and his general behaviour give the earliest clues about him. A number of these are properly the province of the so-called occult and divinatory arts, all of which were anciently studied for hints and signs of character and disposition.

Physiognomy is the study of the face, notably its shape, the type of features, and the expression. Some of these form special separate studies, such as *oculomancy* (the eyes), *rhinomancy* (nose), *otomancy* (ear), *metoposcopy* (forehead), *mentumomancy* (chin).

Phrenology studies the head, especially the 'bumps', which allegedly reveal the psychological and social 'faculties' that predominate in a person's character.

Palmistry studies the shape, size and markings of the hand and fingers. More specifically, *onyxomancy* studies the nails.

Podomancy makes readings from the markings on the soles of the feet.

Sternutometry studies the strength of the sneeze and determines the person's physical constitution, and whether he is socially expansive or restrained.

Gelosology (Gk. *gelōs*, 'laughter') studies the jokes made by the individual, and things that amuse him, his own reaction to the jokes and puns of others.

Stoleomancy (Gk. *stolē*, 'dress') makes a character study from the clothes he wears, and his manner of wearing them.

Horoscopy (Gk. *horos*, 'hour'), from the time of his birth, forms the basis of astrology.

Pateomancy (Gk. *pateō*, 'to walk'), from the gait and manner of walking.

Gesturology (Lat. *gestus*, 'gesture'), from his gestures, particularly the movements of his hands and head.

Statiomancy (Lat. *statio*, 'to stand'), from the stance or the passive position of the individual, whether sloppy, alert, tense, anxious, relaxed.

Graphology (Gk. *graphein*, 'to write'), from the formation of the letters in a person's handwriting.

Laliognomy (Gk. *laleō*, 'to talk'; *gnōmōn*, 'judge'), or speech analysis, judging from the expressions, phrases, words, grammar, pronunciation.

Phonognomy (Gk. *phōnē*, 'voice'), from the sound of the voice, its softness, harshness, speed, whether high-pitched or low.

Typology deduces from one or more traits the category to which a person belongs, whether introvert or extravert, restrictive or permissive, jovial or saturnine, optimistic or pessimistic, leader or led, and so on.

Modern psychologists have proposed several new methods of delving into the deeps of a person's mind. Thus, in *parapraxis* (Gk. 'near-action'), the faulty performance of an action, mistakes, slips, 'Freudian errors', all conceal important clues that can be interpreted to disclose some facet of character, some preoccupation or problem, some obsession or phobia of the individual.

In *xenoanalysis* note is taken of a person's unguarded words and actions when he is under the influence of drink, drugs, hypnotics (*narcoanalysis*), 'truth-pills', shock, pain, sickness, and other xenophrenic*, or strange-minded, states.

A special department of this is *oneiromancy* (Gk. *oneiros*, 'a dream'), the age-old art of dream interpretation, which is now once again an important branch of psychodiagnosis.

In what is called *imagogy*, an analysis is made of the mental or fanciful 'pictures' produced in conditions of automatism as in trance and somnambulism. It also studies the doodles one draws while otherwise preoccupied.

In *projectivism*, a person's spontaneous response to something he sees or imagines is analysed. In the Rorschach test he gives his interpretation of a set of meaningless inkblots.

In the thematic apperception test (TAT) he relates a story about a series of drawings presented to him. Or he is asked to describe a house, then its rooms, then the attic, and finally the contents of an old trunk in the attic. All these disclose his strong and weak qualities, his interests, his fears, his aspirations.

Ordinary intelligence tests are often included, for they gauge not only intelligence, but emotional maturity and general attitudes to people and events.

Word association tests judge a person from his instant verbal response (or hesitation, or silence) when certain key words are uttered by the psychologist.

Free association is used in psychoanalysis. Here a person is encouraged to talk freely and at length, with as little interruption as possible, on any subject he chooses, or on anything that springs to mind.

Psychologists believe that a great deal can be learned about a person from his response to and relationship with others in a group* situation, more specifically his parents, marriage partner, children, boss, subordinates, equals.

Equally, from his reaction in talk and discussion to emotive subjects like religion, race, communism, capitalism, youth, drugs, loyalty, punctuality, obedience, permissiveness, the Establishment, war, responsibility, punishment, examinations, euthanasia, old age, women, men, sex, pornography, homosexuality, marriage. Does he freeze up? Does he react with cynicism, sympathy, scepticism, anger?

His behaviour under conditions of stress is extremely important. Can he stand criticism? Can he stand being contradicted? Can he stand provocation, abuse, threat, ridicule?

A great deal can also be learned in the course of various therapies: drama, art, psychodrama, encounter therapy.

In addition, much useful information may be gleaned from a physical and medical examination that might contribute to an understanding of a person's disposition. Stomach ulcers, migraine, asthma or a heart condition could give one an idea of the degree of stress to which a person is subjected. Helpful in such physical analyses are the various biotelemetric devices such as those that measure heartbeats, respiration, skin resistance and brain activity. The complete and comprehensive data obtained as a result of psychodiagnosis are called a psychogram, a portrait of the inner man.

Books

Anastasi, A., *Psychological Testing*, New York, 1954.
Freud, Sigmund, *The Psychopathology of Everyday Life*, Hogarth Press, London, 1960.
Jung, C. G., *Psychological Types*, Kegan Paul, Trench, Trubner, London, 1923.
Krantz, H., *Die Narkoanalyse*, Tübingen, 1950.
Kretschmer, Ernst, *Physique and Character,* Kegan Paul, Trench, Trubner, London, 1936.
Rabin, A. (ed.), *Projective Techniques in Personality Assessment*, New York, 1968.
Semeonoff, Boris (ed.), *Personality Assessment*, Penguin Books, Harmondsworth, 1949.
Sheldon, William *et al.*, *The Varieties of Human Physique,* Harper, New York, 1940.
Wyss, D., *Depth Psychology: a Critical History*, London, 1966.

PSYCHODRAMA

A technique of group therapy* in which individuals enact certain roles in a drama or play. The acting out of certain emotional situations appears to be a universal and spontaneous activity. Play and games have been the child's own way of role-playing and growing up. Girls play with dolls, and boys with make-believe implements of work and war.

Play-acting in a ritual context is found in all primitive and tribal societies in the world, and every civilized society has its tradition of dramatic ceremonial with a religious purpose. Egyptian drama arose from the worship of Osiris; Greek drama from the Dionysian rites; the medieval mystery plays from the great themes of the Bible.

Drama has always provided both emotional expression and emotional outlet. Aristotle (d. 322 BC) spoke of drama, more specifically tragedy, as the imitation (Gk. *mimēsis*) of an action that arouses feelings of pity and terror in the audience and thereby effects a cleansing (Gk. *katharsis*) or purging of these emotions from the psyche. In modern times the direct association of drama with therapy was first put forward in 1931 by the Rumanian-born American psychologist Jacob L. Moreno (b. 1892), who set forth the basic principles of psychodrama, upon which others have subsequently expanded.

There are no fixed rules in psychodrama, but it is always performed in groups, which usually include a therapist who takes note of everything that happens. Each person (patient) may pick a solo part, a recitation, monologue or mime and spontaneously and without prompting act out any situation that comes into his head. The role he takes will usually give some indication of his problem to the therapist.

More commonly several persons take part in the drama, the therapist perhaps joining in. In some cases a brief outline of the plot is given and the actors choose the parts they wish to play. Such miniature dramas are often specially conceived by the therapist for his patients, but a great deal of freedom of action and speech is allowed. The plot may be changed or reconstructed by the players as they go along. Roles may be changed in the middle of the play. Such role reversal again provides valuable clues. So do any masks used in the play.

The purpose of psychodrama is twofold: it helps the therapist to diagnose the hidden causes of illness, and it helps the patient to effect his own cure. Although speech is permitted the emphasis is on action. Deep-seated problems, concealed and repressed, are given symbolical expression, and an insight is gained into the underlying causes of seemingly irrational behaviour.

In psychodrama the patient has the limelight and is provided with that one crowded hour of fame and glory that each one craves. It helps him, without his being consciously aware of it, to act out his problems. It provides relief from his inner tensions through spontaneous self-expression. Sometimes its effects are immediately abreactive, or releasing, as when a scene from a past experience is actualized to discharge a repressed emotion or revive a painful memory. By thus reliving the original traumatic experience the patient is set free from its pathological influence, and this helps in the integration of his personality.

In a way, modern psychodrama provokes an Aristotelian, cathartic response in the patient. It is essentially a mode of imitation, which, by the self-representation of fear and anxiety situations, drives them out.

Books

Blatner, H., *Psychodrama, Role Playing and Action Methods*, Thetford, 1970.
Greenberg, Ira A. (ed.), *Psychodrama: Theory and Therapy*, Souvenir Press, London, 1975.
Klapman, J. W., *Group Psychotherapy: Theory and Practice*, Grune, New York, 1946.
Moreno, J. L., *Psychodrama*, Beacon, New York, 1946.
Schutzemberger, A. A., *Précis de psychodrame*, Éditions Universitaires, Paris, 1966.
Wethered, Audrey, *Drama and Movement Therapy*, Macdonald & Evans, London, 1973.

PSYCHOGENIC DEATH

Psychogenic, or 'mind-induced' death, is brought about without any detectable material or external cause; it results from a purely psychic or mental operation. Here, a person's life is brought to an end (a) through the deliberate command of another, either with the victim's knowledge (death by suggestion) or without his knowledge (death by the will of another); (b) through the victim himself relinquishing his will to live and willing himself to die (autosuggestive death, or dying by will); (c) through the unconscious operation of the death wish that is inherent in all human beings (*see* thanatophilia).

Some people seem to have the natural power of deliberately willing themselves to die. Frequently quoted is the case recorded in a book by Dr Cheyne, an eighteenth-century physician and relative of Gilbert Burnet (d. 1715), bishop of Salisbury. It concerned the Hon. Colonel Townshend, a squire held in high regard in the country, who claimed the gift of being able to 'die' at will, and then after a short time to return to life. He gave a demonstration in the presence of three men of integrity and standing: the physicians Dr Bayard and Dr Cheyne, and a local squire, Mr Skrine. He lay down, composed himself and shut his eyes, and in a little while it was noticed by the two physicians present that his pulse grew feebler and heartbeats less distinct, until both ceased completely. A mirror held by Mr Skrine to his mouth and nose showed no signs of breath. Townshend remained in this state of suspended animation or clinical death for half an hour, and then slowly came back to life. That same evening Townshend, having previously put his business and private affairs in order, calmly and composedly expired, never to return to life again.

The desire to live can often be imperceptibly eroded by various external factors; and without actively willing to bring death on himself, the victim can unconsciously surrender himself to the forces that lead to death. A typical example is provided in the case of a symbiotic relationship, such as that of a man and wife who have been very close for many years, and when one dies the other falls into a state of apathy, and follows soon after.

Psychogenic death frequently occurs among primitive people, with intimate links with their community or tribe. If a tribal Aborigine has contravened a taboo regulation, even inadvertently, or transgressed a tribal law, or believes he is under the power of demons, or that he has been put under a curse by a witch-doctor, or that a sorcerer has pointed a bone at him, or perhaps unloosed an invisible arrow in his direction, he is stricken with mortal terror, and the awful nature of the situation he is in firmly grips his imagination. He is convinced that there is no escape from his predicament and that he must die. His will to live cannot contend against the inexorable power of the curse that is upon him. The strength seems to run out of him and his energy is sapped; he frets, loses his desire to eat or sleep. His mind is obsessed without respite with the one thought of his impending doom. He falls into a decline and fades away, and literally nothing can save him. In such cases of 'voodoo death' there may be no fever, no pain, no symptoms of any disease, although a very rapid pulse is often present.

The ethnologist Alfred Haddon (d. 1940) quotes the story of a young and healthy Congo tribesman who died of panic within 24 hours of being told that he had eaten the flesh of a tabooed hen. Sir James Frazer (d. 1941) relates cases of Maoris 'dying of sheer fright' on discovering that they had inadvertently eaten the remains of a chief's dinner or touched some tabooed object that belonged to him. Loederer quotes an observer who had lived for forty years in Haiti, who stated that he once saw a strong and healthy man fall to the ground and 'writhe out his death agonies', while at the same time a voodoo priest many miles off was wrapt in silent concentration, cursing the man's life away.

In Mexico the superiority of rival magicians was often resolved by a battle of wills. They would sit opposite each other fully accoutred with the paraphernalia of their craft, and silently project their will towards the other, until one of them, feeling the rival's power impossible to contend against, would forsake the ground, creep away to his lodge and lie down to die.

The rite of praying people to death is another time-honoured method widely practised in many societies. Intense concentration on the victim, with a desire for his death, accompanies a fervent prayer to the gods or demons to take away his life. Generally the victim is informed that he is being 'prayed to death', which greatly strengthens the force of the death rite. In the same way, powerfully directed curses can, it is commonly believed, also be instrumental in causing death.

Mind-induced death is by no means confined to savage or illiterate peoples, and there are many instances of this type of thanatomania* in the Western world. People who have been responsible for unjustly sending others to their death, have been 'summoned' by their victims as they were about to die, and thereafter have been unable to shake off the remembrance of the dread command, and have died soon after. A graveyard ceremony, performed with all the trappings of religion for someone who is alive, can be very effective in causing death. Such requiems for the living are included among the black masses of the satanists.

Books

Barker, J. C., *Scared to Death*, Frederick Muller, London, 1968.
Cannon, W. B., 'Voodoo Death', *American Anthropologist*, 44, 2, 1942, 169.
Cheyne, Dr G., *Hypochondriacal Distempers*, London, 1723.
Franklyn, J., *Death by Enchantment*, Hamish Hamilton, London, 1971.
Frazer, J. G., *Psyche's Task*, London, 1909.
Haddon, A. C., *Magic and Fetishism*, London, 1906.
Loederer, R. A., *Voodoo Fire in Haiti*, Jarrolds, London, 1935.
Meerloo, J. A., 'Shock, Fright and Psychic Death', *American Practitioner*, 12, 1961, 43.
Wickwar, J. W., *Witchcraft and the Black Art*, Herbert Jenkins, London, 1939.

PSYCHOPATHY

A mental disorder not necessarily amounting to insanity, characterized by antisocial behaviour, often leading to acts of aggression and violence. The victim, known as a psychopath, is to be distinguished from the psychotic, who is commonly treated as insane. Psychopathy also refers to the study of the psychopath, and this again is to be distinguished from psychopathology, an ambiguous term for the study of mental disorders in general.

Psychopathy as a mental illness falls into a class of its own, and currently receives much attention from psychologists and behavioural scientists the world over. It is largely a phenomenon of our times and is likely to bulk large in the diagnosis of individual and social ills.

The psychopath is not usually subnormal in intelligence. Often his intelligence is above average. Callous and selfish he lacks the emotional qualities that make for normal interpersonal relationships, such as altruism, affection, empathy, concern for others. But he may show a fanatical attachment to one person, animal or object.

A layabout and cadger, he is a predator who lives off others, whether parents, girlfriends, boyfriends or casual associates. Plausible in speech he will glibly rationalize all his mistakes and shortcomings. A habitual and compulsive liar he pretends to feel affection without actually feeling any. He is fickle, erratic and undependable, totally lacking in loyalty. He indulges in fantasies of power, sexual success, wealth and bravery. His habitual lying (pseudolism) and his erotic daydreams make the psychopath with literary talent into the writer of pornography. The less gifted write anonymous lewd letters, make obscene phone calls, and exhibit themselves.

He becomes quickly bored and restless, and needs constant stimulation, hence his predilection for loud music, drugs, sex perversion. Because he has a low temptation threshold, he easily succumbs to any sensual lures, and is often promiscuous and hedonistic. Impatient and impulsive he must have what he wants, at once and without question, whether it be sexual gratification or money, without regard to consequences, and can be dangerous when frustrated. Although he is extraverted and forms subcults like other degenerates*, he can bear with solitude and go his own way.

The principal characteristic of the psychopath is his social insensitivity, his lack of feelings of guilt, shame, embarrassment, contrition, remorse, anxiety, in situations that would normally arouse these feelings in others. He is a sociopath, opposed to society in general, undisciplined and antisocial in his behaviour, and apparently devoid of conscience. He has little sense of duty or responsibility, and may be aggressive and violent. Varying degrees of psychopathy are to be seen in the road-hog, the bully, the mob-orator, the wife-beater, the baby-basher, the football hooligan, the vandal, the terrorist, the hi-jacker, the 'psychopathic killer'. His class form the greater proportion of the population of remand institutions and prisons.

Research has shown that he is not put off by painful situations, nor deterred from crime by the thought of punishment. He is reckless, and shows a negative reaction in situations that arouse fear, stress and anxiety, in normal people, and hence does not avoid danger. His apparent courage, however, is not normal but pathological, due to a defect in his make-up. Because his moral sense is so far below normal, the psychopath's condition has been described as one of moral insanity, or moral imbecility.

A number of reasons have been advanced to account for this type of disorder. It is sometimes due to chromosomal aberration, for example, an additional X-chromosome; or again to a deficiency in the adrenalin secreting mechanism. Laboratory tests indicate a characteristic abnormality in the EEG of many psychopaths. Emotional isolation in childhood; a broken home; lack of parental guidance; bad company, have all been blamed. Many show signs of psychopathic tendencies from early childhood: in theft, truancy, lying, disobedience, lack of shame and guilt, sexual misbehaviour.

It is generally agreed that such individuals require medical care, though at present no adequate remedy is available. The psychopath is the most difficult of all types to cure, and almost every therapeutic technique used on him has proved ineffective. The rehabilitation of the psychopath is an almost hopeless task. He is the perpetual recidivist. Because of his lack of moral sense he sees nothing wrong in his conduct, and he cannot be made to accept standards that differ from his own, since he sees no reason to change. His life, he finds, is fulfilled and rewarding, at whatever cost to others he does not care.

Many psychologists feel that at its deepest levels the psychopathic malaise flourishes in the wider area of sociopsychosis*. The individual is sick because the society that breeds him is sick.

Books

Aichorn, August, *Wayward Youth*, Viking Press, New York, 1935.
Andry, R., *Delinquency and Parental Pathology*, London, 1960.
Aronfreed, J., *Conscience and Conduct*, New York, 1968.

Craft, M., *Ten Studies in Psychopathic Personality*, Bristol, 1965.
Eissler, Kurt (ed.), *Searchlight on Delinquency*, International Universities Press, New York, 1949.
Hare, R., *Psychopathy: Theory and Research*, New York, 1970.
Lynd, H. M., *On Shame and the Search for Identity*, Science Editions, New York, 1958.
McCord, W. and McCord, J., *The Psychopath: An Essay on the Criminal Mind*, Princeton, New Jersey, 1964.
Piers, G. and Singer, M. B., *Shame and Guilt*, Thomas, Springfield, Illinois, 1953.
Robins, L., *Deviant Children Grown Up*, Baltimore, 1966.

PSYCHOSOMATICS

The study of the influence of thought and emotion on the body, with special reference to the pathogenic or disease-producing power of the mind. Of many an ailment it has been said that 'it's all in the mind', suggesting the controlling influence of mind over body. Many of the major diseases that afflict mankind cannot be explained simply in terms of a person's exposure to infection, since germs are only one of a number of complex factors, of which the emotions are among the most important.

The causes of psychosomatic disorders can be personal, familial, social and environmental, and can reach beyond the individual to the nation as a whole (*see* sociopsychosis). On a personal level they may be due to powerful and active passions like hatred, anger, jealousy, envy, greed, lust, hostility, resentment and aggression. They may arise from the more passive kinds of emotion such as grief, depression, insecurity, guilt, humiliation, disappointment, fear, anxiety homesickness, boredom, loneliness. In other words, they could be expressed in terms of emotional conflict at home, at work and in society. In loss of love, unrequited love, sexual frustration, social ostracism.

In a more general sense many contributing factors can be traced to status-seeking, the pace of life, the rat-race, the human condition, living up to the Joneses, travel, change and all other causes of anxiety* and stress*. They may be connected with the uncertainty of one's role in life, with the feeling of not belonging, and of rootlessness, with the search for identity and purpose, with the collectivization of man, and with the anonymization and loss of identity of the individual.

Any of these factors, alone or in combination with others, can result in physical illness. Stress and tension stimulate reflex actions in the autonomic nervous system, which in turn affect the endocrine system (the output of the pituitary, adrenal, thyroid and other glands), the circulation and breathing, and trigger remote reflexes in various parts of the body. A brief catalogue of the conditions to which they give rise will indicate the wide ramifications that emotional disturbances have on the physiological system.

Respiratory ailments: colds, feelings of suffocation, pains in the chest, rapid breathing, and such diseases as rhinitis, asthma, tuberculosis. *Digestive*: indigestion, heartburn, vomiting, constipation, gastrointestinal troubles, colitis and colonic disorders, peptic ulcer, duodenal ulcer. *Cardiac*: palpitations, heart pains, hypertension or high blood pressure, and cardiovascular, coronary and arterial diseases. *Cerebral*: thrombosis, stroke. *Endocrine*:

239

thyrotoxicosis, diabetes. *Skin*: sweating especially of the palms, itching, rashes, dermatitis, eczema, urticaria. *Muscular*: spasms, cramps, rheumatism, arthritis. *Sexual*: impotence, frigidity, menstrual troubles. *General*: headache, migraine, allergies, lassitude, inability to do any physical or mental work, general aches and pains, nausea, backache, insomnia, dry mouth, frequency of urination, tension and unease.

Books

Hill, O., *Psychosomatic Medicine*, Butterworth, London, 1970.
Pierloot, R., *Recent Researches in Psychosomatics*, Wylie, London, 1971.
Simon, A. (ed.), *The Physiology of the Emotions*, C. C. Thomas, Chicago, 1961.
Walker, Benjamin, *Encyclopedia of Esoteric Man*, Routledge & Kegan Paul, London and Stein & Day, New York, 1977.

PSYCHOTHERAPY

Psychotherapy covers all types of treatment for mental maladjustment and emotional disturbance by purely psychological means, and is thus to be distinguished from psychiatry*. According to Rycroft, it is any form of talking cure. A simple reassurance to an anxious person is the most obvious form of psychotherapy.

Psychotherapy has a long history. Its earliest and very skilful practitioners were the witch-doctors, medicine-men and shamans of tribal societies. The writings of the Egyptian, Greek, Roman and Chinese physicians contain many passages of remarkable psychological insight into mental disorders and their treatment by psychotherapeutic methods.

Medieval Europe produced no significant advance on ancient therapies; on the contrary the treatment of the mentally sick was often barbarous. The first real breakthrough seems to have been achieved with the work of the magnetizers in the eighteenth century (*see* biomagnetic therapy). Subsequently the systematic study of psychotherapy on scientific lines was undertaken by Jean Charcot (d. 1893), Pierre Janet (d. 1947) and others, culminating in the work of Sigmund Freud (d. 1939), founder of psychoanalysis. Freud did not consider that a medical degree was essential for the analyst. It is of interest to note that Freud did his most important work, and perhaps gained his shrewdest insights into the workings of the sick mind while he himself was suffering from a psychoneurosis.

Although there are many kinds of psychotherapy, the term is still specifically applied to the system of psychological cure undertaken by a trained psychoanalyst. But there have been major heresies from the early days of the psychoanalytic movement. Chief of the schismatics are Adler and Jung, with Ferenczi, Rank and Reich on the fringes. The claims of these and other seceders are bitterly repudiated by the Freudians. Some Freudians, indeed, regard the recalcitrants as disturbed types. Why else should they rebel against the doctrine?

Alfred Adler (d. 1937) believed that emotional disturbance sprang from feelings of inferiority, because of some physical defect, and the basic drive in man was to overcome or compensate for this deficiency.

Carl Gustav Jung (d. 1961) disagreed with Freud's pansexualism, flatly denied his theory of dream interpretation, and introduced new concepts like the archetypes, the collective unconscious, and introversion and extraversion.

Sandor Ferenczi (d. 1933) developed a type of privation philosophy, making his patients limit as far as they possibly could such activities as eating, drinking, defecation, urination and sexual activity, but had to abandon it in the face of violent opposition. He then tried caressing and kissing his female patients and encouraged them to reciprocate, much to the annoyance of Freud. The opportunities open to therapists in transferential* relationships with their patients are not always resisted.

Otto Rank (d. 1939) laid emphasis on feelings centring around the birth' trauma, which according to him was more significant than the Oedipus complex.

Wilhelm Reich (d. 1957) disagreed with Freud over the death instinct, and developed new ideas about the structure of character (*see* kinesiotherapy).

The main criticism of the anti-Freudians has been directed against certain specific concepts that form the basis of psychoanalytical theory and practice. They question the need for the long-drawn-out, and lucrative, free association process recommended in the Freudian scriptures, which only the idle and bored are tempted to try and only the affluent can afford. They object to 'Freudian archaeology', which laboriously attempts to trace every mental illness back to childhood trauma. They dispute the pretensions of the Oedipus complex, which raises the commonplace fact of intrafamily rivalry to the status of a mystical dogma.

But the primary target has been the pansexualism of Freud, and his 'plug-and-hole' theory of humanity, that is, its preoccupation with penis and vagina, and the attribution of a sexual motivation to any muscular activity or sense experience, from simple rocking movements to munching chocolates. This leads to the prurient delving into the sex life of the patient, which in their view is reminiscent of the medieval witch-hunter's insatiable curiosity about the intimate erotic practices of his victim. The zealous theologian of the past, who saw everyone as basically sinful, has been replaced by the zealous psychologist, who sees everyone as basically sexual.

Freudian axiomatics has discouraged any fresh theorizing, and no significant step forward has been taken in psychoanalytic theory since 1930, so that for about a half century psychoanalytic exegesis has been an endless threshing of old straw.

The hard core of orthodoxy in modern psychotherapy is still represented by the Freudians. But besides the main heresiarchs mentioned above, there have been numerous other deviations from the original stream. One authority listed no less than 36 schools of psychotherapy, and that was in 1959. The newer therapies, which are quite distinctive and barely acknowledge the Freudian ancestry, now run into dozens more, mostly centring around encounter and other forms of group therapy*. There are also considerable ramifications of schools in subordinate studies. During a conference in

Geneva in 1968 on the psychotherapeutic application of image experience, representatives of about 400 methods were present.

Much of the criticism directed as psychiatry is also directed at psychotherapy in general, both with regard to the methods of cure and to their success. As far as their success is concerned, Professor H. J. Eysenck, after a review of statistics, concluded that untreated neurotics recovered in the same proportion as neurotics subjected to psychotherapy. Spontaneous remission, in fact, occurred more frequently if a patient were untreated.

Books

Beloff, John, *Psychological Sciences: a Review of Modern Psychology*, Crosby, Lockwood, Staples, London, 1973.

Brown, William, *Psychological Methods of Healing*, University of London Press, 1938.

Eysenck, H. J., *The Effects of Psychotherapy*, International Science Press, New York, 1966.

Ford, D. H. and Urban, H. B., *Systems of Psychotherapy*, New York, 1963.

Goldstein, A. P. and Dean, S. J. (eds), *The Investigation of Psychotherapy*, Wiley, Chichester, 1966.

Harper, Robert A., *Psychoanalysis and Psychotherapy*, Prentice-Hall, New Jersey, 1959.

London, P., *The Modes and Morals of Psychotherapy*, New York, 1964.

Rycroft, Charles, *A Critical Dictionary of Psychoanalysis*, Penguin, Harmondsworth, 1972.

Szasz, Thomas S., *The Ethics of Psychoanalysis*, Basic Books, New York, 1965.

Wolberg, Lewis R., *The Techniques of Psychotherapy*, Grune, New York, 1967.

QUACKERY

Quackery is healing by those who pretend to have the knowledge and qualifications. The pseudohealer is known as a quack, shortened from 'quacksalver', one who quacks, or boasts, about his salves. Terms of derision and denigration are applied to many professions, more especially to healers. Thus we have 'sawbones' for surgeon, and 'headshrinker' for psychiatrist.

During the sixteenth century the quack was also called an 'empiric', because he had no theoretical knowledge of medicine but practised only on the basis of his experience. Alternative terms were 'mountebank', because he used to mount on his bench (Italian, *banco*) to announce his skills; and 'charlatan', because of his boastful chatter (Italian, *ciarlatano*). Associated with him in the seventeenth century was an obsequious assistant who used to swallow, or pretend to swallow, allegedly poisonous toads, after which the quack would give him an antidote. From this comes the term 'toad-eater', or 'toady', for a cringing and sycophantic parasite.

The itinerant quack dentist likewise had an assistant from whose mouth he would pull out worms that were supposed to be causing him toothache, indigestion, consumption and other ills.

Throughout history quacks have run a parallel course with professional physicians. The Persian physician Rhazes (*c.* 925) gives a vivid description of the quacks of his day, some of whose dodges are still current. They are glib and quick at repartee; possess a sharp commercial instinct; make capital out of partial recoveries and remissions; claim to use secret remedies of the past (Peruvian balsams, Himalayan roots, Indian snake-oil, Chinese elixirs); and make a great pretence of being up to date in their methods. They are always quick to exploit any current fears. At the time of the great Lisbon earthquake of 1755, one quack compounded pills that were 'good for the earthquake'. When in 1910 a comet appeared and caused great consternation, another quack made a pile of money selling comet pills. They make much use of magnetism, electricity, radium and sundry invisible rays. Their alleged cures usually cover cases that other doctors 'refuse to treat'.

In spite of the opprobrium attached to their activities, the history of medicine shows that quacks preserved many valuable remedies of primitive medicine*, and made important medical contributions that were often taken over by the orthodox physicians. And above all that they were much more concerned with the welfare of the poor. The *Thesaurus Pauperum* of Petrus Hispanus (fl. 1200) was a collection of cheap prescriptions with readily available ingredients, for poor people who often had to prescribe for themselves. Paracelsus (d. 1541), whose genius is only now beginning to be recognized, said that whatever he had learned of value about medicine came not from the learned works of Galen and Avicenna, but from sage women, peasants, gypsies, shepherds, barbers and farriers, who never failed to show a deep concern for the poor, the wretched, the needy, who had no provision made for them.

In England and Europe treatment was long in the hands of old wives, lay healers, priests and herbalists, who generally followed old-established folk-methods. The early history of medicine contains many chapters that reflect adversely on the professional conduct of the orthodox healer. The doctor treated only the rich. The surgeon was similarly preoccupied only with those who could afford to pay him. The ordinary man, therefore, had to depend entirely on the folk-healer.

In 1540 an Act of Henry VIII granted special privileges to the surgeons. The immediate effect was that the surgeons claimed a monopoly, and declared the folk-healers illegal, so that the poor were left without attention. The situation became so scandalous that another act had to be passed by the king in 1542, withdrawing some of the privileges from the surgeons, who,

> minding only their own lucre, and not the welfare or ease of the diseased, have troubled and vexed many honest persons whom God hath endowed with the knowledge of nature . . . and who have not taken anything for their pains, but have ministered the same to the poor for God's sake and from pity and charity.

This withdrawal of the monopoly from an avaricious clique was promptly dubbed by them the Quack's Charter.

QUACKERY

Orthodox practitioners have always scorned the work of unorthodox healers. Over a thousand years ago, Ar-Razi (d. 925), Arab physician of Baghdad, wrote a treatise entitled, 'The reason why illiterate common folk and women are more successful than learned physicians in treating certain diseases, and the excuses which physicians make for this'. To this day the medical fraternity continues to brand as quacks all those who do not pass through the accepted channels of their profession. Many physicians have been struck off the medical register for attempting to introduce unorthodox innovations.

Again, the orthodox physician does not like to acknowledge that some-one outside his profession is able to cure a disease that is beyond his competence, and tends to attribute all the miracle-cures of the 'quack' to mistaken diagnosis, mistaken prognosis, spontaneous remission, alleviation of symptoms or the simultaneous use of other, approved, remedies. Such a doctor could well sympathize with the reaction of the Harley Street specialist who, on meeting a patient who has long stopped consulting him, greets him with: 'You still alive! What quack has been treating you?' As Ackerknecht points out, quackerish behaviour can be combined with the possession of an MD diploma.

The title of quack has been repeatedly bestowed on those stepping outside the established order who are ahead of the times and whose methods have since been given the nod of respectability. The early advocates of antisepsis, anaesthesia, immunization and other innovations were so branded. The mesmerism of the eighteenth century is now hypnosis or psychosomatic sleep, and standard practice in many conventional therapies. The massagist and bone-setter of earlier days has now graduated to the more respectable physiotherapist. But many still remain on the borderline: the homoeopath, the naturopath, the herbalist, the acupuncturist and radiesthetist.

Oliver Wendell Holmes (d. 1894) lists a few of the items acquired by the medical profession from its lay brotherhood: from a monk, the use of antimony; from a soldier, how to treat gout; from a friar, how to cut for the stone; from a sailor, how to keep off scurvy; from a postmaster, how to sound the Eustachian tube; from a dairy maid, how to prevent smallpox; from an old market woman, how to catch the itch insect.

The famous scientist Alexis Carrel (d. 1944) said, 'More than half the great remedies known to medical history have come from empiricists, that is from "irregulars", men and women of no or little scientific training.'

Books

Ackerknecht, Erwin H., *Therapeutics: From the Primitives to the Twentieth Century*, Hafner, New York, 1973.
Carrel, Alexis, *Man the Unknown*, Harpers, London, 1939.
Cramp, A. J., *Nostrums and Quackery and Pseudo-Medicine*, American Medical Association, Chicago, 1936.
Fishbein, Morris, *Fads and Quackery in Healing*, London, 1932.
Gardner, Martin, *Fads and Fallacies in the Name of Science*, Dover, New York, 1957.
Holbrook, S. H., *The Golden Age of Quackery*, Macmillan, London, 1914.
Jameson, Eric, *The Natural History of Quackery*, Michael Joseph, London, 1961.

Lawrence, E., *Primitive Psychotherapy and Quackery*, Constable, London, 1910.
Maple, Eric, *Magic, Medicine and Quackery*, Robert Hale, London, 1968.
Minty, Marchant, *Medical Quackery*, Heinemann, London, 1932.
Pettigrew, T. J., *Superstitions Connected with the History and Practice of Medicine and Surgery*, London, 1844.
Zilboorg, G., *The Medical Man and the Witch Doctor During the Renaissance*, Johns Hopkins Press, Baltimore, 1935.

R

REJUVENATION

The recovery of youthful appearance, health and vigour in old age. Men seek it chiefly with the object of reactivating their sexual vigour, and women to restore their youthful beauty. Essentially, all rejuvenatory processes are concerned with the prolongation, as far as possible, of the period of greatest maturity between puberty and old age. The subject is connected with longevity (as distinct from senility) since those who are naturally long-lived are thought not merely to live long, but to retain their vigour as well.

From classical times, exceptional longevity was always attributed to the Seres (Chinese). For centuries taoist alchemists endeavoured to produce an elixir of immortality. It was the dream and death of more than one Chinese emperor. The great semi-legendary sages of other countries were also alleged to have lived an indeterminate number of years. In Europe the rosicrucians, alchemists and other medieval mages made similar claims, and were believed at one time or another to have distilled or discovered the universal medicine, the philosopher's stone, the tincture of the physicians, potable gold and other powders and potions of immortality. In fact, many alchemists were known to have lived well into their sixties, seventies and even eighties, at a time when the average expectation of life was 38 years.

In folklore and legend numerous colourful characters were reputed to have survived the ravages of time by various means. Among them, Aristaeus (fl. 570 BC) claimed to subsist on the 'celestial dew' from the atmosphere. Hermippus (c. AD 50) lived by shunamism*, or the exhalation of virgins. The Wandering Jew, a contemporary of Jesus, is reputedly still alive, denied the solace of death for his lack of compassion. Simon Magus, a wonder-worker who died in a battle of wills with St Peter, was said to have lived for over a century by methods taught by his demon aids. Apollonius of Tyana (d. AD 120), another wonder-worker and philosopher, sustained himself by magical means for two centuries. Artephius (d. 1150), hermetic sage, survived for three centuries on psychic vampirism*. The Count de Saint-Germain (d. 1784), an historical figure, lived as a kind of everlasting man. The German writer Johannes Heinrich Cohausen (d. 1750) in his *Hermippus Redivivus*, subtitled, 'The Sage's Triumph Over Old Age and the Grave', gives many other instances, both legendary and historical, of longevity and rejuvenation.

The causes of physical and mental decline and the reasons underlying prolonged vigour and radiant health are still being sought. It is generally agreed that longevity and vitality are hereditary. There appears to be a definite correlation between the ages reached by parents, and the life expectancy of their children. It is also observed that children of young mothers live longer. Again, certain countries, because of their climate, air, soil or water, are conducive to long life.

Innumerable régimes have been advocated for the attainment of the ideal of a long, healthy and active life. It is suggested that the first thing is to stop exposing oneself to agents of 'shortevity' and 'dejuvenation'. Among these, one should avoid excesses of all kinds: overeating, overexertion, overindulgence in alcohol and sex, and completely abstain from drugs and smoking. Psychologically, the emotions to be particularly shunned are jealousy, envy, hatred, malice, lust, anger and any others provoking stress*. More precisely what should be aimed at is a positive mental attitude (*see* mind cure), relaxation, a naturopathic* régime, and moderation in all things.

Methods to be recommended only with caution include injections of glandular and gonadal extract, aphrodisiac drugs, ultraviolet light, cryotherapy, blood-letting, blood transfusion, surgical operations. Unfortunately, most of the modern exponents of rejuvenation therapy seem to have concentrated on these methods, and their results have not had any enduring success, as the following brief outline will show.

In 1889 Charles Brown-Séquard (d. 1894) at the age of 72 gave a lecture before the French Society of Biology describing how he had prepared a solution by grinding up the testicles of young dogs and guineapigs, and after preliminary animal experiments gave himself subcutaneous injections of the solution. He concluded by saying that he had rejuvenated himself by 30 years, and that very day was able to 'pay a visit' to his young wife. His lecture created a sensation, but the success of his treatment was of short duration. His young wife left him, and he died shortly after of a cerebral haemorrhage.

Eugen Steinach (d. 1944) of the Biological Institute of Vienna, grafted the testicles of young rats on to old male rats, and young ovaries on old females, and noted signs of rejuvenation. In 1910 he performed the operation known as vaso-ligation, tying off the vas deferens, or sperm ducts, through which semen leaves the testicles, to increase the blood supply to the testicular cells, and noted a short period of increased vigour. Among the patrons of Steinach's method was Sigmund Freud, father of psychoanalysis.

The Russian surgeon Serge Voronoff (d. 1951), while serving at the court of the khedive of Egypt, noticed that the court eunuchs seemed to age quickly, and concluded that it was because they received no rejuvenating secretion from the male sex glands. On his return to Europe in 1920, he took the testicles from a chimpanzee and grafted them into the groin of a 73-year-old man. Unfortunately this 'monkey-gland' treatment also had only a temporary effect.

Paul Niehans (b. 1884) of Vevey, Switzerland, uses 'fresh-cell therapy' (or cellular therapy) and holds that fresh embryonic genital cells from the organs of a newly-killed animal foetus can revitalize ageing and degenerate tissues of the corresponding organs in human beings. Among his patients were Pope Pius XII, Ibn Saud, Konrad Adenauer, Somerset Maugham, the Aga Khan and Thomas Mann.

The scientist Professor Ana Aslan (b. 1910) of Bucharest advocates the virtues of the drug procaine, which is the scientific name for novocain, the dentist's anaesthetic. She increased the acid content of procaine, which she now calls H3 or Gerovital, and is said to have achieved remarkable results in rejuvenation. Her patients included Mao Tse-tung, Nikita Khrushchev and Bernard Montgomery.

New hope came with the manufacture of synthetic sex hormones in the 1930s. The male sex hormone, testosterone, was found to be beneficial in those deficient in the male hormone, but it could not be widely used in male rejuvenation for fear that it might give rise to cancer as well. The female sex hormone estrogen is given to alleviate distressing changes during the menopause and has only marginal rejuvenative effects.

But hope is far from dead, and like the alchemists of old, today's scientists continue to believe that they will some day produce the 'youth-pill' that will really work.

Brief list of famous long-lived people (from AD 1800)
Adams, John Quincy (d. 1848 aged 81), American president.
Adenauer, Konrad (d. 1967 aged 91), German chancellor
Bessemer, Henry (d. 1898 aged 85), English engineer and inventor
Booth, William (d. 1912 aged 83), founder of the Salvation Army
Buber, Martin (d. 1965 aged 87), Jewish religious philosopher
Carlyle, Thomas (d. 1881 aged 86), Scots writer
Churchill, Winston (d. 1965 aged 91), British Prime Minister
Clemenceau, Georges (d. 1929 aged 88), French Premier
Croce, Benedetto (d. 1952 aged 86), Italian philosopher
Crookes, William (d. 1919 aged 87), English chemist
Degas, Hilaire Germain Edgar (d. 1917 aged 83), French painter
De la Mare, Walter (d. 1956 aged 83), English poet and novelist
Eddy, Mary Baker (d. 1910 aged 89), founder of Christian Science
Edison, Thomas Alva (d. 1931 aged 84), American inventor
Eiffel, Alexandre (d. 1923 aged 91), French engineer
Emerson, Ralph Waldo (d. 1882 aged 80), American essayist and poet
Evans, John Arthur (d. 1941 aged 90), English archaeologist
Fabre, Jean Henri (d. 1915 aged 90), French entomologist
Fechner, Gustav (d. 1887 aged 86), German physicist and philosopher
Forster, Edward Morgan (d. 1970 aged 91), English novelist
Galton, Francis (d. 1911 aged 89), English scientist and eugenist
Gide, André (d. 1951 aged 82), French novelist and literary critic
Gladstone, William Ewart (d. 1898 aged 89), English statesman
Goethe, Johann Wolfgang (d. 1832 aged 83), German writer
Goya, Francisco (d. 1828 aged 82), Spanish painter
Hardy, Thomas (d. 1928 aged 88), English novelist

Herschel, William (d. 1822 aged 84), German-born English astronomer
Hokusai (d. 1849 aged 89), Japanese painter and print-maker
Hooker, Joseph (d. 1911 aged 94), English botanist and explorer
Hoover, Herbert (d. 1964 aged 90), American president
Housman, Laurence (d. 1959 aged 84), English writer
Hugo, Victor (d. 1885 aged 83), French poet and novelist
Humboldt, Alexander von (d. 1859 aged 90), German naturalist
Inge, William Ralph (d. 1954 aged 94), English prelate and scholar
Jefferson, Thomas (d. 1826 aged 83), American president
John XXIII (d. 1963 aged 82), pope
Jung, Carl Gustav (d. 1961 aged 86), Swiss psychologist
Kant, Immanuel (d. 1804 aged 80), German philosopher
Lister, Joseph (d. 1912 aged 85), English surgeon
Maeterlinck, Maurice (d. 1949 aged 87), Belgian dramatist
Mann, Thomas (d. 1955 aged 80), German novelist
Matisse, Henri (d. 1954 aged 86), French painter
Maugham, Somerset (d. 1965 aged 91), English novelist and playwright
Nash, John (d. 1835 aged 83), English architect
Newman, John Henry (d. 1890 aged 89), English cardinal
Paderewski, Ignacy (d. 1941 aged 81), Polish pianist and statesman
Pavlov, Ivan (d. 1936 aged 87), Russian physiologist
Pétain, Henri Philippe (d. 1951 aged 95), French general
Picasso, Pablo (d. 1973 aged 92), Spanish painter
Planck, Max (d. 1947 aged 89), German physicist
Powys, John Cowper (d. 1963 aged 91), English writer
Rubinstein, Artur (b. 1889), Polish-born American pianist
Ruskin, John (d. 1900 aged 81), English writer
Russell, Bertrand (d. 1970 aged 98), English mathematician and philosopher
Samuel, Herbert (d. 1963 aged 93), English Jewish statesman
Shaw, George Bernard (d. 1950 aged 94), Irish playwright
Sherrington, Charles (d. 1952 aged 94), English neurologist
Sibelius, Jean (d. 1957 aged 92), Finnish musician
Spencer, Herbert (d. 1903 aged 83), English sociologist
Strauss, Richard (d. 1949 aged 85), German musician
Stravinsky, Igor (d. 1971 aged 89) Russian-born American musician
Trevelyan, George (d. 1928 aged 90), English historian
Truman, Harry (d. 1972 aged 88), American president
Verdi, Giuseppe (d. 1901 aged 88), Italian operatic composer
Watt, James (d. 1819 aged 83), English inventor
Webster, Noah (d. 1843 aged 85), American lexicographer
Wells, Herbert George (d. 1946 aged 80), English writer
Williams, Ralph Vaughan (d. 1958 aged 86), English composer
Wordsworth, William (d. 1850 aged 80), English poet
Wright, Frank Lloyd (d. 1959 aged 90), American architect.

Books

De Ropp, Robert, *Man Against Aging*, St Martin's Press, New York, 1960.
Ettinger, R. C. W., *The Prospect of Immortality*, Macfadden, New York, 1964.

Goetz-Claren, Wolfgang, *Cellular and Genetic Therapy*, New York, 1966.

Gruman, Gerald, *A History of Ideas About the Prolongation of Life*, American Philosophical Society, Philadelphia, 1966.

Guillerme, Jacques, *Longevity*, Walker, New York, 1957.

Harrington, Alan, *The Immortalist*, Panther Books, London, 1973.

Leyel, C. F., *Elixirs of Life*, Stuart & Watkins, London, 1970.

McGrady, Patrick, *The Youth Doctors*, Arthur Barker, London, 1969.

Maury, Marguerite, *The Secret of Life and Youth*, Macdonald, London, 1964.

Prehoda, Robert W., *Extended Youth: the Promise of Gerontology*, Putnam, New York, 1968.

Trimmer, Eric J., *Rejuvenation: the History of an Idea*, Robert Hale, London, 1967.

Wilson, Robert, *Feminine Forever*, Evans, New York, 1960.

RELIGIOUS THERAPY

Religious therapy is based on the concept of personal reconciliation with a transcendent power that is the ultimate source of holiness, wholeness and healing. There is said to be a religious instinct immanent in the human being, and the repression of this instinct is more detrimental to his wellbeing than the repression of his sexual instincts. Sigmund Freud (d. 1939) spoke of religion as the universal obsessional neurosis of mankind. Man is a dependent and worshipping animal, and if he displaces God, he replaces him with some human and fallible ideal.

Although religion is said to alleviate depression, conflict and a sense of spiritual emptiness, it does not necessarily free a person from unhappiness, or secure him from suffering. Indeed, suffering often forms part of the religious life. Saints have suffered, as we see from the story of their lives.

The factors that disturb men are not such as can be cured by drugs or psychotherapy. They involve the profound perturbations arising from spiritual loneliness and the soul's separation from its source. It is not sufficient to take pills that will restore the balance of the neurohormones, nor to indulge in reveries of free association before a psychoanalyst. Nor even to devote oneself to good works.

Ethics and morality are of Caesar's world, and religion is not a value-system in this sense. The function of religious therapy is not health of mind through better morals, but the restoration of a lost connection. Its ultimate foundations are not human knowledge but tradition, not human understanding but revelation, not reason but faith.

Many modern psychologists believe that much of our mental illness springs from the lack of a religious motivation in life, an absence of spiritual meaning, which manifests in abulia* and angst*. C. G. Jung (d. 1961) said that he had never had an adult patient whose illness was not due to lack of religion.

If religion means reconciliation with God, then what is needed is a conversion, in the New Testament sense of *metanoia*, a 'change of mind', leading to a change of direction Godwards. Religious therapy or counselling takes charge of the conversion process, and involves a reversion to prayer and a return to worship.

249

Books

Braceland, J. (ed.), *Faith, Reason and Modern Psychiatry*, Kennedy, New York, 1955.

Freud, S., *The Future of an Illusion*, Hogarth Press, London, 1961.

Godin, A., *The Pastor as Counsellor*, Holt, Rinehart & Winston, New York, 1965.

Hostie, R., *Pastoral Counselling*, Sheed & Ward, London, 1966.

James, William, *The Varieties of Religious Experience*, Longmans, Green, New York, 1902.

Jung, C. G., *Modern Man in Search of a Soul*, George Routledge, London, 1932.

Mowrer, O. H., *The Crisis in Psychiatry and Religion*, Van Nostrand, New Jersey, 1961.

O'Doherty, E. F. and McGrath, D., *The Priest and Mental Health*, Alba House, New York, 1963.

Rumke, H. C., *The Psychology of Unbelief*, Rockliff, London, 1952.

White, V., *Soul and Psyche*, Collis & Harvill, London, 1960.

Wise, C. A., *Religion in Illness and Health*, New York, 1942.

SCATOTHERAPY

Scatotherapy (Gk. *skatos*, 'filth', 'dung'), is healing by the ingestion or application of substances obtained from or exuded by the body, like faeces, urine, mucus, saliva, sweat, tears, semen, blood, hair, nails, the caul, secundine, afterbirth, and such parts and organs as would normally be regarded as disgusting. Like borboric therapy*, it can amount to a perversion, but sometimes forms part of recognized healing methods, like organotherapy*.

Many aphrodisiacs*, fertility drinks, pregnancy recipes, love philtres and magical remedies of the past and present contain scatological ingredients. Today we know that the bacteria living in all animal bodies release their excretory products into the faeces and urine, which are therefore rich in antibiotic substances. Dung possesses genuine healing enzymes; urine contains an important sex hormone; saliva is known to be prophylactic; sweat has healing, rejuvenating, aphrodisiac and other virtues; tears contain lysozyme, an enzyme which dissolves bacterial colonies.

Every animal produces different antibiotic substances, which are found in its excreta. It has been established that the tiger and the cow differ not only in their appearance and character, but in the hormones they generate and the products they excrete. From earliest times animal dung was used, and still is used, in many parts of the world, for medicative purposes. Externally, ass dung was applied for inflammation; hen dung for burns; hare dung for sagging breasts. Goat dung was rubbed on for teething troubles; crocodile dung applied to the phallus to increase its size; camel dung rubbed into the scalp to make the hair wavy; cat dung to prevent hair loss. Internally, cowdung was taken with wine or water for tuberculosis; goose dung for urinary complaints;

horse dung to aid childbirth; sheep dung for measles and gonorrhoea; wolf dung for catarrh.

Man has his own kind of excrement, which animals can easily distinguish from that of other species. And each individual has his own characteristic stool, with variations in odour, colour, consistency, frequency and timing, depending on race, age, sex, health and diet. As a dog can pick out the bodily smell of its master among millions of other individuals, so it would be possible to distinguish the characteristic discharge of one individual from that of another as surely as a fingerprint, had we the requisite knowledge.

Through the ages human excrement has been widely used in medicinal treatment. The faeces of holy lamas and other revered personages were dried and used as snuff in cases of illness, just as the water in which the guru has washed his mouth is sometimes drunk by his followers. The Ebers papyrus (c. 1630 BC) of ancient Egypt prescribes no less than 50 remedies containing human and animal faeces and urine for various complaints. Such scatotherapeutic prescriptions were recommended by Greek, Roman and medieval physicians for barrenness, impotency, snake-bite, toothache and swellings.

Urine, too, was put to many uses. There is an extensive tradition about the virtues of animal urine. Thus: dog urine restored the colour of one's hair; horse urine, or stale, thickened the hair; cow urine taken internally purified the whole system.

Human urine was said to be particularly valuable, because of its many wonderful properties. Lant, or urine kept in a vessel for a day or two, was applied externally for chilblains. Fresh, it was free from bacteria, and a good antiseptic, and if rubbed into the gums it relieved toothache. Taken internally it was a restorative, purgative, stimulant and tonic, as well as a mild intoxicant. The ammonia in it neutralized acids, and it was therefore good for acid-forming diseases. For men, the drinking of urine was believed to improve virility, a belief that may have been substantiated by Dr Butenandt's discovery in 1931 that male urine contains the active male hormone androsterone. For girls, a cupful of urine induces menstruation. Women used to be given a draught of their own urine for hysteria*, and during childbirth would drink the urine of their husbands to hasten delivery.

Until the end of the last century urine used to be drunk all over Europe for malaria; and until the middle of the present century in parts of rural England it was taken as a prophylactic against boils and carbuncles (Rawcliffe, 1959, p. 213). Lye tea, made of human urine diluted with lime water, was until recently a popular remedy for colds. Indeed, some naturopaths still recommended a wineglassful of urine before meals for arthritis and rheumatism (Powell, 1975, p. 258).

The Biblical verse, 'He that believeth on me, out of his belly shall flow rivers of living water' (John 7:38) has sometimes been interpreted as scriptural authority for the virtues of urine as a vitalizing element second only to blood. Following this interpretation, the murderer John George Haig (hanged 1949) used to drink the blood of his victims as well as his own urine.

Although blood is not strictly a scatological substance, it is, like saliva and semen, treated as such once it leaves the body. Blood has a deeply mystical significance; it is regarded as the quintessence of all the 'wet elements', and its presence is assumed in many situations. Thus wine is the blood of the grape; fruit-juice or sap is the blood of the tree; milk is blood filtered through the breasts; semen is blood filtered through the testes.

Warrior tribes in ancient days made it a practice to drink the blood of their foes, especially fallen chieftains, in order to imbibe their valour and courage. In a number of primitive communities blood is still given to the weak and ailing to restore them to vigour. Here again, belief in the vitalizing potency of blood might appear to have received confirmation in the blood transfusion of modern surgical and hospital practice.

The smell, taste and substance of blood are supposed to be highly aphrodisiac. Blood heightens sexual excitement, increases male potency, and ensures female fertility. We are told that Faustina, wife of Marcus Aurelius, anxious to have a child, drank the warm blood of a dying gladiator and then shared her husband's bed. She at once became pregnant, bringing forth Commodus (b. AD 161), who later as emperor became notorious for his cruelty.

In ancient Rome human blood was prescribed as a cure for epilepsy and was best taken while still warm. Epileptics were, therefore, stationed near the exit gates of the public arena and drank the blood of slain gladiators as they were dragged out. In medieval Europe epileptics were made to drink a draught of warm blood caught gushing from the neck of a decapitated victim.

According to the physicians of the schools of Salerno in Italy (founded AD 860) and Montpellier in France (founded 1130), the two most famed seats of European medical learning in the early Middle Ages, human blood, especially the blood of virgins, of which only a few drops were sufficient, was excellent for a wide number of ills. The French king Lois XI (d. 1483) and Pope Innocent VIII (d. 1492) in their old age were both said to have been restored by drinking wine mixed with an ounce of blood taken from young men (see shunamism). Even the smell of blood was considered effective. The medieval hermetic philosopher Artephius (d. 1150) used to distil a spirit made from the blood of boys and inhale the fumes, and it was to this that he ascribed his long life.

Menstrual blood, however, was regarded as defiling, poisonous and deadly for crops, vineyards, orchards and all foods. At the same time it was thought to have certain curative properties. Pliny (d. AD 79) said that the application of menstrual blood cured gout, warts, lumbago, sore throat and erysipelas. Mixed with bread and eaten, it cured tertian fever. Baths with menstrual blood added to the water cured leprosy*.

But above all it was regarded as an extremely potent elixir that could be absorbed either by penile imbibition during intercourse, or orally. A woman's menstrual blood added to a man's drink, was supposed to strengthen his sexual drive and arouse in him strange lusts for that woman. Until the eighteenth century it was not unknown in Germany for a woman to mix some of her menstrual blood into the food and drink of her husband or lover to kindle the amorous flame.

The most potent and indeed dangerous of all menstrual blood was the menarche, the first day's flow of the first menstruation of a virgin girl. It was never to be used for any purpose except by a person who knew how to handle it. Next in potency came the first day's flow of any woman, the potency decreasing after that, with the blood of the fourth day being very mild.

Another widely prevalent form of scatotherapy is spermepotation (Lat. *epoto*, 'suck up, swallow'), the drinking of the male sperm. The semen of bulls, horses, donkeys, rams, goats and other animals noted for their virility figured in many religious and social ceremonies of ancient Egypt, India, Africa and Australia. It was generally obtained by masturbating the animal.

Human semen, the vital essence of the male, has been recognized in all occult lore as a highly charged liquid, replete with magical substances and sinful to waste. Fresh human semen was said to be eagerly sought by vampires, witches and succubae, who would extract it during *congressus subtilis*. In Europe the semen ejaculated by a man at the moment of his hanging was believed to be particularly powerful, and was sometimes collected straight after emission, to be used as an ingredient in magical potions. If it fell to the ground it was said to produce the mandrake plant.

Human semen was also often used in love philtres. From it were prepared a variety of potions and elixirs which, when given to a woman, threw her into an inextinguishable frenzy of love for the man yielding it, having on her the same effect as a woman's menstrual blood was supposed to have on a man.

Drinking semen for strength was very common in all countries. Australian Aborigines regarded it as a supernatural 'medicine', which they administered to the feeble members of the community. It was best obtained fresh, before exposure, whence the practice of penilingus or penis-sucking. In France and Germany fresh semen was held to be a specific for wasting diseases and epilepsy*, and for the restoration of flagging vitality. Fresh semen was also reported to be a wonderful beauty aid for the complexion. This notion was once so widespread that in the fourteenth century Bishop Burchard inveighed against all women who swallowed their husband's semen to make themselves sexually attractive and exciting.

Men sometimes injest their own sperm, and this practice too has an ancient lineage. An Egyptian papyrus records how the god Atum concluded an act of masturbation with the words, 'I ejaculated into my own mouth.' Hindu tantric texts emphasize that one's own semen should not be wasted but absorbed: 'The plough (penis) and the bulls (testes) the wise man will use for ploughing his own land and sowing his own seed, so that he can eat his own fruit.' Sperm can be absorbed internally by encratic practices such as asceticism or *coitus reservatus*, or by concentrating to ejaculation during certain yogic asanas, such as variations of the headstand, which have been devised specially for this purpose.

John Hunter (d. 1793), a famous Scottish surgeon, observed that semen when held for a time in the mouth produces a warmth similar to that of spices, a fact which may have strengthened belief in its stimulant properties. Some authorities, including Havelock Ellis (d. 1939), consider semen to be a nourishing substance.

Yet another scatological medicament was obtained from mummy, the material derived from a dried or embalmed human corpse, the most valuable being that imported from Mizraim (ancient Egypt). The custom of using mummy prevailed from very early times in many parts of the world, and survived in Europe till at least the eighteenth century. Sir Thomas Browne (d. 1682) in his *Hydriotaphia* makes a reference to it: 'Mummy is become merchandise, Mizraim cures wounds, and Pharaoh is sold for balsams.' There is still a demand among witches and the like for genuine powdered Egyptian mummy, and it can be obtained, among other places, in certain New York pharmacies, at 40 dollars an ounce (Harris and Weeks, 1973, p. 92).

Books

Bourke, J. G., *Scatologic Rites of All Nations*, Lowdermilk, Washington, DC, 1891.

Dawson, W. R., 'Mummy as a Drug', in *The Bridle of Pegasus*, London, 1930.

Eisler, Robert, *Man Into Wolf: an Anthropological Interpretation of Sadism, Masochism and Lycanthropy*, Routledge & Kegan Paul, London, 1951.

Harris, J. E. and Weeks, K. R., *X-Raying the Pharaohs*, Macdonald, London, 1973.

McLaughlin, Terence, *Coprophilia, or a Peck of Dirt*, Cassell, London, 1971.

Powell, Eric, *The Natural Home Physician*, 2nd edn, Health Science Press, Hengiscote, North Devon, 1975.

Rawcliffe, D. H., *Illusions and Delusions of the Supernatural and the Occult*, Dover, New York, 1959.

Seeman, Bernard, *The River of Life: the Story of Man's Blood from Magic to Science*, Museum Press, London, 1962.

Thorwald, Jürgen, *Science and Secrets of Early Medicine*, Thames & Hudson, London, 1962.

Walker, Benjamin, *Hindu World: an Encyclopedic Outline of Hinduism*, Allen & Unwin, London and Praeger, New York, 1968.

Wall, O. A., *Sex and Sex Worship*, London, 1919.

SCHIZOPHRENIA

(Gk. *schizein*, 'to split'; *phrēn*, 'mind'), a form of mental illness embracing a wide variety of incapacitating psychotic conditions. It was formerly called *dementia praecox* (insanity of youth), because it usually makes its appearance in young people and commonly afflicts the shy and oversensitive type. A person suffering from dementia praecox was known as a precocious dement, and his deterioration was thought to be irreversible. Today one variety of schizophrenia is still called *hebephrenia* (Gk. *hēbē*, 'youth'), because it begins in late childhood, its symptoms being arrested mental development, silly and senseless mannerisms and carelessness in personal appearance. Such cases are often tube-fed and have to be carried.

Other symptoms, which indeed are said to characterize different types of schizophrenia, are *paranoia*, in which the patient has delusions of grandeur (popularly called megalomania) or of persecution. He may speak and behave quite lucidly, but what he says and does indicates that another world has intruded quite distinctly into the rational world in which he lives. In still another form of the illness the patient develops *catatonia*, when he is plunged into a state of stupor, repeatedly performs strange actions for hours on end; or sits and stares into space, and remains frozen in peculiar attitudes. It has been remarked that the bizarre poses of catatonia seem to possess an archetypal character, and often resemble the more extravagant asanas or fixed postures of yoga. Paranoia is sometimes regarded as the active form, and catatonia the passive form, of schizophrenia. Because schizophrenia can come on suddenly and develop in a few days, it was earlier thought to be a type of possession.

The main characteristics of schizophrenia are withdrawal from normal contact with people; extreme introversion; autistic thought, or fantasizing; a loss of drive and initiative; and a total lack of emotional involvement with the outside world of reality. Sometimes the behaviour is completely irrational, as when the patient laughs for no reason, or smiles as if at some private joke. He is inclined to echopraxia, in which he imitates the actions of others. He fails to respond to questions and has a compulsion to echolalia, that is, he tends to repeat a word or phrase heard by him or that occurs to him, often with rhyming or onomatopoeic variations. Hallucinations are common. He is assailed by strange, often menacing voices. His food tastes strange. His time-sense becomes distorted. He has feelings of physical and mental interference going on inside him, and a sense of depersonalization*. Thoughts refuse to obey his will; logical thinking becomes difficult or impossible. Sometimes he is overcome by irrational, nameless and overwhelming fear*. There is an awful sense of inner tension.

Often there is an obsessional monomania*. Physicians of earlier times reported symptoms in their patients that clearly indicated schizophrenia. Celsus (fl. AD 50) wrote of a man who was afraid to drink because he thought he was a clay brick and that the liquid would dissolve him. Galen (d. AD 201) describes an obsessed person who thought he was Atlas bearing the burden of the world on his back. Alexander of Tralles (c. AD 360), a philosopher and physician of Lydia, describes one of his patients who bound up her middle finger fearing that the world would collapse if she bent it. Fridericus Flacht (d. 1630), of the university of Basel, gave the case of the man who imagined his buttocks were made of crystal, and as far as possible he did whatever he had to in a standing position, fearing that if he inadvertently sat down too quickly his buttocks would splinter into a thousand pieces. In our own day we have cases of patients who imagine that people are trying to blow poison gas at them from another planet, or that someone in a far-off country is conspiring to carry them off to the moon. There are also the classic cases of those who believe they are Cleopatra or Napoleon.

Like hysteria* and epilepsy*, there is no generally accepted definition of schizophrenia. A well-known psychiatrist, Dr Thomas Szasz, held that schizophrenia is 'a pseudoproblem such as that of ether in yesterday's physics'. The important questions concerning the diagnosis*, prognosis, aetiology* and therapy* are still largely unanswered. Schizophrenia is a disintegration of the psychic functions. The disease resists pharmacological or empirical treatment. It is a functional disturbance of the mind, not readily amenable to physiological, biochemical, histopathological or bacteriological treatment. But treatment continues to be rather drastic, and includes brain surgery, electric shocks, and drugs of high potency (see asylum).

It is said that schizophrenia and epilepsy are 'opposite'* diseases, and a person suffering from one never suffers from the other. Again, schizophrenia being a disease of introversion, is the opposite of hysteria, a disease of extra-version.

Occultists believe that the roots of schizophrenia rise from a pathological condition of the etheric double.

Books

Arieti, Silvano, *Interpretation of Schizophrenia*, Brunner, New York, 1955.

Auerback, Alfred (ed.), *Schizophrenia: An Integrated Approach*, New York, 1959.

Bellak, Leopold (ed.), *Schizophrenia*, Logos, New York, 1958.

Bleuler, Eugen, *Dementia Praecox or the Group of Schizophrenias*, International Universities Press, New York, 1958.

Jackson, Don (ed.), *The Etiology of Schizophrenia*, Basic Books, New York, 1960.

Kasanin, Jacob S. (ed.), *Language and Thought in Schizophrenia*, University of California Press, 1944.

Kraepelin, Emil, *Dementia Praecox and Paraphrenia*, London, 1919.

Roheim, Geza, *Magic and Schizophrenia*, International Universities Press, New York, 1955.

Rosen, George, *Madness in Society*, Routledge & Kegan Paul, London, 1967.

Searles, H., *The Non-Human Environment in Schizophrenia*, International Universities Press, New York, 1960.

Sullivan, H. S., *Schizophrenia as a Human Process*, Norton, New York, 1962.

Szasz, Thomas, *The Myth of Mental Illness*, Harper, New York, 1961.

Wing, J. K. and Brown, G. W., *Institutionalism and Schizophrenia*, Cambridge, 1970.

SEXOPHOBIA

Sexophobia, or the fear of the opposite sex, and especially of sexual relations in any form (coitophobia), is found in individuals, communities and religions. It springs from the idea that sex is dirty, sinful and dangerous. It can cause pain and mutilation, lead to venereal disease and endanger one's spiritual welfare.

In the man, it may be associated with the *vagina dentata*, 'toothed vulva', which will bite off the male organ during intercourse, and manifests in misogyny or hatred of women, and can cause impotence. In woman, it may be due to an earlier experience of rape, resulting in fear of the *penis aculeatus*, 'pointed phallus', which will tear and prick during defloration and sexual intercourse, and manifests in misandry or hatred of men, in frigidity and in symptoms like vaginismus, in which muscular spasms develop in the vagina making coitus difficult and painful and often impossible.

Like eating, the act of coition is regarded in many communities as bristling with all kinds of occult hazards and full of pitfalls. Many primitive peoples think that coitus weakens a man and exposes him to attack by spirits. Certain ascetic sects have taught that coition, which naturally leads to ejaculation and the expenditure of seminal fluid, is weakening. Aristotle (d. 322 BC) said that every act of coition was a step towards baldness and general debilitation. Zoroastrians and Moslems are enjoined to call on the name of God before attempting the act of intercourse, as a safeguard against its many perils. In Finland certain people believe that a man after copulation is infected with an emanation issuing from the woman, termed *pezh*, which is not only harmful but highly contagious. Even today there are individuals who believe that sexual intercourse impairs the eyesight, weakens the spine, dilutes the blood, enfeebles the system and shortens life.

The idea that sex is morally reprehensible and spiritually injurious and sinful, is found in various sects among the Jews, Christians, Moslems, Hindus and others. Intercourse is a matter of shame, and tolerated only because it is procreative. Some indeed care little about progeny, and abhor children as the fruit of sin. Ascetic communities, past and present, have believed that sexual relations are contaminating and should be avoided. Jain yogis of India say that sex desire is like a fever that brings delirium and can never result in true satisfaction. It only leads to more desire, destroys tranquillity and soils the purity of the soul.

An old Tibetan tradition says that in the beginning men and women were without sexual desire, but were oppositely charged with an inner light. Desire for union was satisfied by looking, and the light from the male entered and impregnated the female womb. But men degenerated and sought to obtain satisfaction by touch, thus creating the sexual instinct, which immediately extinguished the inner light, for the two are incompatible. Sexuality is now a material and animal activity, far removed from its spiritual origin and destiny.

A number of gnostic and neo-Platonist sects of the early centuries of the Christian era regarded the sexual act with revulsion, because in their view it brought man to the level of the beast and, worse still, jeopardized his future life. Woman was a degraded being, and man's contact with her in this intimate fashion thoroughly polluted his spirit. The encratites held that a married woman could not enter the kingdom of heaven. In the apocryphal *Acts of St John*, a gnostic work, it is said, 'Union between man and woman is a crime, and a woman should rather seek death than perform such an abomination.'

Among the church fathers, Origen (d. 254) felt very strongly in the matter, and declared, 'Matrimony is impure and unholy; a means of sensual passion'; and in order to escape the lure of sensual temptation he castrated himself. Another theologian, Gregory of Nyssa (d. 395), lamented Adam's disobedience, but for which, he said, we would have lived in virgin purity, and some simple mode of vegetation would have been the means of peopling the earth.

From earliest Christian times down to recent days, original sin was believed to be the sexual union of Adam and Eve. According to St Augustine (d. 430), the consequence of original sin was carnal desire (*concupiscentia carnalis*), the lust of the flesh. 'If Adam and Eve had not sinned,' said St Augustine in his *City of God*, 'they would still have procreated children, but without lust. Their genital organs would have followed the dictates of their will, just like their limbs.'

Certain theologians of the early church taught that sexual intercourse even for the married was an odious expedient. The act was necessary to fulfil the divine ordinance to increase and multiply, but the pleasure accompanying it was condemned as inspired by Satan. Contact with the female body, therefore, had to be reduced to the minimum. In the Middle Ages one result of this extreme view was the invention of the *chemise cagoule*, a sort of heavy nightdress with a suitably placed hole, through which the husband could impregnate his wife while avoiding all other contact.

In his *Religio Medici*, Sir Thomas Browne (d. 1682) wrote:

I could be content that we might procreate like trees, without conjunction, or that there were any way to perpetuate the world without this trivial and vulgar way of coition. It is the foolishest act a wise man commits in all his life; nor is there anything that will more deject his cooled imagination, when he shall consider what an odd and unworthy piece of folly he hath committed. I speak not in prejudice, nor am I averse from that sweet sex, but naturally amorous of all that is beautiful.

The German philosopher Arthur Schopenhauer (d. 1860), who in later life became a confirmed misogynist, thought that sexual intercourse was 'an act which on sober reflection one recalls with repugnance and in a more elevated mood even with disgust'. The famous Danish thinker and existentialist, Søren Kierkegaard (d. 1855), agreed with Origen:

It is an abominable lie to say that marriage pleases God. From the Christian viewpoint it is a criminal act, and what makes it even more odious is that by this very crime an innocent being is brought forth into that community of criminals which is human life.

William Thomas Stead (d. 1912), a well-known writer of the last generation, felt that the sexual act was 'monstrously indecent' and he could not understand how any self-respecting man and woman could face each other in the daylight after spending the night together.

Allan Bennett (d. 1924), a Scots occultist and Buddhist adept, expressed the opinion that a god who devised such a bestial and degrading method of propagating the species was a god delighting in loathsomeness and not a god worthy of being worshipped.

Books

Eisler, Robert, *Man Into Wolf*, Routledge & Kegan Paul, London, 1951.
Eliade, Mircea, *The Two and the One*, Harvil Press, London, 1961.
Fielding, W. J., *Strange Customs of Courtship and Marriage*, London, 1961.
Hirsch, E. W., *Sexual Fear*, New York, 1950.
Lacarrière, J., *The God Possessed*, Allen & Unwin, London, 1963.
Ploss, H. H. and Bartels, M. and P., *Woman*, 3 vols, ed. by E. J. Dingwall, London, 1935.
Stern, Karl, *The Flight From Woman*, Allen & Unwin, London, 1966.
Tabori, Paul, *Secret and Forbidden*, New English Library, London, 1969.
Vaerting, M., *The Dominant Sex*, Allen & Unwin, London, 1923.

SEX THERAPY

The treatment of diseases, especially nervous and mental maladies, by means of sexual activity, familiar to Chinese, Hindu, Greek and other physicians from very early times. The underlying idea was that continued quiescence of the sex organs, and prolonged retention and immobility of semen and other sexual fluids, the absence of orgasm and the general denial of organic release, were deleterious to health and wellbeing. Any form of sex activity was better than none for the normal individual, although the most satisfying therapeutically was heterosexual coitus.

Sigmund Freud (d. 1939) records how once when Jean Charcot and Josef Breuer, the psychologists, and Chrobak, one of the most eminent gynaecologists in Vienna, were discussing their patients, they all agreed that their disturbed mental conditions were due to sexual frustration. Breuer spoke of them as secret desires; Charcot had said, 'C'est toujours la chose genitale, toujours' ('It is always the genital thing, always'); Chrobak concurred, adding that the prescription for such a malady, which however could not be ordered was, 'Penis normalis dosim repetatur' ('a normal penis in repeated doses').

Love-making has been described as 'an exchange of electricity', and such an exchange is a fundamental aid in reducing mental tension. Men and women need to be sexually stimulated at regular intervals, as this keeps them healthy both physically and mentally. Normal people need the vital exchange they find from contact in each other's bodies, in each other's auras, in the contact of lips and sexual organs, in the exchange of sexual and other fluids. Men need the release that comes from emission, and women from orgasm. Women, in the occult view, derive great benefit from semen, and men from the emissions of the female sex glands.

Early texts on the subject prescribe various methods of intercourse that bring specific benefits, and warn against the dangers of using the wrong techniques and postures at the wrong times. Chinese, Hindu and Arab sexologists recommend different methods of intercourse at different times of day or night and different seasons of the year. There are specific benefits to be derived from face to face and rear to face intercourse; from a woman mounting the man; from oral and anal intercourse.

According to the Chinese, the best time for intercourse is during the waxing moon, especially from the new moon to the first quarter. Intercourse should be performed at night, and the erect penis should be left in the vagina for at least fifteen minutes before the usual coital movements begin. This causes the skin of both partners to glow, gives vitality to the man and great beauty to the woman, increases the dimensions of the virile member, and makes the woman's breasts firm and round. Skin diseases and eye ailments disappear with continued practice of this mode of intercourse.

Hindu sexologists prescribe different methods of coitus and coital postures for different ailments. All men over 21 are advised to be careful during intercourse with a young woman, as young females tend to vampirize and absorb a great deal of male energy without giving anything in return. Men suffering from a plethora of blood and excessive fatness may use young girls but with great caution and in moderation. The fluids of young girls are sharp and hot and weaken the sexual potency of the partner, and can cause a number of mental and physical maladies. For every occasion and for all types of men, a mature woman is the best sexual companion. The ideal is a woman between 30 and 40.

According to the Arab expert Sheikh Nefzawi (d. 1520), intercourse performed while standing affects the knee-joints and causes nervous shivering; performed sideways it predisposes the system to gout and sciatica. Allowing a woman to bestride you affects the heart. Nefzawi further adds that one should not mount a woman fasting as it causes backache, reduces vigour and weakens the eyes. One should not leave the member inside after ejaculation or the result might be gallstones, softening of the spine and inflammation of the lungs. Cancer will result if one washes the member immediately after ejaculation.

Books

Bakan, David, *Sigmund Freud and the Jewish Mystical Tradition*, Van Nostrand, New York, 1958.
Chaklader, H. C., *Studies in Vatsyayana's Kamasutra*, Calcutta, 1929.
Gillan, Patricia and Richard, *Sex Therapy Today*, Open Books, London, 1976.
Gulik, R. R. van, *Sexual Life in Ancient China*, Brill, Leiden, 1961.
Walker, Benjamin, *Encyclopedia of Esoteric Man*, Routledge & Kegan Paul, London, and Stein & Day, New York, 1977.
Walton, A. H. (ed.), *The Perfumed Garden of Shaykh Nefzawi*, Pantheon Books, London, 1963.

SHUNAMISM

Shunamism, or shunamitism, is the restoration of an old person's vigour by close association with young people. It is named after the girl who ministered to King David in his old age in order to rejuvenate him. The Bible relates that the king was stricken in years and 'gat no heat', and his physicians decided to get a virgin for him 'to lie in his bosom that he may get heat'. They searched for and found a fair damsel, Abishag the Shunammite, who cherished the king and served him, but the king did not have intercourse with her (1 Kings 1:4).

The idea behind this story is one of great antiquity, based on the belief that the breath, perspiration, heat, body odours and physical contact of the young can restore the vitality of the aged. This notion was current among the Egyptians, Babylonians, Greeks, Romans and Chinese. Roman chroniclers speak of a man named Hermippus (L. Claudius Hermippus), who when he reached the age of 70, and feeling that the years were beginning to tell, cut himself off completely from all his aged companions, surrounding himself and mixing and playing only with active and healthy youngsters. The inscription on his marble tombstone, long extant and long commented upon, declared, after dedication to Aesculapius and Sanitas, that he lived 115 years and 5 days by the 'perspiration (exhalations) of young virgins, causing great wonder to all physicians'.

Laurent states that 'practically every important king and noble from medieval up to modern times has at some time or other essayed this elixir of life'. Frederick Barbarossa (d. 1190), Hohenstaufen emperor, in his old age embraced young boys and held them close to his stomach and hips in order to savour and absorb their energy. Rudolf I (d. 1291) of Hapsburg in his illness enjoined his nobles and courtiers to bring him their daughters whom he would hold in his arms for a few moments and kiss, declaring that he thus drew unto himself some of their energy and youthful spirits. It is recorded that when Pope Innocent VIII (d. 1492) lay dying at the age of 60, a Hebrew physician proposed to rejuvenate him, and selected three healthy boys to stay near him and stroke him. The Italian historian Rodocanachi said that the pope had a transfusion from the lads who were paid a ducat each for the blood.

The Renaissance physician Marsilio Ficino (d. 1499) held that if men are refreshed and fortified by the sight and smell of flowers, how much more would they be rejuvenated and their drooping spirits revived by association with young girls through imbibing the fragrant odours and healthy aura given out by them. He suggested that aged people should drink blood 'in the manner of leeches' from the freshly opened veins of young volunteers.

Francis Bacon (d. 1626) in his *Sylva Sylvarum* says:

> The spirits of young people can restore vitality to an aged body and keep it in good health for a long time. It has been observed that old men who spend much time in the company of youths live long, for their spirits emerge strengthened from such contacts.

His contemporary, Robert Burton (d. 1640) wrote:

> The heat of love can thaw the frozen affections of ancient men, dissolve the ice of age, and so far inable them, though they be sixty years of age above the girdle, to be scarce thirty beneath.

Thomas Sydenham (d. 1689), 'the English Hippocrates', 'warmed' his patients with young boys and kittens. The Dutch physician Hermann Boerhaave (d. 1739) saved the life of a German prince by advising him to sleep between two young girls. It is said that Mohandas Gandhi (d. 1948), the Indian politician and reformer, sometimes 'slept chastely in bed with young girls' to give him strength during his long fasts (Garrison, 1972, p. 65).

Among the aristocracy of eighteenth-century Europe, recourse to what is now called gerocomy was in vogue, both in Paris and London, for the rehabilitation of the victims of old age. In Paris the most notorious house for this purpose was kept by Madame H. Janus, as she was called. Special agents were sent out of Paris into the provinces to recruit the girls, and there were always about forty to fifty virgins available for her clients. In her palatial establishment Madame Janus's 'pupils' lived in their own rooms, ate the healthiest food, took daily physical exercise, and above all had to remain virgin. They were very well paid.

The clients consisted mainly of old men and impotent young men, but also others who felt jaded and in need of freshening up, among them dukes, marshals and merchant princes. Each client was required to deposit a large sum of money which was forfeited if he deflowered any of the girls put at his disposal. He was given an aromatic bath, then massaged and dried, his mouth muzzled, and he was then put into bed with two nude virgins, one blonde and one brunette, so placed that their bodies were in contact with his.

The girls served him thus for one week, and were then replaced by a fresh pair. The first pair were allowed to replenish their energies by resting for two weeks, after which they were brought into service again. Usually three couples of virgins were necessary for one man. A girl lasted for only three years, after which she was returned intact to her parents with her large earnings.

By the middle of the eighteenth century London, too, had such resorts, of which the best maintained was that of Miss Anna Fawkland. It consisted of three 'temples' named Aurora (served by virgins between 11 and 16), Flora (for regular prostitutes) and the Mysteries (for 'secret and unheard-of debaucheries'). The temple of Aurora received only impotent men over 60, and was conducted in almost the same manner as the Parisian establishment, except that the girls graduated in time to the temple of Flora and then to the temple of the Mysteries. Lord Cornwallis and Lord Buckingham were among the regular visitors to this temple of platonic love, sleeping nude beside the girls and 'absorbing their virgin nourishment'.

Occultists reject the claims of shunamism. The attempt to rejuvenate King David failed, for the king died soon after the experiment. Turkish sultans and oriental monarchs surrounded themselves with youthful beauties and yet were impotent before they reached the age of 40, and could hardly rise to any occasion without the aid of powerful aphrodisiacs. Close contact with virgins can only arouse the final spark in a dying ember.

Besides, shunamite practices have their hazards. Growing boys and girls have a natural faculty for taking in energy from their surroundings, and old men who are in close proximity with them, far from absorbing the vigour of youth, are themselves vampirized by the strong indrawing powers of youth (*see* psychic vampirism). Older people who are in constant close contact with teenagers show rapid signs of debilitation.

But it is not only a dangerous practice, it is a shameful one, and an aged man should think twice before he attempts to batten on the youthful vigour of juveniles. As Robert Burton (d. 1640) concludes, 'It is most odious when an old acherontic dizard, that hath one foot in the grave, shall flicker after a lusty young wench that is blithe and bonny.'

Young and immature people are like unripe and sour fruit, and certainly not the proper diet for an aged person. Besides, young people who are aware of the purpose for which they are being used would loathe and despise the old and probably be revolted at the sight of their sagging flesh and doddering limbs. Whatever benefits might accrue from association with fresh beauties would be more than offset by this humiliating knowledge.

There is indeed a psychological benefit in being surrounded by beauty, but this can be attained by less obnoxious means than using a living bridge in an attempt to cross the gulf from senility to vigour.

Books

Abse, Dannie, *Medicine on Trial*, Aldus Books, London, 1967.
Bloch, Iwan, *Odoratus Sexualis*, Panurge Press, New York, 1934.
Bloch, Ivan, *Sexual Life in England*, Corgi Books, London, 1965.
Comfort, Alex, *The Process of Ageing,* Weidenfeld & Nicolson, London, 1965.
Garrison, Omar, *Tantra: the Yoga of Sex*, Academy Editions, London, 1972.
Laurent, E. and Nagour, P., *Magica Sexualis*, Falstaff Press, New York, 1934.

SLEEP THERAPY

Although we spend about a third of our lives in sleeping, very little is known about the true cause and purpose of sleep. In the words of Dr Gustav Eckstein, 'Eighty sleep theories have come and gone.' Some have suggested that we sleep because our brain manufactures a hypnotoxin which makes us sleep. If so, this substance has not yet been found. The nearest the psychologists have got to an interpretation is that we seem to need the safety-valve of dreams to release the tensions built up while we are awake.

A régime of good sleep is a certain remedy for a great many mental ills. Long-lived people sleep well, and it is thought that a proper quota of sleep can stall the ageing process. Sleep stimulates the natural restorative processes in the body, and so postpones the advent of ageing. The findings of the Soviet Academy of Medical Sciences after long experiments on animals, confirmed that prolonged sleep may play a paramount role in warding off senility. Several old-age symptoms, such as lowered muscle-tone, loss of the sex instinct and falling hair, were eliminated by artificially induced sleep.

Sleep is essential to wellbeing, and continued sleeplessness will eventually lead to physical illness and ultimately to insanity. One of the worst forms of punishment inflicted in the Middle Ages was tortura insomnia or enforced sleeplessness, still used in modern brainwashing techniques.

It has been found that when a person stays awake or is forced to stay awake, after 24 hours he becomes irritable, his head aches, his eyes burn and itch. After 48 hours he becomes touchy, takes offence at imaginary slights, feels a tight band about the head. After 65 hours his vision becomes blurred, he begins to hallucinate and see things. One subject felt cobwebs on his hands and face and vainly tried to wipe them off; another saw hair in his milk and refused to drink it; a third felt the floor heaving and undulating. Objects shift, their size expands and contracts; haloes and fogs appear around things. After 80 hours there are thinking disorders, and strange auditory hallucinations, as of someone muttering, whispering or jabbering, and also visual hallucinations of forms that are not present. After 96 hours psychotic symptoms develop, together with a sense of depersonalization*. The record for staying awake for a normal person is 10 days. Much of the data on the effects of insomnolence has been obtained at wakathons, where volunteers are kept awake for experimental purposes.

When a person misses his sleep, he makes up for it when he does have a chance to sleep, by a spate of dreaming, much more so than usual. If he is forced to keep awake, he tries to restore the loss by fleeting stolen naps called 'lapses' or 'microsleeps'. Each lapse lasts a fraction of a second, but in that time, as in regular sleep, the eyelids droop, the heartbeat slows down and there is a brief period of blankness with wisps of dream. Such microsleeps cannot be a substitute for real sleep, but are better than no sleep at all.

In an effort to improve the quality of sleep and allow patients with chronic insomnia to get more rest, all kinds of experiments have been tried with the aid of drugs, gas, music, electrical manipulation, and so on. One method is sleeping while immersed in warm saline water to achieve a kind of weightlessness to counteract the stressful efforts of gravity. Still another is an 'equalizing pressure chamber', which permits the muscles employed in breathing to relax, while allowing the physiological concomitants of breathing to be continued.

But all such methods are inferior to, and no substitute for, natural, restful sleep, in quiet surroundings, without noise or music, and emphatically without drugs, the reason being that all induced methods interfere with the natural dream cycle.

Modern sleep therapy is especially concerned with dreams, about which we know even less than we do about sleep. But the close connection between dreaming and mental health is very clearly established. We do not understand the 'crazy' nature of our dreams, but we do know that the distortion is part of the dreaming process. As one scientist put it, sleeping permits us to go safely insane for a short time every night of our lives.

Dreams rest the brain, for paradoxically the brain is extremely active when we are not dreaming. And natural sleep provides us with the opportunity for dreaming. The effect of drugs is disastrous, since all drugs, including sleeping-pills, barbiturates, alcohol, tranquillizers, reserpine, amphetamine and LSD inhibit dream periods. They are dream-depressants and, therefore, harmful. It is virtually impossible to get more than two or three hours of natural, dreamful sleep while under the influence of such chemical aids. Whereas sleep eliminates certain brain toxins, drugs put them back. Anxiety*, fear* and tension also reduce dreaming periods, and, like drugs, both symptomize and accelerate mental illness.

Books

Eckstein, Gustav, *The Body Has a Head*, Collins, London, 1971.

Giles, L., *Sleep*, Bobbs-Merrill, New York, 1938.

Kleitman, O. N., *Sleep and Wakefulness*, University of Chicago Press, 1963.

Koella, W. P., *Sleep, Its Nature and Physiological Organization*, Thomas, Springfield, Illinois, 1967.

Korth, Leslie, *The Healing Sleep*, Health Science Press, London, 1964.

Murray, E., *Sleep, Dreams and Arousal*, New York, 1965.

Wolstenholme, G. E. W. and O'Connor, M. (eds), *The Nature of Sleep*, Churchill, London, 1960.

Zubek, J. P. (ed.), *Sensory Deprivation: Fifteen Years of Research*, Appleton-Century-Crofts, New York, 1969.

SOCIOPSYCHOSIS

Sociopsychosis reflects the spiritual malaise that permeates society as a whole. It is the pathology not of individuals, but of communities, nations and, indeed, historical epochs. Alternative terms are socioneurosis, ethnopathology, sociatry (now used principally for the study of institutions for social care, like hospitals and asylums) and sociopathology (not to be confused with the study of the sociopath or psychopath).

Although starting as an investigation into personality disorders of the individual in society, sociopsychosis has now developed into a vast study of the unhealthy attitudes communicated to individuals by a sick society. This is based on the belief in the reciprocal relationship between the ills of the individual and of the society in which he lives. According to certain psychiatrists, a hospital, for example, can be treated as a sick organization, and modern society has many features of a hospital writ large. Individuals become almost helpless victims of a combination of circumstances, political, national and sociological, that are no longer within their power to change. In the words of a London graffito: 'Do not adjust your common sense; there is a fault in society', and it is this fault that represents the sociopsychosis with which we are now becoming familiar.

The chief sociopsychotic symptoms may be indicated by a brief analysis of the main areas of social collapse. Statistics for this purpose are mostly taken from America, and sometimes more specifically from California, on the ground that the problems of California today become the problems of the rest of the USA tomorrow, and of Europe the day after.

About 30 murders are committed in the United States every day. Lesser crimes of violence, such as kidnapping, assault and mugging, and crimes not necessarily involving violence, such as burglary and shoplifting, occur at the rate of 10 every second. In 1972 over 2 million guns were legally sold in the USA, 75,000 of them in California alone.

Growing alcoholism, drug addiction and drug abuse are an almost universal problem in the developed countries. The highest users are to be found among women with high family incomes and with two or three children. America has 7 million confirmed alcoholics and 50 million occasional or part-time drinkers. There are 100,000 acute alcoholics in England and Wales, and about 2 million on the borderline. Of the 7500 people killed on British roads every year a substantial proportion are the victims of drunken drivers.

There is no evidence that the developed nations are becoming markedly more healthy. The last five years have shown that the life expectancy of the average adult American male has declined, and is expected to decline still further. Health improvement appears to have reached its peak and has now levelled off. The trend applies to the rest of the Western world as well. People are no longer getting healthier. Coronary heart disease, the direct result of stress, is the largest single cause of death and disablement in the West. Mental illness remains endemic and depression epidemic in the affluent society. Suicide is high among the causes of death.

The problems of ergonomics, of man and his working conditions, are increasing rapidly. These centre around job satisfaction, labour—management relations, absenteeism, alcoholism, strikes, social levelling and class envy. As machines take over and more and more working men become redundant, the problem of what is to be done with them will increasingly engage the thoughts of governments. Along with the benefits of expanding production and prosperity loom the problems of the general environment which are important contributory factors in sociopsychosis: environmental pollution, overpopulation, overcrowding, noise.

Entertainment, once a rare and occasional part of life, is now the daily pabulum of the people, giving them their needed quantum of sports, violence and pornography. There is no relationship between entertainment and morals. The culture heroes of today are the entertainers, many of whom lead lives of sordid glamour, and who are often drug addicts, psychopaths and sexual perverts. Advertising is blatantly sex-oriented. Fashions are designed to keep sexual tensions very near the surface. Some types of clothes with tight

265

pressure on the sexual and anal regions are a constant stimulus to mild eroticism.

In most Western countries today abortions are fast becoming commonplace and may soon be had on demand. It is usually done by having the uterine contents aspirated under strong negative pressure, or suction. Where the operation cannot be legally performed, illegal 'back-street' abortions continue. In the USA about 1 million women undergo illegal abortion every year, of whom about 5000 die as a result. In Western Europe (excluding the UK), some 350,000 illegal abortions, and in the UK about 100,000 cases, are carried out annually. In addition about 200 dead babies are left in London dustbins each year.

Moralists point out that the increasing recourse to abortion is symptomatic of a sociopsychosis, forming part of the pattern of permissiveness, pornography, obscenity and sexual degradation of a decadent culture. Abortion caters mainly for the promiscuous. In the advanced countries, half the number of women involved are unmarried. Those who are well off usually request abortion for trivial social or cosmetic reasons. There is, say the moralists, obviously a growing cynicism and a hardening of personality in the woman who seeks on demand what amounts to virtual infanticide, and who submits to having the growing entity within her 'extracted by a vacuum cleaner', 'squeezed out like a boil', 'slaughtered in a conveyor-belt abattoir', or 'thrown into the w.c. like a piece of disposable tissue'.

Promiscuous sexual relations, pre-marital and extra-marital sex, adultery, wife-swapping and homosexuality are now accepted as part of the pattern of society. The number of unmarried mothers and illegitimate children is rising steeply. About 7 per cent of all children born in the USA today are illegitimate. One-fifth of all brides and one-third of all teenage brides in the USA are pregnant before marriage. 1 in 4 US marriages ends in divorce: in California the ratio is 1 in 2.

The first casualties of this situation are the children. In the break-up of family life the children suffer most. Every hour 5 infants in the USA receive severe injuries at the hands of their parents. Every day 2 or 3 children under five are killed by their parents. In the UK 12 children suffer non-accidental injuries inflicted by their parents every day, as a result of which at least 1 dies and 1 is permanently injured.

Teenage affluence has not improved the quality of the young. There is growing conflict with parents and society. In the past five years the incidence of hooliganism, mugging, sexual violence, burglary and shoplifting, mainly among adolescents, has risen by more than 50 per cent. There are Teenagers Alcoholics Anonymous in several major cities in the USA, and over 1 million youthful users of marihuana, LSD and similar drugs. Unaccountable depression is rampant in certain strata of youthful society. More than 2000 college students, and 1000 boys and girls of high-school age in the USA commit suicide each year.

VD (venereal disease, chiefly syphilis and gonorrhoea) has had a phenomenal rise in recent years. Its effects on the individual are so widespread that almost any disease subsequently acquired will be aggravated because of it. It is a permanent guest once it gains entry, and when the obvious external symptoms vanish, its ghost continues to haunt the individual, and by blood-spread is the ultimate cause of many groups of symptoms that continue to smoulder underground and crop up in one form or other throughout life.

During the period immediately following the Second World War it was thought that VD had been brought under control, but by the mid-1960s there was a sudden and inexplicable reversal which caused widespread alarm. It was found that the prevention of its spread became impossible, because in a permissive society contact tracing of infected persons was a virtually endless task. Every minute of the day two people in the USA were catching VD. Over 1 million new cases of syphilis and gonorrhoea were being reported annually. It has now become pandemic there.

The situation continues to deteriorate both in the USA and elsewhere, and some authorities doubt if its spread can ever be arrested now. The antibiotics that were once successful in the treatment of VD are gradually becoming ineffectual because both the gonococcus, the microbe causing gonorrhoea, and the spirochaete of syphilis are acquiring resistance to them. Teenagers constitute a third of all cases of gonorrhoea in the USA, UK and Scandinavia, largely because of the relaxation of moral codes, the spread of indiscriminate, irresponsible, and misleading sex information, which tends to arouse curiosity, allay fears and appease conscience.

Since 1970 the control of infectious syphilis in all parts of the world has been eroded by a great resurgence of new cases. On a world scale the incidence of gonorrhoea has also risen, from 60 million cases recorded in 1957 to an estimated 230 million in 1972. A WHO report states that gonorrhoea has 'reached almost epidemic proportions in Europe'. In the middle of 1976 a new strain, causing 'beta' gonorrhoea, appeared in the USA and UK, which is totally immune to penicillin. At present it seems to respond to the more potent antibiotic, spectinomycin, but doctors warn that in time it may develop resistance to this too. If so, we have as yet no drug to cope with the situation. The hope of 'conquering' VD has now virtually faded.

The generation gap has produced an unprecedented generation conflict, in which the adult world has capitulated all along the line. Many elders envy the permissiveness of youth and imitate or attempt to imitate their lifestyles and mores. One of the slogans of the early youth brigade was: 'Don't trust anyone over 25', later advanced to 30 as the slogan-makers grew older themselves. Little attempt is made by elders to counter arguments against morality. The upshot is a growing absence of parental and social disapproval of wrong behaviour. According to sociologists of so-called advanced thought, obedience is demeaning, authority is tyrannical and all feelings of guilt and shame, for whatever reason, are festering sores. The real four-letter concepts in their view are discipline, self-control, morality, duty, self-respect.

Throughout history a rapid decline in moral standards has been one of the evils of affluence. Men it would seem are unable to cope with material prosperity. Confronted with a bewildering choice of contradictory values and a multiplicity of standards, people find themselves in a state of confusion and turmoil. Many thinking people become disenchanted with material progress, and regret the loss of faith in a great spiritual reality. But no solution of the downward trend is at present in sight, and according to them the prognosis is gloomy.

Books

Felstein, Ivor, *Sexual Pollution: the Fall and Rise of Venereal Disease*, David & Charles, London, 1974.
Frank, L. K., *Society as the Patient*, Rutgers University Press, 1948.
Halliday, J. L., *Psychosocial Medicine: a Study of the Sick Society*, Norton, New York, 1948.
Hordern, Anthony, *Legal Abortion: the English Experience*, Pergamon Press, Oxford, 1971.
Morton, R. S., *Venereal Disease*, 2nd edn, Penguin Books, Harmondsworth, 1972.
Rapoport, R. N., *Community as Doctor*, Tavistock Publications, London, 1960.
Rogow, Arnold, *The Psychiatrists*, Allen & Unwin, London, 1971.
Ruesch, J., *Social Psychiatry*, Routledge & Kegan Paul, London, 1970.
Whiteley, C. H. *et al.*, *The Permissive Morality*, Methuen, London, 1964.
Wootton, B., *Social Change and Social Pathology*, Allen & Unwin, London, 1959.

SOMNAMBULISM

(Lat. *somnus*, 'sleep'; *ambulare*, 'to walk'), a xenophrenic* state of deep sleep in which a person, dominated by some strong inner impulse, may move about, perform various tasks, talk and write, although he is not afterwards conscious of having done so. Hypnotized subjects, especially those under deep hypnosis, are in a similar state of somnambulistic trance, and in the past were referred to as somnambules. But strictly speaking somnambulism is spontaneous and not induced by hypnosis. Nor does it occur during an REM (dream) phase of sleep.

The somnambulist may have his eyes closed, or open, but he does not seem to be aware of his surroundings; he sees, hears and feels nothing, but blindly obeys the compulsion that rules him, perceiving only that which bears relation to it. He is often insensible to pain. He will perform complicated, difficult and at times highly dangerous feats. While in a state of psychological dissociation, the somnambulist has driven cars through city traffic, walked on high perilous ledges and even committed murder (Luce and Segal, 1967, p. 102). Normally when the impulse that moves him has passed, he returns to bed and sleeps calmly till he awakens at his usual hour, and has no remembrance of what has transpired. But he will be able to recall it in every detail during the next period of somnambulism.

Frequently the somnambulist does things he could not normally do. Mathematicians find solutions to problems which they have vainly sought before; persons devoid of poetic talent compose good verse; authors struggling over difficult passages write whole chapters of novels, which on the following day they have no recollection of having done. The inspiration apparently comes from the unconscious mind. James Braid (d. 1850), a Scottish physician, recorded an often quoted case of a woman who in a state of somnambulism recited long Hebrew passages from the Bible, although she did not know a word of the language. It was eventually discovered that she was simply repeating what she had heard from a priest who had been in the habit of reading his Hebrew Bible aloud, and in whose house she had worked as a girl. The French physician Charles Richet (d. 1935) cites the case of a woman who while in this state sang whole arias from the opera *Africana*, although she had only heard it once, and when awake would have been incapable of singing a single note of it.

It is said that somnambulism reveals a man's potentiality, for it shows what he is capable of doing when the inhibitions normally placed upon him by his conscious mind are in abeyance. Some think it represents an attempt to re-enact a situation, or to complete something left undone, or seek something that is missing. Although somnambulism is latent in everyone, spontaneous sleep-walking usually indicates some morbid condition of the nervous system. In the occult view it may be described as the domination of the body by one's own etheric double during trance.

Many famous people have been sleep-walkers. To take two examples from recent times: Franklin Roosevelt and Adolf Hitler both walked in their sleep.

Books

Didier, Adolph, *Animal Magnetism and Somnambulism*, London, 1856.
Haddock, J., *Somnolism and Psycheism*, London, 1849.
Luce, G. C. and Segal, J., *Sleep*, Heinemann, London, 1967.
Tuke, D. H., *Sleepwalking and Hypnotism*, London, 1884.
Van Pelt, S. J., *Hypnotism and the Power Within*, London, 1950.

SPIRITUAL HEALING

A general term covering many forms of unorthodox healing without the use of drugs, usually through psychic power, or through the mediation of supernatural agencies. Medicine-men, witch-doctors, shamans, village wart-charmers, faith-healers, trance-healers, distant-healers, and those who practise mind cure* based on right-thinking, or divine healing by prayer and the laying on of hands, are all included among the practitioners of spiritual healing. In fact, some element of spiritual healing enters even into the most sophisticated medical practice.

In *spirit healing* the healer has the aid of discarnate entities. As a rule he is a medium through whom the spirit doctor or guide in the other world sends healing power, prescribes medicines and other means of cure, and even performs operations. Often the medium goes into deep trance and the spirit speaks or operates through the 'sleeping doctor'. Spirit healing is well documented. Among the better known names was Miss Rose (*c*. 1925) through whom the spirit of a certain Dr Beale of Hulham House used to diagnose and cure the sick. George Chapman of Aylesbury, Buckinghamshire, heals through the dead Dr William Lang, by performing 'etheric surgery', that is, he passes his hands over the affected area without cutting or penetrating the body. The best known 'psychic surgeons'* operating today are in Brazil and the Philippines.

What is called *trance healing* differs somewhat from spirit healing, for the latter does not always require spirit mediation. While in trance, the healer may suggest a cure drawn from his own unconscious, or, as is sometimes believed, he may get the information from the astral sphere which he himself supposedly visits while in trance. Shamans and tribal healers frequently go into such trance, and return to prescribe treatment for those who are sick. A remarkable trance-healer was the American 'Sleeping Lucy' (d. 1901). Born Lucy Ainsworth, in Vermont, she had received a modest education and no medical training. She was twice married, first to a Mr Cooke, and after his death to a Mr Raddin. Her gifts were first discovered when she was only 14 years old, and she subsequently helped to cure hundreds of people. Other famous trance-healers were the Americans, Andrew Jackson Davis (d. 1910), the 'Poughkeepsie seer', and Edgar Cayce (d. 1945), the 'sleeping prophet'.

Healing may be effected without the patient being physically present. This is known as *distant healing*, also called absent or telepathic healing, or tele-therapy. Treatment is administered even though the subject be many miles away, perhaps in another country. Sometimes it is not even necessary for the patient to write to the healer, it is sufficient for a friend to send details of the illness. The healer may employ prayers, sympathetic concentration, heal-ing thought-waves, or radiesthesia. In the latter case he may send the patient some object, such as a drawing sketched by him, so that the patient might expose himself to its radiations and speed up the natural healing processes of his body.

There are also various kinds of *psychic healing*, a term applied to those methods supposedly dependent for their success on clairvoyance, intuition or other paranormal faculty. Medical clairvoyants diagnose and describe the nature of their own ailments by autoscopy, or psychic 'self-inspection', or the ailments of their patients by scanning their aura, and prescribe cures accord-ingly. Some diagnose by psychometry, when they hold some personal object belonging to the patient and suggest treatment.

In *faith healing*, cures are largely dependent on the faith of the practitioner in himself, or on the faith of the patient in the practitioner, or the faith of either one or both of them in a divine or spiritual power. Suggestion is believed to be basic to most types of faith healing. Many remarkable faith cures have taken place at the tombs and shrines of saints and holy persons. Such were the miracles around the tomb of the Abbé François de Paris (d. 1727) that precipitated an outbreak of convulsionism; also the cures at Lourdes, and at Holywell in Wales. Pentecostalists and other ecstatic Chris-tian sects heal by faith and the laying on of hands. The Earl of Sandwich (d. 1916) is said to have cured many organic and functional diseases by prayer and faith.

Divine intervention is sought by most faith-healers. The celebrated Zuave Jacó, in France, achieved cures by prayer and blessings in the name of God. Antoine of Belgium, who also cured by faith, founded a new cult which by 1934 had 27 churches in Belgium and 1 in France dedicated to Antoinism. A famous Japanese spiritual healer, Miss Tosie Osanami, received help from Shinto deities. Patients would bring their own empty bottles which she would place on the family shrine with Shinto prayers. The bottles were said to fill up with liquid or ointment in the presence of all. When taken to court for fraud, she managed to produce the phenomena before the astounded judge and jury and was acquitted.

Faith healing is perhaps the commonest of all forms of spiritual healing, and dozens of modern healers practise their art in Europe and America. In 1934 John Maillard, vicar of the church of St Stephen in Brighton, received permission from the Anglican bishop of Chichester to practise faith healing because of his remarkable powers in this direction, and cured hundreds by this means. He used to say: 'Illness is frequently a consequence of sin; piety affords believers physical well-being as well as moral health. All sick people, even those whom medicine has failed, can be cured by faith, piety and prayer.'

Another remarkable faith-healer was Dorothy Kerin (d. 1963), once a chronic invalid whose case was known to several medical establishments, including St Bartholomew's Hospital, London. At the age of 23 she was like a living skeleton. She had lost her sight and lay dying of tuberculosis, complicated by peritonitis and meningitis. While sunk in semi-consciousness, she had a vision: an angel took her hand and said, 'Your sufferings are over. Get up and walk.' She called for her dressing-gown, and although she had not walked for five years, walked steadily down the corridor. Her sight was restored, and in 12 hours her bones began to be covered with firm and healthy flesh. She survived to become one of Britain's most famous faith-healers by laying on of hands.

Probably the best known of all recent spiritual healers in England was Harry Edwards (d. 1976). Originally a printer by occupation, he served in the Royal Army Medical Corps during the First World War and was posted to India. There he became interested in occultism, and later turned to psychic research and spiritualism. At one of the séances he attended, the following message was received through the medium: 'Harry Edwards, why don't you use your gifts of healing?' This was the beginning of an outstanding career. He started practising in 1935 through healing spirit guides, and carried on until his death. He described his work as 'a continuation of the work which The Master commenced'. In all, he treated over 1 million patients, mainly at his sanctuary at Burrows Lea.

Orthodox physicians tend to account for cases of spiritual healing as the result of wrong diagnosis or spontaneous remission. In 1960 the British Medical Association granted permission for faith and spiritual healers to work in hospitals, provided they had the consent of the medical staffs concerned.

Books

Edwards, Harry, *The Healing Intelligence*, Herbert Jenkins, London, 1965.
Holzer, Hans, *Beyond Medicine*, Abelard-Schuman, London, 1974.
Jones, D. C., *Spiritual Healing*, Longmans, London, 1955.
Kiev, Ari (ed.), *Magic, Faith and Healing*, Free Press, New York, 1975.
Rae, J. B., *Spiritual Healing and Medical Science*, SPCK, London, 1934.
Rose, Louis, *Faith Healing*, Gollancz, London, 1968.
Turner, Gordon, *An Outline of Spiritual Healing*, Parrish, London, 1963.
Watson, Lyall, *The Romeo Error*, Hodder & Stoughton, London, 1974.

Weatherhead, L., *Psychology, Religion and Healing*, London, 1951.
Worrall, Ambrose, *Miracle Healers*, New American Library, New York, 1968.

STIGMATA

Stigmata (Gk. 'marks') are wounds, burns, blisters, scratches or other scars that appear on the body, not caused by ordinary physical means. The term is frequently confined to the marks found on the body of saintly persons corresponding to the 5 wounds inflicted on Jesus during the Crucifixion, and also the 32 marks around the head corresponding to the scars left by the crown of thorns.

Occasionally the saintly stigmata are accompanied by the *ferita*, the lance-wound in the side of the heart, brought on by the spiritual 'transverberation of the heart'. Montague Summers says, 'In some rare instances autopsy has revealed in the heart characters and symbols, or flesh formations of the Instruments of the Passion.' The stigmata never produce pus, and the blood of stigmatics vanishes in many cases; the skin remains clean and the bed-clothes unsoiled. Sometimes the wounds are luminous and exhale a scent.

The first recorded stigmata were those of St Paul, who wrote, 'I bear in my body the marks of the Lord Jesus' (Gal. 6:17). After him, the best known case was that of St Francis of Assisi (d. 1226) who was stigmaticized while in deep contemplation of the Crucifixion, on Mount Alverno in 1224, two years before his death. His hands and feet appeared to be pierced through the middle with nails. These marks endured till his death, frequently bled, and hurt so much that he was unable to walk.

It has been remarked that once Roman Catholic mystics were provided with this concrete evidence of stigmatization, they unconsciously reproduced the example, and since St Francis's time some 340 cases of the phenomenon have been recorded, mostly among women, mostly fraudulent, but a few apparently authentic. About 50 stigmatics are alive today.

Among the better-known instances in recent times are the following. Anna Katherine Emmerich (d. 1824), a nun of Dülmen, Germany, who bore the marks of the Cross on her head and breast, and wounds on hands and feet, which bled. Her body remained incorrupt for many years after her death. Rosette Tamisier (d. 1863), a devout French girl with mystical leanings, whose body became marked by the stigmata during an illness. The case was investigated by the archbishop of Avignon, who declared the stigmata fraudulent, but many others, including high church dignitaries, believed they were genuine. To the end of her life she asserted that 'the miracles were true, true, true'. St Gemma Galgani (d. 1903) underwent many extraordinary ecstatic experiences, and after 1889 intermittently received the stigmata on her hands and feet. She was canonized in 1940. Teresa Neumann (d. 1962), a Bavarian peasant, first manifested the phenomenon, which was accompanied by bleeding, in 1925. From 1926 she almost totally abstained from solid food. Francesco Forgione (d. 1968), better known as Padre Pio, Italian Capuchin friar, first received the stigmata in 1918, which thereafter remained with him always. He was also regarded as clairvoyant, and as possessing the power of bilocation (being in two places at the same time) and the gift of healing.

Apart from divine or diabolical agency, stigmáta have variously been attributed to hysteria*; to suggestion by self or others; to freakish menstruation; religious devotion combined with strong emotion; intense concentration on the Crucifixion; ascetic contemplation; sudden shock.

A diseased condition of the skin has often been mistaken for stigmatic marks. Such, for instance, is ecchymosis, a discoloration of the skin due to the extravasation of subcutaneous blood; erythema, a subcutaneous congestion resulting in inflammation and redness of the skin surface; haemetidrosis, or sweating blood, where the blood seems to percolate through the skin; chromidrosis, where the sweat may be coloured red, pink or yellow. Besides these, fraud has frequently been detected, where bleeding was caused by self-inflicted wounds, the use of dye, and similar expedients.

Stigmata also include the curious phenomenon of *dermography*, 'skin writing', in which letters, pictures or other intelligible marks appear on the skin. It can be fraudulently produced by tracing such marks lightly on the skin, which in very sensitive persons develop into weals along the tracings some minutes later. Skin writing may also appear as a result of mental concentration and can be induced by hypnosis. Spiritualists believe it can be caused by spirit agencies operating on a medium. Unlike other stigmatic marks, this writing does not stay for more than a few hours.

Books

Amadeo, Father, *Blessed Gemma Galgani*, Burns & Oates, London, 1935.
Carty, Charles M., *Two Stigmatists: Padre Pio and Teresa Neumann*, Veritas, Dublin, 1956.
Garçon, Maurice, *Rosette Tamisier*, Paris, 1929.
Summers, Montague, *The Physical Phenomena of Mysticism*, Rider, London, 1950.
Thurston, Herbert, *The Physical Phenomena of Mysticism*, Burns & Oates, London, 1952.

STRESS

A term borrowed from the physical sciences, it is the bodily and mental strain a person is subjected to in the course of his reactions and adaptations to the threats, challenges and pressures of life. As a clinical condition it covers all forms of response to fear*, anxiety*, conflict, frustration, arousal and tension.

In the Hippocratic writings we find the earliest attempt to explain stress symptoms from the medical point of view, as the painful modification of certain physiological processes to meet a threatening situation, and an attempt on the part of the body to restore its equilibrium.

Stress afflicts men in all walks of life and all circumstances, even those who are free from the tensions of civilized existence. It has been found from a study of primitive peoples in Africa, New Guinea and the Amazon basin, that anxiety leading to stress prevails as commonly with them as it does in more advanced societies, and that they react as frequently with peptic ulcers, heart conditions and other stress symptoms as their more industrially advanced brethren.

As understood today stress is a syndrome of post-Freudian psychology, which has assumed great importance as a result of many years of animal research by the Austrian-born Canadian, Dr Hans Selye (b. 1907) of McGill University, Montreal, and others who have followed in his footsteps.

Life has many stressors, or stress-producing agents, broadly divided into two categories, physical and psychological. These include heat, cold, hunger, disease, loss of health, injury, shock; threats to life and security, financial worry; sensory deprivation, annoyances, anger, change; facing interviews, examinations, competition, travel; dealing with the bureaucracy, keeping up with the Joneses; noise, pop music, films of sex and violence; going to school, puberty, intercourse, a new job, marriage, pregnancy, childbearing, becoming a parent, divorce, retirement, death in the family; and scores of others. Stress situations arise as frequently from promotion as from demotion, from success as from failure. A sudden access of wealth or good fortune can prove acutely stressful.

A person's physical and mental condition alters when undergoing stress. The progress of the stress syndrome often passes through certain distinct phases. First, the initial alarm or shock phase, associated with instantaneous responses of the autonomic nervous system, and all the ensuing neurohormonal, glandular and other biochemical changes. Then come the defence and resistance phases; and finally, the phase of exhaustion. All these can trigger numbing reactions: paleness, trembling, stammering, sexual incapacity, and a desperate yearning to play possum and give up the struggle. Depression* is one way of responding to stress.

People under stress show most of the following physiological reactions: overall increase in the metabolic rate of the body; increased perspiration, and decreased skin resistance; decrease in the alpha-wave activity of the brain; higher lactate-ion concentration in the blood; increase in blood sugar; change in the acid-base balance of the body; increase of arterial pH (acidity); increase of base excess; retention of sodium and excretion of potassium; deposit of large amounts of calcium salts to certain organs resulting in their progressive petrification.

Also, increase in the activity of the neurohormones, especially the adrenal and pituitary glands, and in the secretion of cholesterol; a rise in the level of the cortico-steroids, the hormones found in the adrenal glands; accelerated heart rate and cardiac output, manifested in the pounding of the heart. Stress, thus, contributes to cardiovascular disease such as hypertension (high blood pressure); accelerated respiratory rate and consumption of oxygen; more rapid breathing and difficulty in breathing; increased production and elimination of carbon dioxide (CO_2); a tendency to asthmatic attack; muscular tension, trembling, weakness of the limbs, lassitude, faintness, giddiness; dry throat, nausea, heartburn, headache, hot flushes; abdominal discomfort, an urge to urinate and empty the bowels; a sense of suffocation; backache; insomnia; tightness of abdominal muscles; colitis and peptic ulcer.

Books

Appley, M. H. and Trumbull, R. (ed), *Psychological Stress: Issues in Research,* New York, 1967.

Basowitz, H. *et al.*, *Anxiety and Stress*, McGraw-Hill, New York, 1955.

Broadbent, D. G., *Decision and Stress*, Academic Press, London, 1971.

Butterfield, W. J. H., *The Nature of Stress Disorder*, London, 1959.

Galton, Lawrence, *The Silent Disease: Hypertension*, Crown, New York, 1973.

Janis, I. L., *Psychological Stress*, Wiley, New York, 1958.

Lazarus, R. S., *Psychological Stress and the Coping Process*, McGraw-Hill, New York, 1966.

Liebman, S. (ed.), *Stress Situations*, Lippincott, Philadelphia, 1955.

Nottidge, P. and Lamplugh, D., *Stress and Overstress*, Angus & Robertson, London, 1974.

Selye, Hans, *The Stress of Life*, McGraw-Hill, New York, 1956.

Sigerist, Henry E., *Civilization and Disease*, University of Chicago Press, 1970.

Wolf, Harold, *Stress and Disease*, Thomas, Springfield, Illinois, 1953.

Wolf, S. C. *et al.*, *Life Stress and Essential Hypertension*, Baltimore, 1955.

SUICIDE

Suicide is the active expression of the death wish, or thanatophilia*. Because it involves murder, albeit murder of self, it was, and still is, from the standpoint of most religions, condemned as a sin. Until recently in most countries attempted suicide was regarded as a criminal offence, but it is now treated as a symptom of mental unbalance, and in some cases as a symbolic cry for help.

The reasons for suicide and attempted suicide are many and varied. Lack of love, unrequited love or unfulfilled love perhaps contribute to the greatest number of suicides the world over. Take away love and hope from a man and he is prepared to die; also, marital or sexual conflict, inadequacy and failure. Apathy or lack of interest in life sometimes makes a man give up. Grief over the death of a loved one, especially a spouse, when the emptiness and loss seem irreparable, is another cause.

There are, of course, many other precipitating factors: physical pain, in the case of chronic ill-health, painful or incurable disease; adverse fortune and financial loss, coupled with humiliation and inability to maintain previous standards of living – the suicide rate usually rises in times of financial crisis; failure in an examination, loss of career or employment; failure to get a promotion; feelings of humiliation, inferiority, discouragement and depression.

Also, physical deformity, sexual deviation and a sense of being different and abnormal; remorse and shame over some public exposure, involving one's private life, morals, honour and consequent inability to face one's associates and peers; a sense of guilt over some delinquency or habit, and a compulsion to punish the sinning self – a means of forgetting the past; sometimes, a desire for revenge, to make others feel sorry that one is dead, to spite one's enemies, to create anguish in the hearts of loved ones.

In addition, isolation, ostracism, being sent to coventry and social punishment in which one is treated as an outcast, shunned and despised by friends; old age, the knowledge of being a burden on others, an inability to support oneself and a sense of helplessness when one is unable to do things one could do before; feelings of being in the way, unwanted, abandoned, lonely.

Some people commit suicide because they are happy, either from a sense of guilt at their happiness or because they do not have the spiritual strength to stand up to the emotional onslaught. Others may want to die at a time of idyllic happiness, 'that the moment might be eternal'. Strangely, great waves of financial prosperity, contentment and security often also result in an increase in the suicide rate. In 1963 the year that the Prime Minister, Harold Macmillan, said that the man in the street had never had it so good, well over 5,000 people took their own lives in Britain.

There is no doubt that the suicide rate has risen enormously since the two world wars. But wars are only partly responsible, for the whole tenor of modern life tends to unhinge and unbalance the individual. According to observers, as men seek physical stimulation and satisfaction, and rely more and more on gadgetry, machines, pills and external aids, and less and less on the things of the spirit, they tend to succumb more rapidly to the stress of life.

Suicide is more frequent than murder. According to recent WHO statistics, more than 1,000 persons commit suicide every day. In the USA alone someone is killing himself, or trying to kill himself once every minute. There are an estimated 65,000 unofficial suicides annually, of which 30,000 are official. This includes some 2,000 college students, 1,000 boys and girls of high-school age, and about 100 of 14-year-olds and below. And the USA is only twelfth on the list, since several other countries have higher suicide rates. The highest are found in Hungary, Sweden, Switzerland, Austria, Finland, West Germany (West Berlin has the highest suicide rate in the world), Japan, England (about 14 a day), Czechoslovakia and Denmark. Comparatively low rates are recorded in Holland, Norway, Scotland, Spain, Eire, Chile and Egypt.

Statistics suggest that there are more suicides among those living in dry climates than in humid; more in spring and summer than in autumn and winter; more on Mondays and Tuesdays than other days; more in large cities than in small; more in urban areas than in rural; more among the unemployed than employed; in peacetime than in wartime; in the afternoons than mornings. There is more suicide among Protestants than Catholics; among the single than the married; more among those who are widowed or divorced than not; more in small families than large; more among whites than non-whites; among soldiers (especially officers) than civilians; among the aged than the young; among psychiatrists (the highest in the world), doctors, lawyers and businessmen than among clergymen, miners and teachers.

Books

Alvarez, A., *The Savage God: a Study of Suicide*, Weidenfeld & Nicolson, London, 1972.

Durkheim, Émile, *Suicide: a Study in Sociology*, 1897, London; Routledge & Kegan Paul, London, 1950 edn.

Hillman, James, *Suicide and the Soul*, Hodder, London, 1964.

Landsberg, P. L., *The Experience of Death: the Moral Problem of Suicide*, London, 1953.

Meerloo, J. A., *Suicide and Mass Suicide*, New York, 1962.

Menninger, K. A., *Man Against Himself*, London, 1938.

Stengel, E., *Suicide and Attempted Suicide*, Penguin Books, Harmondsworth, 1964.

SYPHILIS

Syphilis appears to have plagued man since prehistoric times. A syphilitic human bone dating from about 2500 BC was found in the Gobi desert. Ancient Egyptian papyri refer to an illness called *uchedu*, whose symptoms resemble syphilis, which was already known for many centuries. There are similar references in the early Mesopotamian inscriptions, and an Assyrian record tells of a woman named Ukhat ('whore') who died of a venereal complaint. In Hindu legend, the god Shiva, whose symbol is the phallus, himself suffers from a venereal disease. In the classical world, Hippocrates (d. 359 BC) describes a disease whose symptoms include the rotting of the genitals, and four centuries later the Latin physician Celsus (fl. AD 50) also mentions a venereal disease for which mercury, an early cure for syphilis, was prescribed. In many of these regions syphilis was regarded as a punishment sent by the Crab-god.

Some authorities, however, hold that syphilis was unknown to Europe and Asia at this time, and that these early descriptions correspond to a form of soft sore (chancroid) or yaws. If it was syphilis it was probably only a very mild variety, for its virulence was not recorded till true syphilis was brought over from the New World in the fifteenth century.

Syphilis was said to have been endemic among the Amerinds, and was regarded as a disease of the nobility among the Aztecs. There was even an Aztec god of syphilis named Nanahuatzin (or Nanahuatl). It was widespread in the Caribbean region, and was introduced to Europe by the crew of Columbus (d. 1506), who contracted it from the promiscuous Arawak or Haitian women. Later the conquistadors received their own strain of the disease from central America and Mexico.

When a local epidemic swept Barcelona in 1493, the people could not think of a commonplace cause, and thought of it as a blight sent from heaven. Astrologers attributed it to the conjunction of the four major planets in the constellation of Scorpio, although some thought it might have been brought by the gypsies who migrated to Western Europe in the fifteenth century, or by the Moriscos or Christianized Moors expelled from Spain. Later other theories were advanced. Jean Baptiste van Helmont (d. 1644) believed it all started as a result of an act of intercourse between a man and a mare suffering from glanders. Others thought it came from congress with a monkey; or with a leper. In fact, syphilis may be contracted in many ways, including contact without copulation. It is transmissible to a child in the womb.

The disease broke out in truly epidemic proportions in Naples in the army of Charles VIII (d. 1498) of France, shortly after he took the city in 1495. It spread rapidly among the troops, and then all over Italy, France and the rest of Europe. Everyone disowned it. The French of Provence called it the Spanish disease; the Spaniards called it the Bordeaux disease; the Parisians called it the *morbus germanicus* (German illness); the Florentines called it the Naples sickness. The English spoke of it as the French pox, or the great pox (to distinguish it from the small pox) or simply 'the pox'. When it reached the Far East the Japanese called it the Chinese disease.

The name syphilis comes from a poem (1530) by Girolamo Fracastoro of

Verona, in which Syphilus, a Greek shepherd is struck with the disease as a punishment for defying and abusing the sun. It was a hideous and deforming chastisement. When it first appeared in Europe, syphilis was a far more acute, virulent and fatal condition than it is today. Uninterrupted transmission from one person to another in the course of about five centuries has led to a gradual tolerance, one result being an increasing mildness. But it mimics many other diseases, hence the old maxim, 'If you know syphilis, you know medicine.'

The cures prescribed for syphilis were wide-ranging. The people of the Caribbean used the greenish resin from the guaiacum tree found in the West Indies. The Aztecs made a decoction of a plant containing the drug ephedrine. Its use spread over a wide area from Mexico to Colorado and survived into the period of the first American colonies. It was adopted as a popular beverage by the new settlers in Salt Lake City at the time of Brigham Young (d. 1877) and so came to be known as Brigham tea or Mormon tea. In Europe, when Cesare Borgia (d. 1507), son of Pope Alexander VI, contracted syphilis, his doctor prescribed treatment that included getting the sores sucked by 'someone of worthless estate', poulticing them with live frogs cut in half, and then lying in the freshly disembowelled carcass of a mule. Other cures recommended for the disease were: intercourse with a virgin, the application of mule dung to the male organ, washing with horse urine, and the inductance of fever*, especially malaria.

The use of mercury as a cure for syphiloid diseases was long known to the ancients, and was revived during the Renaissance, when it was known as 'salivation', because of the large quantities of saliva produced by the mercury. The use of this remedy continued until the discovery in 1907 by Paul Ehrlich (d. 1915), a Jewish pathologist, of a compound of arsenic which he called salvarsan. It was also known as '606', because it happened to be the 606th substance tested by him. The latest cure is penicillin and other antibiotics. But in spite of these drugs syphilis has never been wiped out, and it seems that a more tenacious breed of spirochete is evolving that resists even antibiotics.

Many eminent people have had syphilis. Among rulers there were several Roman emperors, including Caligula (d. AD 41), Nero (d. AD 68), and Heliogabalus (d. AD 222). Charles VIII of France (d. 1498), Francis I of France (d. 1547), Philip II of Spain (d. 1598), and Ivan the Terrible (d. 1584), czar of Russia, were all known to have been afflicted by the disease. The New World virus came to England in 1496, probably brought by English mercenaries who fought under Charles VIII of France. But as some scholars suggest, there are indications that it existed in England in a milder form before that date, as John of Gaunt (d. 1399), son of Edward III of England, appears to have had it.

Henry VIII (d. 1547) was syphilitic, and all his children were congenital syphilitics. Edward IV (d. 1553), his son, died of syphilis in boyhood. Mary I (Mary Tudor, or Bloody Mary) (d. 1558) and Elizabeth I (d. 1603), daughters of Henry VIII, also had it. Mary Queen of Scots (d. 1587) got it from Lord Darnley, and they bequeathed it to their son James I (d. 1625).

Among the great dictators, Napoleon Bonaparte (d. 1821), Benito Mussolini (d. 1945) and Adolf Hitler (d. 1945) all had syphilis.

Several popes and prelates were known to have been afflicted with the disease: Urban VI (d. 1389), Sixtus IV (d. 1485), Alexander VI (d. 1503) and Cardinal Wolsey (d. 1530).

Among philosophers, Socrates (d. 399 BC) might have had a syphiloid affliction. Descriptions of his features suggest venereal disease, and the famous bust in the Louvre reveals in the 'saddle-nose', or collapse of the nasal septum, what has been called 'a definitely syphilitic nose'. In more recent times we have Søren Kierkegaard (d. 1855), Arthur Schopenhauer (d. 1860), and Friedrich Nietzsche (d. 1900).

Among musicians: Ludwig van Beethoven (d. 1827), Franz Schubert (d. 1828), Nicolo Paganini (d. 1840), Robert Schumann (d. 1856), Hugo Wolf (d. 1903) and Frederick Delius (d. 1934).

Artists: Albrecht Dürer (d. 1528), Benvenuto Cellini (d. 1571), Rembrandt (d. 1669), Francisco Goya (d. 1828), Edouard Manet (d. 1883), Henri Toulouse-Lautrec (de. 1901) and Paul Gauguin (d. 1903).

Notable among the physicians claimed by syphilis was John Hunter (d. 1793) founder of modern scientific surgery. But he acquired it as a result of his zeal for understanding the disease. He deliberately inoculated himself with the germ and became a victim of syphilis.

Many poets and writers have been syphilitic. Ulrich von Hutten (d. 1523), Lutheran poet and polemist, suffered from the disease. The monstrously large nose of Cyrano de Bergerac (d. 1655) was a syphilitic deformity. John Milton (d. 1674) suffered from congenital syphilis. Jonathan Swift (d. 1745) was attacked by it and this could account for the general bitterness of his writings. John Keats (d. 1821) contracted syphilis while on a visit to Oxford. Heinrich Heine (d. 1856) was also afflicted. Charles Baudelaire (d. 1867) died a lunatic, paralysed and speechless, and poisoned by drugs, drink and syphilis. Jules de Goncourt (d. 1870), Guy de Maupassant (d. 1893) and Alphonse Daudet (d. 1897) are also to be numbered among the victims of the disease, as are Oscar Wilde (d. 1900) and August Strindberg (d. 1912). Among politicians, Randolph Churchill (d. 1895), father of Winston Churchill, died from general paralysis of the insane as a result of syphilis.

Syphilis has a traumatic effect on its victims. There is something about this type of venereal disease in particular that profoundly affects the victim as though he were aware that the very well-springs of his being were corrupted. D. H. Lawrence (d. 1930) wrote that no one could contract syphilis 'without feeling the most shattering and profound terror go through him, through the very roots of his being'.

It has been claimed that the sensitive minds of writers, artists, poets and musicians have often been stimulated by the cerebral irritation of an early general paresis, and that many brilliant men who have contracted syphilis have benefited from it. It would seem that some of the world's greatest achievements in the cultural field have been formulated by syphilitic brains. Aleister Crowley (d. 1947), who also had the disease, held that syphilis was the basis of genius, and that 'it would be salutary for every male to be impregnated with the germs of this virus in order to facilitate the culture of individual genius'.

Books

Bett, W. R., *The Infirmities of Genius*, Christopher Johnson, London, 1952.
Bloch, J., *Der Ursprung der Syphilis*, 2 vols, Jena, 1901, 1911.
Cartwright, Frederick, *Disease and History*, Hart-Davis, London, 1972.
Fournier, A., *Les Affectiones parasyphilitiques*, Paris, 1894.
Frazier, C. N. and Li, H. C., *Race Variations to Syphilis*, London, 1948.
Holcomb, R. C., *Who Gave the World Syphilis?*, Froben, New York, 1937.
Lawrence, D. H., *Pornography, Obscenity and All That*, London, 1929.
L'Étang, Hugh, *The Pathology of Leadership*, Heinemann, London, 1969.
Proksh, J. K., *Die Geschichte der venerischen Krankheiten*, Bonn, 1895.
Pusey, W. A., *History and Epidemiology of Syphilis*, Baltimore, 1933.
Rosenbaum, J., *Histoire de la syphilis dans l'antiquité*, Brussels, 1847.
Shrewsbury, J. F., *The Plague of the Philistines*, Gollancz, London, 1964.
Sudhoff, K. and Singer, C., *The Earliest Printed Literature on Syphilis*, Florence, 1925.
Symonds, John, *The Great Beast: the Life of Aleister Crowley*, Macdonald, London, 1971.
Turner, David, *Syphilis: a Practical Dissertation on the Venereal Disease*, London, 1717.
Wykes, Alan, *The Doctor and His Enemy*, Michael Joseph, London, 1965.

T

THANATOMANIA

Thanatomania (Gk. *thanatos*, 'death') is a term used for any morbid preoccupation with death, or obsessive curiosity about matters relating to death, such as the desire for death, the fear of death, including psychogenic (or mind-induced) death*.

The fear of death, or thanatophobia, comes to the surface in the feeling of acute anxiety during one's own sickness, or that of a loved one, or in periods of great gloom and depression. A sense of the impending end, and fear of extinction, known as *angor animi*, 'anguish of the spirit', is found in patients with critical diseases like angina pectoris, asthma, thrombosis; in those who are dying of sickness or any other cause; and in those who are under sentence of death.

The desire for death, or thanatophilia* — a much more common phenomenon than is generally supposed — manifests in what has been called the 'death wish', the deep-seated desire for extinction which is said to be inherent in the psyche of all living beings.

In a more general sense thanatomania expresses itself in the urge to witness scenes of horror and death. There is a strange element of pleasure in watching someone else's danger, or even his pain, as seen in the popular craze for boxing and wrestling, bull-fighting, cock-fighting, hunting and other blood sports. In centuries past, executions and hangings were carried out in public and were always crowded with sightseers, including women and small children. Until quite recently morbid crowds used to hang around prison gates on execution day. There can be little doubt that, if public executions were reintroduced today, people in civilized countries would flock to them and find immense gratification from the spectacle.

Many people can watch with inner gloating, hearts beating fast with excitement, even with ecstasy, and with eyes bright with unnatural passion, the struggles of some living thing expiring in agony before their eyes. They are hushed in silence as they watch the blood flow, and realize that that intangible entity called life is rapidly ebbing away. Film directors tend to cater to this perverse feeling, by dwelling, often in slow motion, on scenes of stabbing, shooting and protracted death.

Thanatomania also comes to the surface in the unwholesome interest shown by people when they crowd around the scene of an accident or fire, or watch a trapeze artist in the circus, or a motor race, perhaps with a vague thought, almost hope, that they might witness a fatal outcome. Also, in the general hunger for stories of violence, murder and carnage.

Thanatomania finds its pathological extreme in necrophilia* and related perversions.

Books

Aries, Philippe, *Western Attitudes Towards Death: From the Middle Ages to the Present*, Johns Hopkins Press, Baltimore, 1974.
Brown, Norman O., *Life Against Death*, Wesleyan University, Connecticut, 1959.
Choron, J., *Death in Western Thought*, Collier, New York, 1966.
Feifel, Herman (ed.), *The Meaning of Death*, McGraw-Hill, New York, 1965.
Frazer, J. G., *The Fear of Death in Primitive Religion*, 3 vols, London, 1936.
Freud, Sigmund, *Beyond the Pleasure Principle*, Hogarth Press, London, 1955.
Harrington, Alan, *The Immortalist*, Panther, London, 1973.
Herzog, Edgar, *Psyche and Death*, Hodder & Stoughton, London, 1966.
Kastenbaum, R. and Aisenberg, R., *The Psychology of Death*, Springer, New York, 1972.
Kubler-Ross, Elisabeth, *On Death and Dying*, Tavistock Publications, London, 1970.
Lifton, R. J., *Death in Life*, Penguin, London, 1971.

THANATOPHILIA

(Gk. *thanatos*, 'death'; *philia*, 'love'), a facet of thanatomania*, in which the victim seeks a way to personal extinction. According to psychologists, such a death wish, as it is called, is inherent in the psyche of all living things. This does not deny the existence, at the same time, of a will to live. But the urge towards survival is not the over-riding one in all circumstances, and a longing for the peace of oblivion may often supervene.

All things, animate and inanimate, if left to themselves, naturally tend towards a state of inertia, so that it might be said that the terminal condition, and one that lies behind all activity, is perfect stillness. The inanimate precedes the animate, and the animate longs to return to its original state, which is one of peace, quiescence and repose.

Introducing this concept of the 'death instinct', Sigmund Freud (d. 1939) said that the tendency of instinct is to repeat an earlier condition, and that the desire to return to the inanimate and the inorganic is ever-present. Apart from the self-preservation (ego) and reproductive (sexual) instincts, there are those that seek death. Later psychologists subdivided these latter instincts into *destrudo*, destructive or aggressive, directed at others, and *mortido*, directed at oneself.

The centre of our troubled situation lies in our consciousness, which manifests itself in our individuality and self-assertion. And deep down we all desire to obliterate this exasperating state of affairs. Existence is an effort that disturbs our rest. Life, as the existentialists have it, is a fever in matter, and we unconsciously wish to extinguish it and surrender to the sluggish drift of things, the termination of which is the oblivion of death.

This is exemplified in man from the moment of birth when, as an infant, he is torn from the warm maternal nest and makes stridently manifest his desire to 'return to the womb'. It has been pointed out that everyone has a suicide potential, and if science did find a drug to extend the human life span, we should need another drug to fortify our will to live.

The death wish shows itself in a number of ways, a few of which are listed here.

(a) In suicide* plain and simple, where a person finally and without equivocation takes the way out by ending his life.

(b) In 'psychogenic death'*, or death-by-suggestion, where a person does not commit violence against himself, but simply surrenders his will to live.

(c) In murder and violence, since criminal tendencies betray the urge to fulfil one's own death, rehearsed by killing another, and dramatized in the ensuing trial and execution. The murderer really wishes to kill himself.

(d) In war, which provides for many people a manner of suicide without the moral or religious guilt attaching to it. It affords a chance for the fulfilment of the death wish on a national scale. When men fight, they secretly court death.

(e) In the prevalence of certain religious, philosophical and political beliefs, such as atheism, agnosticism, humanism, existentialism, nihilism and anarchism. For example, atheism, which does not admit a belief in life after death, is the death wish *par excellence*.

(f) In socialism and other forms of misplaced humanitarianism, which by monetary largesse and prodigal disbursement of social benefits lead to a huge increment of dysgenic* factors in the community.

(g) In science and scientific progress, which appear to move towards death. Some people see science as a relentless current carrying the whole of civilization into the abyss by way of moral and spiritual decadence which are the concomitants of materialistic ways of thought.

(h) In the choice of death-defying professions, sports and activities, such as mountain-climbing, performing on the high trapeze, automobile-racing, parachuting, sky-diving, pot-holing. The attendant hair-raising risks have been compared to the forepleasure that precedes orgasm, that is, death.

(i) In insanity, which veils full consciousness with its burdening responsibilities; in hysteria*, which provides a cloak under which to conceal the breakdown of one's ability to cope with life's situations.

(j) In sickness, which provides another chance of escape to the death-wisher. Doctors have found that many patients do not want to get well. Malingerers who pretend to be ill; addicts to polysurgery (repeated surgical operations, either on demand or induced by pretending); neurotic invalids, all make a tentative reconnaissance of death's perimeters and seek to enter it.

(k) In various miscellaneous categories, such as alcoholics, drug addicts, those who are accident prone, those with chronic bad luck (in most cases unconsciously sought); in suicidal patriotism, fanatical devotion to a cause, martyrdom, asceticism, all of which are fundamentally life-abnegating.

(l) In pleasure, which can also be a means of escape from the hard realities of life. Behind even the desire to 'live, laugh and love' lies concealed, the psychologist tells us, a strong element of self-destruction.

Books

Alexander, Franz, 'The Need for Punishment and the Death Instinct', *International Journal of Psychoanalysis*, 10, 1929, 260.
Barker, J. C., *Scared to Death*, Frederick Muller, London, 1968.
Dublin, Louis and Bunzel, Bessie, *To Be or Not to Be: a Study of Suicide*, New York, 1933.
Freud, Sigmund, *Beyond the Pleasure Principle*, Hogarth Press, London; 1955 edn.
Landsberg, P. L., *The Experience of Death: the Moral Problem of Suicide*, London, 1953.
Menninger, Karl, *Man Against Himself*, New York, 1938.

THEOMANIA

(Gk. 'god-madness'), a general term for all types of excessive religious or devotional fervour, where a person reaches a condition of frenzy and exalta-tion, as if inspired or possessed by a deity. It often manifests in physical symptoms and unusual phenomena, such as convulsions, hysterical contor-tions of the limbs, immunity to pain, gifts of healing, apparent clairvoyance, and xenoglossis or 'speaking in tongues'. Theomania can be brought on by prolonged preoccupation with religion, by prayers, asceticism, music, danc-ing, singing, drugs or any of the agents that precipitate xenophrenia*.

In ancient times theomania was listed with the furors*, and was regarded as akin to madness. The *furor divini*, 'divine frenzy', is distinguished by some authorities from ecstasy, a state of mental and physical exaltation which, however, does not manifest the divine presence; and from possession*, where a person is possessed, not by a god, but by a demon or spirit. But the distinc-tions are not always clear, and the various forms of exaltation manifested by shamans, witch-doctors, medicine-men and other hierophants in primitive communities are also commonly grouped under the heading of theomania.

In its most extreme form theomania implies a belief in one's own divinity, so that the victim imagines that he is God. The asseverations, 'God and I are One' or 'I am God', constantly intoned by certain Hindu mystics, and the concept of the identity of the individual soul with the Universal Soul, are basic to the teachings of the Upanishads, the philosophical section of the

Vedas. The early sufis, notably Mansur al-Hallaj (d. 922), also identified themselves with the deity.

In some cases of theomania the victim falls into a state of *theolepsy* (Gk. 'god-seized'), when it is believed that a divine being has taken hold of him and is responsible for his inspired utterances. Another variety of theomania, described as *telestic* (Gk. *telos*, 'rite'), was the delirium that possessed a person during the performance of certain religious ceremonials, and applied specifically to those overcome with ecstasy during the Eleusinian and other early mysteries.

During the Dionysia of ancient Greece theomania was progressively whipped up by wild religious revels, reaching its climax in the rite of *sparagmos* (Gk. 'convulsion'), when an animal representing the god was torn apart and its raw flesh eaten, as a result of which the worshipper became *entheoi*, 'en-godded', and believed himself to be possessed by the deity. From this pagan usage we have the term *enthusiasm*. When the worship of the Phrygian goddess Cybele was introduced into Rome in 204 BC, the maniacal behaviour of the *fanatici*, or those who worshipped at her shrine (Lat. *fanum*, 'temple'), became a matter of wonder to the Romans. From the excesses of these devotees we get the word 'fanatic'.

At various times in Europe theomania reached epidemic proportions, as among the medieval Flagellants of Germany, Poland and Hungary in the thirteenth century, who lashed themselves and others in penance for their sins; among those stricken with the Dancing Mania in Holland, Belgium and Germany in the fourteenth century; and among the Convulsionaries of France in the eighteenth century, and several other bands of religious enthusiasts.

In the seventeenth century in England the term 'enthusiasm' came to be applied in a derogatory sense to the extravagant display of religious piety, excessive zeal and emotional fervour manifested by many sects who claimed to act under the inspiration or guidance of the Holy Spirit, which was said to descend upon them, and who gave expression to their 'enthusiasm' in prophecies, speaking in tongues, and bodily convulsions. Such 'enthusiasm' was detected among the Shakers, the early Quakers, the Methodists, Revivalists, Pentecostalists, Adventists and Messianists.

Books

Delatte, A., *Les Conceptions de l'enthousiasme chez les philosophes présocratiques*, Paris, 1934.

Grattan, T. C., *Civilized America*, London, 1859.

Hecker, J. F. C., *The Epidemics of the Middle Ages*, London, 1844.

Knox, Ronald, *Enthusiasm: a Chapter in the History of Religion*, Oxford University Press, 1950.

Leuba, J. H., *The Psychology of Religious Mysticism*, Kegan Paul, London, 1929.

Mackay, A., *The Western World*, London, 1849.

Stinstra, John, *Essay on Fanaticism*, Dublin, 1774.

Taylor, Isaac, *The Natural History of Enthusiasm*, London, 1823.

Taylor, T., *A Dissertation on the Eleusinian and Bacchic Mysteries*, New York, 1875.

THERAPY

The art concerned with the relief of suffering in its broadest sense. The more common term 'medicine' (Lat. *medicare*, 'to heal') devotes itself to the curing of disease. Therapy as a whole embraces a great many skills and subordinate studies, of which the chief are mentioned below.

*Aetiology** is concerned with the causes of disease. *Semeiology* or *symptomatology* studies symptoms. *Diagnostics* is the art of diagnosis. *Pathology* treats of the underlying processes of diseases. *Nosology* names and classifies disease. *Prognosis* forecasts the course of an illness. The *materia medica* classifies the various substances used by physicians for medical purpose. *Pharmacology* studies drugs. *Posology* or *dosology* deals with the exact quantity of a drug or the size of a dose to be administered to a patient. *Toxicology* deals with poisons. *Prophylaxis* treats of methods of guarding against disease, and includes all forms of preventive medicine, vaccination, immunology, preventive hygiene. *Public health* is concerned with safeguarding the health of the whole community by sanitation and vital statistics. *Epidemiology*, a branch of public health, devotes its attention to the prevention and control of epidemics.

Therapy can be referred back to prehistoric times when primitive man, following his own instincts and occasionally the lead given him by animals, evolved methods of treating himself and his fellows in time of illness. The mineral, plant and animal worlds provided him with remedies, and he sought from his own experience those situations that had therapeutic value, from dieting to rest.

Today it is beginning to be realized that almost every activity can serve as a method of healing. At the World Congress of Alternative Medicine held at San Remo, Italy, in May 1973, delegates representing more than 135 different therapies put forward their views. The conclusion would appear to be that ultimately therapeutics cannot be separated from mental and, indeed, spiritual wellbeing. Health and healing are bound up with wholeness and with holiness.

Books

Ackerknecht, Erwin, *Therapeutics: From the Primitives to the Twentieth Century,* Hafner, New York, 1973.

Atkinson, D. T., *Myth, Magic and Medicine*, Fawcett, London, 1956.

Dawson, G. G., *Healing: Pagan and Christian*, Macmillan, London, 1935.

Hartmann, Franz, *Occult Science in Medicine*, Theosophical Publishing House, London, 1893.

Ledermann, E. K., *Philosophy and Healing,* Tavistock Publications, London, 1970.

Precope, J., *Medicine, Magic and Mythology*, Heinemann, London, 1954.

Sigerist, H. E., *A History of Medicine*, Oxford University Press, 1961.

Singer, C. and Underwood, E. A., *A Short History of Medicine*, 2nd edn, Clarendon Press, Oxford, 1962.

THERMOSOMATICS

The study of temperature in relation to the body, including the body's adaptation to extremes of heat and cold, and temperature changes in certain mental and mystical states. It is known, for instance, that during conditions of suspended animation, including hibernation, the metabolism is greatly decreased, and breathing and temperature drop considerably.

Dr Walter B. Cannon coined the term *homeostasis* for the inbuilt regulating system that maintains the balance of such automatic functions as the heartbeat, hormonal activity and body temperature. When for any reason the homeostatic process is temporarily disrupted, the body can for a time endure, without succumbing, the changed internal economy until normal conditions are restored. The homeostatic balance is very resistant to change in a healthy person, and is closely connected with an individual's sense of wellbeing and even his life. During fever*, when the temperature rises a few degrees, a person has a sense of malaise, but if raised only one or two degrees more will result in his death.

Some individuals and even certain ethnic groups have a natural faculty that enables them to endure climatic extremes. Certain psychological states such as religious exaltation also render a person immune to temperature changes. Training can do the same, as we see in the case of those who break the river ice in mid-winter for their daily swim. Hysteria* and hypnosis* can likewise induce a degree of immunity to heat and cold.

It is known that a man can accelerate or slow down his heartbeat at will, and that cold feet can be made warm by concentration. Hypnotized hysterics can have their temperatures raised or lowered by suggestion. J. A. Hadfield, of London University, described how he was able to produce changes in the temperature of a patient's arm by waking suggestion; and A. Macey records how in an internment camp in Berlin on a winter day when the snow lay thick on the ground, he managed by hypnotic suggestion to bring on a violent outbreak of perspiration in a freezing subject.

The human body has its own highly efficient cooling system: perspiration and mucus secretions; but there are limits to its normal operation. In India certain yogis by long practice keep cool even in the hottest weather. This is helped by concentration on a cool, snow-filled landscape. Similarly fire-walking and other demonstrations of heat immunity are, to some extent, possibly due to training and autosuggestion. In the course of US government-sponsored tests conducted at the University of California by Dr Craig Taylor, a physiologist and engineer, it was found that human beings could withstand 'hot-box' temperatures until the heat passed the boiling-point of water ($212°F$). Professor Taylor himself stayed in an experimental cylinder till the atmosphere rose to $262°F$, and endured it for over 15 minutes. While he was inside an egg fried on a metal frying-pan in front of him.

A lowering of temperature, like the slowing down of the breathing rate, is generally held to aid the preservation of body cells and tissues. The eighteenth-century Scottish physician John Hunter (d. 1793) came up with the idea that it might be possible to prolong life 'by freezing a person in the frigid zone', so that all action and waste would cease until the body was thawed, say, after an interval of 100 years. It occurred to him that by such alternate oblivion and activity, it might be possible to prolong life to 1,000 years. He gave up the idea after he froze two live carp in 1776 and found the fish were dead when he thawed them out.

But today scientists envisage the possibility of lowering the temperature of the body to a point just before death supervenes, and preserving it in special refrigeration vaults in a state of virtual suspended animation, to be resurrected at some time in the future. They suggest also that reproductive cells, both male and female, could be maintained deep-frozen in banks for future use.

Hypothermic sleep, or artificial hibernation after the body temperature has been lowered to 86°F, results in a slowing down of all physiological and metabolic processes and thus reduces the speed of ageing. Hypothermy below that level cannot be sustained under normal conditions, but if the heart could be regulated to beat by mechanical means, then a temperature of 80°F or slightly less could be maintained without damage to the living body. A method of healing known as cryotherapy (Gk. *kruos*, 'ice') consists in freezing a sick organ or limb before treatment or surgery. This facilitates the operation and greatly speeds up the healing process.

The body's normal resistance to cold is quite astonishing. The physiological mechanisms of many animal species inhabiting the Arctic regions instinctively react to the onset of winter. Blood is drawn away from the extremities, and the temperature sinks to a level close to freezing-point. Among such species is the husky, caribou, seal, polar bear and the seagull.

Certain peoples by some inherent bodily quality, or through long training in special methods, can withstand a considerable degree of cold. The Patagonians go about bare-bodied in winter, where Europeans in the same place have to wear woollen undergarments and heavy overcoats. A scientific research team was sent out to study why desert Aborigines of central Australia do not suffer from the intense cold at night, which sometimes reaches freezing-point, and how, for instance, they are able to sleep out in the open quite comfortably with only one blanket. The scientists returned convinced that these primitives have 'an inherent hardiness to withstand cold' which other peoples do not possess. Similarly scientific expeditions to the Himalayas have reported seeing completely naked hermits living high up among the permanent snows. This faculty has been ascribed to the secret of *tummo*, a heat-generating technique practised for centuries by certain Tibetan lamas, who are able to live in caves through the coldest winters, wearing only a single cotton garment.

The biographies of Christian saints contain many examples of such immunity to cold and heat. One curious phenomenon associated with the *unio mystica*, the 'mystical union' of the soul with God, is known as the *incendium amoris*, 'fire of love', which arises from the mystic's love of God. It manifests in feelings that are often akin to erotomania* and in extraordinary changes in bodily temperature. St Catherine of Genoa (d. 1510) and St Mary Magdalene of Pazzi (d. 1607), who both experienced the incendium amoris, lived in such an increased degree of physical warmth that even in winter they sought for cold places, loved the coldest winds, and applied cold compresses to soothe themselves. St Philip Neri (d. 1595) was often in a state of such high bodily temperature that Cardinal Crescenzi said that the touch of his hand was as if he had a raging fever. During the process for the beatification of Serafino of Dio (d. 1699), nuns declared that in her lifetime it scorched them if they touched her.

Books

Barclay, Glen, *Mind Over Matter,* Arthur Barker, London, 1973.

Bayliss, E. A. *et al.* (eds), *Man in a Cold Environment*, Edward Arnold, London, 1955.

Cannon, Walter B., *The Wisdom of the Body*, Kegan Paul, Trubner Trench, London, 1939.

Hadfield, J. A., 'The Influence of Suggestion on Body Temperature', *The Lancet*, July 1920.

Hannon, J. P. and Viereck, E. (eds), *Neural Aspects of Temperature Regulation*, Fort Wainwright, Alaska, 1961.

Hardy, J. D. (ed.), *Temperature: Its Measurement and Control in Science and Industry*, Reinhold, New York, 1963.

Irving, Laurence, 'Adaptations to Cold', *Scientific American*, January 1966.

Leach, Gerald, *The Biocrats*, Jonathan Cape, London, 1970.

Macey, A., *Hypnotism Explained*, London, 1933.

Newburgh, L. H. (ed.), *Physiology of Heat Regulation and the Science of Clothing*, Saunders, Philadelphia, 1949.

Selle, W. A., *Body Temperature*, C. C. Thomas, Springfield, Illinois, 1952.

Singer, Kurt, *Tales from the Unknown*, W. H. Allen, London, 1970.

TOUCH HEALING

A mode of therapy in which the healer touches, strokes or rubs the diseased part with his hand or, more rarely, his foot. It is of very remote antiquity, the earliest records being of the priest-healers of ancient Egypt and Babylonia, and the imperial physicians of China. The Marsii, Psylli and other Mediterranean tribes cured snake-bite by touching the afflicted spot.

Certain exalted personages, especially in royal and priestly families, were believed to be endowed with the divine gift. Pyrrhus (d. 272 BC) king of Epirus, had the power of curing enlarged spleen and colic pains by simply pressing the big toe of his right foot or the thumb of his right hand upon the area. Vespasian (d. AD 79), Roman emperor, while pronouncing a formula taught him by the hierophants, was able to cure nervous afflictions, lameness and blindness by touch. Another emperor, Hadrian (d. AD 138), cured dropsy in the same way.

In medieval Europe the kings of Hungary were said to cure jaundice by moving the hand over the patient. In like manner, the dukes of Burgundy cured the plague, and the kings of Spain delivered those who were possessed by the devil. In France the tradition was established by Clovis (c. AD 481) after he accidentally discovered that he had the gift. Many later French kings also claimed to have it. In 1686 Louis XIV touched 1600 persons on Easter Sunday alone.

In England the practice appears to have started with the saintly Edward the Confessor (d. 1066) and from him the power descended to all his successors to the throne. The 'royal touch' was said to be particularly effective in the case of scrofula (or struma), tuberculous glands. For this reason scrofula was popularly called 'the king's evil'. From the time of Henry VII it became customary for the monarch to present each person he touched with an angel-noble, a gold coin, and this touch-piece, as it came to be called, used to be pierced and worn around the neck as a talisman to prevent a recurrence. A special service instituted by Henry VII remained in the Prayer Book till 1719. James I reputedly cured the diseased throat of the Turkish ambassador's son by stroking the afflicted area.

Touch healing was carried on by all the English monarchs, although from the time of Charles I silver and then copper coins were substituted for gold. William III (d. 1702), the first open doubter, pronounced it 'a silly superstition', and officiated at the function only once, telling his patients that he hoped God would give them more sense. But Queen Anne revived the rite, and on a historic day in 1714 touched 200 persons, among them the 3-year-old Samuel Johnson, who had been brought from Lichfield by his mother. He was the last person officially 'touched' by an English monarch of whom any record exists.

Apart from royalty, touch healing in England has had numerous lay practitioners, of whom the best known was Valentine Greatrakes (d. 1683). Another healer, James Leverett, claimed to have cured over 600 people. In 1792 James Hallett of Sussex also claimed success with cancer, blindness and the king's evil. Many of these claims were authenticated by reliable witnesses.

The following are among the explanations put forward to account for the phenomenon: the powerful aura or mana of certain persons, especially those who receive the homage of the multitude, like kings and prelates; the particularly strong 'animal magnetism' (bioflux) emanating from the body, especially the hand, of natural healers; faith on the part of the patient.

Touching forms part of certain kinds of spiritual healing. Many modern encounter groups practise mutual touching as a therapeutic exercise.

Touch healing is akin to the ritual laying on of hands, or cheirothesy (Gk. *cheir*, 'hand'; *thesis*, 'placing'), in which a person, duly qualified and consecrated for the purpose, places his hands on another person, usually on the head, in order to transmit power, blessing, grace or other benefit, as in ceremonies of initiation, ordination, healing, exorcism.

In the Bible we read that the apostles were promised the gift of healing through their hands (Mk. 16:18). By the laying on of his hands, the disciple Ananias caused Saul (the apostle Paul) to be filled with the Holy Ghost (Acts 9:17). Timothy was given the gift of prophecy and other spiritual gifts by the same means (1 Tim. 4:14).

Books

Becket, M., *Free and Impartial Inquiry into the Antiquity and Efficacy of Touching for the King's Evil*, London, 1772.
Bloch, Marc, *The Royal Touch*, Routledge & Kegan Paul, London, 1973.
Crawfurd, R., *The King's Evil*, Clarendon Press, Oxford, 1911.
Hutton, J. B., *Healing Hands*, McKay, New York, 1967.
Sorell, Walter, *The Story of the Human Hand*, Weidenfeld & Nicolson, London, 1968.
Thompson, C. J. S., *The Mysteries of History*, Faber & Gwyer, London, 1928.

TRANSFERENCE

Transference in a general sense is the emotional adjustment that takes place in any interpersonal association, in which one of the individuals concerned attributes to the other qualities that are associated with types taken from his or her own early experience, such as father, mother, elder sibling, uncle, schoolteacher. In psychoanalysis it is applied to the process in which a person seeking counselling or guidance sees in the person from whom he seeks it, a larger-than-life embodiment of some character of his past, known or imagined. He transfers to his counsellor some of the feelings, whether of love or hate, associated with the early model, especially those which for some reason have remained unresolved from childhood.

Transference is a phenomenon found in many grades of differential association, as between confessor and female penitent (the subject of earlier anti-Catholic literature), between doctor and patient, doctor and nurse, boss and secretary, guru and female chela, therapist and client. The authority of the one and the 'subordination' of the other often places the relationship on an anomalous footing. The patient, subject, advisee, is psychologically inferior and open to exploitation.

In all forms of psychotherapy it has been found that, although there exists a degree of ambivalence in the attitude of patient to therapist, the more dominant emotions are those of overevaluation. The therapist becomes the object of the patient's gratitude, respect, devotion, love, sexuality. The patient does or says things to gain the esteem, respect, applause and admiration of the analyst, and fears his disapproval. Such transferential involvement can lead to a desire to surrender, to grovel, to give oneself in a physical sense to the superior.

In psychoanalysis transference is regarded as part of the healing process, in the course of which the patient makes a series of personal discoveries about himself. But the abuse of this relationship is not uncommon. The unscrupulous therapist can foster dependence in the patient, and then, as Dr Malcolm Pines says, exploit it for years to his own advantage 'in the form of a steady income, to say nothing of the opportunities for sexual gratification' (Varma, 1974, p. 279).

Sandor Ferenczi (d. 1933), a follower of Freud, introduced a theory of love and permissiveness into his own psychotherapy, and would kiss and caress his female patients, and encourage them to reciprocate. Freud, greatly irritated by these measures, proposed to expel Ferenczi from the position of responsibility he occupied in the Psychoanalytic Association, but the latter died before this could be done.

Subsequently reputable analysts were widely rumoured to be sleeping with their female patients, 'either for therapeutic or for other reasons' (Rogow, 1971, p. 103). Chesler speaks of many New York and Californian analysts who over the years systematically preached and practised sex with their female patients (Chesler, 1974, p. 131).

Introverted and 'deprived' men who become therapists often find it difficult to resist taking advantage of their acquired status as confessors and father figures, with their young female patients lying on a couch, and, as it were waiting to be seduced. In such cases the women are in a vulnerable position, since if they complain or bring legal action it can always be said that they are subject to neurotic delusions, which is why they came for treatment in the first place.

Books

Chesler, P., *Women and Madness,* Allen Lane, London, 1974.
Fairburn, W. R. D., *Psychoanalytic Studies of the Personality*, Tavistock Publications, London, 1952.
Freud, S., *Introductory Lectures on Psychoanalysis*, Hogarth Press, London, 1963.
Rogow, Arnold, *The Psychiatrists*, Allen & Unwin, London, 1971.
Shepard, Mary, *The Love Treatment: Sexual Intimacy Between Patients and Psychotherapists*, Wyden, New York, 1971.
Toman, W., *Introduction to Psychoanalytic Theory of Motivation*, New York, 1960.
Varma, Ved (ed.), *Psychotherapy Today*, Constable, London, 1974.
Winnicott, D. W., *Collected Papers*, Tavistock Publications, London, 1958.

TUBERCULOSIS

Or TB, consumption, phthisis, hectic fever, lupus, scrofula, 'the wasting sickness', 'the white plague'. It was once counted among the leading causes of death. Until its conquest by antibiotics, this disease was responsible for 1 out of 7 deaths from all causes. The rapidly progressive form of the disease, known as galloping consumption, could kill in a few weeks.

Though an infectious disease, TB depends as much on the soil as the seed, as much on heredity as on infection. Not everyone who is exposed to it contracts it. The vast majority of people even in advanced countries have healed TB lesions in their lungs, showing that they have at some time been attacked by and resisted the tubercle bacillus. It is now generally admitted that consumption does not necessarily result from exposure to the bacillus, but that many contributory emotional factors predispose one to it. Hence it has been called a psychosomatic* disease.

Among the countless folk-remedies prescribed for consumption among different nations, the following are a sampling: eat the ordure of a boy, dried and mixed with honey; swallow the gallstones of a monkey; place some dog-fat in a can and hang it across the shoulders; eat snail-slime; swallow baby frogs whole before breakfast; drink distilled laurel water; inhale the fumes of diluted prussic acid; stay as much as possible in the atmosphere of cowsheds so as to inhale the health-giving odour of cows and especially cow dung.

Greek and Hindu physicians of antiquity found a connection between the 'wasting disease' and such mental factors as grief, unrequited love and ungratified desires. Subsequently, the chest specialist René Laennec (d. 1826), who invented the stethoscope to avoid the embarrassment of putting his ear to a woman's breast, wrote that 'profound melancholic passions' produce this illness. Until the beginning of the nineteenth century physicians accepted the *spes phthisica*, the peculiar mental unease, as well as courage and hopefulness, of tuberculous patients, as diagnostic of the disease itself.

Like few other sicknesses, consumption gives one a characteristic turn of mind. Many observers as well as ex-sufferers have noted, among other things, a marked rise in sexual feelings that usually accompanies consumption. Bett was tempted to speculate that the toxins released by the tubercle bacillus perhaps affect the higher intellectual centres of the cerebral cortex, allowing such faculties as imagination, rhythm, colour sense, and poetical instinct to operate with greater freedom. It inclines one both to exaltation and morbidity, and if a touch of melancholy does indeed stimulate the higher faculties, then TB may have been a contributory factor in the evolution of genius. Jacobson said that an almost sure recipe for producing the highest type of creative mind would be 'an initial spark of genius plus tuberculosis'. The disease has claimed a large number of victims among literary, musical and artistic people, as also men and women of outstanding achievement in other fields. The following is a brief list.

Raphael (d. 1520); Albrecht Dürer (d. 1528), German engraver; John Calvin (d. 1564); Cardinal Richelieu (d. 1642); Paul Scarron (d. 1660), French poet; Molière (d. 1673); Baruch Spinoza (d. 1677); Henry Purcell (d. 1695), English composer; Antoine Watteau (d. 1721), French painter; Laurence Sterne (d. 1768); Voltaire (d. 1778); Jean-Jacques Rousseau (d. 1778); Samuel Johnson (d. 1784); Wolfgang Amadeus Mozart (d. 1791); Novalis (d. 1801), German romantic poet; Friedrich von Schiller (d. 1805); John Keats (d. 1821); Percy Bysshe Shelley (d. 1822); René Laennec (d. 1826), French physician; Carl Ernst von Weber (d. 1826), composer; Sir Walter Scott (d. 1832); Johann Wolfgang von Goethe (de. 1832); Nicolo Paganini (d. 1840), violinist; Emily Brontë (d. 1848); Frédéric Chopin (d. 1849); Edgar Allan Poe (d. 1849); Charlotte Brontë (d. 1855); Washington Irving (d. 1859); Elizabeth Barrett Browning (d. 1861); Henry Thoreau (d. 1862); Fyodor Dostoevsky (d. 1881); Sidney Lanier (d. 1881), American lyric poet; Ralph Waldo Emerson (d. 1882); Jules Laforgue (d. 1887), French symbolist poet; John Addington Symonds (d. 1893), literary critic; Robert Louis Stevenson (d. 1894); Aubrey Beardsley (d. 1898), artist and designer; Cecil Rhodes (d. 1902); Paul Gauguin (d. 1903); Anton Chekhov (d. 1904); Francis Thompson (d. 1907); Paul Ehrlich (d. 1915), bacteriologist; Amadeo Modigliani (d. 1920), Italian painter and sculptor; Katherine Mansfield (d. 1923), author; Franz Kafka (d. 1924), Austrian Jewish novelist; D. H. Lawrence (d. 1930); Maxim Gorky (d. 1936); Ernst Ludwig Kirchner (d. 1938), German painter; Simone Weil (d. 1943), French philosophical writer; Adolf Hitler (d. 1945); George Orwell (d. 1950); Eugene O'Neill (d. 1953).

Books

Bett, W. R., *The Infirmities of Genius*, Christopher Johnson, London, 1952.
Brown, Lawrason, *The Story of Clinical Pulmonary Tuberculosis*, Baltimore, 1941.
Burke, R. M., *An Historical Chronology of Tuberculosis*, 2nd edn, Baltimore, 1955.
Castiglioni, A., *History of Tuberculosis*, Medical Life Press, New York, 1933.
Cummins, S. L., *Tuberculosis in History*, Ballière, Tindall & Cox, London, 1949.
Dubos, René and Jean, *The White Plague: Tuberculosis, Man and Society*, Gollancz, London, 1953.
Huber, J. B., *Consumption: Its Relation to Man and His Civilization*, Lippincott, Philadelphia, 1906.
Jacobson, A. C., *Genius: Some Revaluations*, Adelphi Publications, London, 1926.
Kissen, D. M., *Emotional Factors in Pulmonary Tuberculosis*, Tavistock Publications, London, 1958.
Meachen, G. N., *A Short History of Tuberculosis*, London, 1936.
Moorman, L. J., *Tuberculosis and Genius*, University of Chicago Press, 1940.

Munro, D. G. M., *The Psycho-pathology of Tuberculosis*, Oxford University Press, 1926.
Waksman, Selman A., *The Conquest of Tuberculosis*, Robert Hale, London, 1965.
Wittkower, E., *A Psychiatrist Looks at Tuberculosis*, 2nd edn, Baltimore, 1955.

U

URINOSCOPY

Diagnosis of disease by examination of the urine goes back to ancient Egypt, China, India and Greece. The close connection between the kidneys and heart, and by association, between urine and blood, was first set forth by Galen (d. AD 201), who thought that urine was secreted direct by the vena cava. Blood from the kidneys is now known to be carried to the heart by the inferior (or lower) vena cava, the largest vein in the body. It was believed that by examination of the urine it was possible to determine the patient's physical condition in complete detail. Even today urine analysis remains one of the chief methods of medical diagnosis.

The ease and frequency of passing urine; its appearance, smell, taste, quality and density; its weight, quantity and specific gravity; the sedimentation in it; its reaction when mixed with other chemicals, all used to be taken into account. The state of health, the nature of sickness, virility, sterility, the condition of the internal organs, pregnancy, the sex of the unborn child and length of life could allegedly be determined by urinoscopy. Among its most enthusiastic practitioners were the urinarians, water-casters or piss-prophets, as they were dubbed, of medieval Europe. Experts did not trouble to visit patients, but by inspecting a sample of their urine would tell the age, sex and ailment, and prescribe a cure.

The colour of urine was of great importance. If slightly ruddy, it showed a weak stomach; if red, fever; if saffron, jaundice, and if pale, good health. A large collection of proverbial lore was evolved to aid the memory. For example: 'Live right, piss light.' People kept bottles of urine of absent relations and by its changing appearance judged the state of the loved one's health. When it started to turn dark it presaged danger to life, and when it turned black the absent one was believed to be dead.

Legend has it that Sir Thomas More (beheaded 1535) upon hearing of his condemnation by Henry VIII, examined his next urination and remarked with his usual wit that he saw nothing in it that indicated that he might not live, if it so pleased the king.

Books

Bourke, J. G., *Scatologic Rites of All Nations*, Lowdermilk, Washington, DC, 1891.

Brian, T., *The Pisse-Prophet*, London, 1637.
Hart, J., *The Anatomie of Urines*, London, 1625.
Smith, Anthony, *The Body*, Allen & Unwin, London, 1968.

XENOPHRENIA

Xenophrenia (Gk. *xenos*, 'strange'; *phrēn*, 'mind') includes all states of mind other than the consciousness of the normal, waking adult. It extends over a wide range of human experience, from the first shifting of conscious awareness from the things around one, as during a 'brown study', to the total unconsciousness of deep coma. The return from a xenophrenic to a normal state of consciousness may be accompanied by varying states of recall: there may be total recall, as after a brief reverie; partial recall, as of a dream after sleep; or total amnesia or absence of recall, as after a fainting spell.

In occult terms the cause of xenophrenia is a greater or lesser degree of displacement of the etheric body from its alignment with the physical. When the normal adult is awake and functioning in the practical world, his two bodies are in perfect alignment, or 'coincidence'. In xenophrenia the etheric double moves slightly or completely out of coincidence. During slight discoincidence the vision may become blurred, speech slurred, gait unsteady, thought confused and normal consciousness altered, so that some measure of contact is lost with the practical world. Occasionally another dimension supervenes. In extreme xenophrenic states there is total loss of practical awareness, or unconsciousness.

Both infancy and senility are xenophrenic states; so are sickness, drunkenness, drug-intoxication, ecstasy, somnambulism* (sleep-walking), hypnosis*, hypnagogia (drowsiness), blackouts, trance, vertigo, delusions, hallucinations, dissociation, depersonalization*, 'possession'*, multiple personality*, insanity, epilepsy*, narcolepsy (brief unconsciousness), sleep, coma and dying.

Xenophrenia may be precipitated in a number of ways: injury, accident, infection; drugs, alcohol, chemicals, poisons; physical disease; metabolic, glandular or hormonic dysfunction; exhaustion, pain*, shock*; mental disease; hysteria*, migraine*, depression*; overwhelming emotion, panic, terror, rage, jealousy, intense love, grief, intense joy; sensory stimulation, sexual intercourse, orgasm; music, chanting, dancing, whirling, drumming, flickering lights, incense; sensory deprivation, boredom, starvation, thirst, protracted solitude, continence, insomnolence; deep thought, meditation, prayer.

Books

King, C. Daly, *States of Human Consciousness*, University Books, New York, 1963.
Lilly, John, *The Centre of the Cyclone*, Calder & Boyars, London, 1973.
Masters, R. E. L. and Houston, J., *The Varieties of Psychedelic Experience,* Blond, London, 1967.
Singer, J. L., *Daydreaming: an Introduction to the Experimental Study of Inner Experience*, Random House, New York, 1966.
Tart, Charles (ed.), *Altered States of Consciousness*, Wiley, New York, 1969.
Walker, Benjamin, *Beyond the Body*, Routledge & Kegan Paul, London, 1974.

Z

ZONE THERAPY

Zone therapy is based on the belief that the body has distinct zones that can become the focus of infection or disease, and that treatment should be confined to these areas. While admitting that the body works as a unit, the zone therapist points out that in sickness the whole body very rarely goes out of action at the same time; usually it is only one area that is affected by any specific malaise or injury. Diagnosis can as a rule be made from an examination of that area, and treatment can be effective if concentrated on that area as well.

There are many types of zone therapy. According to a belief first formulated in ancient Egypt, the whole physical organism is served by a highly refined network of subtle arteries which operate in the etheric body invisible to the ordinary senses. Because of their intricate ramification through the body the treatment of pain or malaise is not necessarily administered in the region where the symptoms manifest, but often in some other part of the body where the relevant subtle artery can be more easily stimulated.

Chinese acupuncture* is based on a similar idea of subtle arteries, and so are a number of other healing systems both Eastern and Western. One relic of a medieval belief found in England was that a nerve behind the ear (actually a tiny branch of the vagus nerve) controlled digestion. It was called the alderman's nerve and the popular belief was that a drop of cold wine applied behind the ear after a banquet prevented indigestion.

The ancient Greeks divided the body into four regions, each associated with one of the four elements: the aeric with air, centred in the liver; the hydric with water, in the bladder; the telluric with earth, in the intestines; and the pyric with fire, in the heart. Roman and early medieval anatomists spoke of the empyrean region in the head, of the thoracic in the chest, and the elementarium in the viscera.

Early Teutonic medical theory had an arrangement of nine zones, which were sometimes defined as the nine bodily parts, namely, the head, chest, neck, heart, stomach, intestines, sex organs and rectum, arms, legs. These were guarded by nine guardians, each of whom kept off one of the nine venoms, each of a different colour, carried about by the winds.

Chinese and Tibetan zone therapy makes use of the pulses in the hands and the wrists. These are situated in the three phalanges of the thumb, and in three pulses on the wrist, and are believed to control every part and organ of the body. Diseases are diagnosed and healing started by manipulation of the relevant pulse. The study of pulse diagnosis and pulse therapy found many expert practitioners, especially among Muhammadan physicians of the Middle East.

In medieval pathology the abdomen was believed to contain the chief zones of the body, and relics of their demarcation still survive in medical terminology. These were (a) the epigastrium (Gk. 'above the stomach'), from the sternum or breastbone towards the navel, which governed diseases of the liver; (b) the hypochondrium, on either side of the epigastric region; disaffections of this zone were believed to cause hypochondria, melancholia and neurasthenia (*see* neurosis); (c) the lumbar region on either side of the lower abdomen, that is, below the right and left hypochondriac zones; this was the seat of backache, lumbago and kidney disorders; (d) the umbilical or gastric region, around the navel; the seat of most abdominal, gastric, digestive or intestinal disorders; (e) the hypogastric or pubic region, the lower middle part of the abdomen; (f) the inguinal or iliac region of the groin, associated with certain disorders of the lower bowel and sex organs.

Since then a number of new zone therapies have been developed. Thus, in 1881 the Budapest physician Ignatz Peczely invented the science of iridology, based on examination of the iris of the eye. Here, the iris is divided into several zones, each of which is supposed to reflect the condition of the major organs of the body. Various markings show inherent weakness, structural damage, drug deposits, and so on, and diagnosis is made by examining the zones. Iridology continues to have many exponents.

In 1917 Dr William H. Fitzgerald (d. 1925) developed a form of phalange therapy, based on a vertical division of the body into the right and left sides, each side consisting of five zones. On the right side, an invisible etheric artery from the right-hand little finger passes up along the same side of the hand, up through the right arm, shoulder, right side of the neck, right ear, right side of the head, then straight down again through the body to the little toe of the right foot. The little finger of the right hand is believed to control all the areas and organs of the body through which the artery passes. The top phalange of the little finger controls the area of the head and neck; the middle phalange controls the organs of the thorax; and the lower phalange the abdomen, sex organs and legs.

In the same way the ring finger traces a parallel course to the next toe; the middle finger to the middle toe; the forefinger to the long toe; and the right thumb to the big toe of the right foot. Similarly five other lines from the fingers of the left hand pass through the body to the toes of the left foot. Ailments are cured by squeezing, massaging, pinching or rubbing the appropriate phalange of the finger which controls the affected zone.

Another kind of zone therapy called podoscopy or podology traces zones on the soles of the feet. In this system the underside of the big toe governs the brain and nervous system; the ball of the big toe, the neck; the part between the big toe and the second toe controls the eyes; between the second and third toes, the nose; between the third and fourth, the mouth; between the fourth and little toes, the ears. The ball of the foot governs the lungs; the area along the outer margin, the heart; along the inner margin, the spine; the heel controls the sexual organs; and downwards from the heel, the arch of the sole controls the intestines, kidneys, gall bladder and liver. In podoscopy the right side of the body is governed by zones in the left foot, and conversely, the left side of the body by zones in the right foot. Treatment is effected by massaging the related zone of the foot in an upward direction towards the ankle.

Books

Ackerman, A. S. E., *Popular Fallacies*, Old Westminster Press, London, 1923.
Brockbank, William, *Ancient Therapeutic Arts*, London, 1954.
Cutten, G. B., *Three Thousand Years of Medical Healing*, New York, 1911.
Gardner, Martin, *Fads and Fallacies in the Name of Science*, Dover, New York, 1957.
Jensen, Bernard, *The Science and Practice of Iridology*, Hidden Valley Health Ranch, Escondido, California, 1952.
Powell, Eric, *The Natural Home Physician*, Health Science Press, London, 1975.
Rechung, Lama, *Tibetan Medicine*, Wellcome Institute, London, 1973.

Index

Note: figures in italics denote a main article.

abaton, 144
Abishag, 260
abortion, 74, 81, 100, 266
aboulia, *see* abulia
Abraham, 157
Abrams, Albert, 62
abreaction, 235
absent healing, 270
absent-mindedness, 77
abulia, *1*
accident(s), 7
accident-prone, 283
accidie, 1
acclivity, 231
acedia, 1
acetylcholines, 130, 131
acetylcholinesterase, 132
Achilles, 192
acids, 9
acrobatics, 154
acrophobia, 182
ACTH, 130
acting, 164, 234
actinic rays (actinotherapy), 79, 191
Acts of St John, 257
acupuncture, *3*, 211
acute, 200
Adam, 257
Adam's apple, 130
Adams, John Quincy, 247
Adenauer, Konrad, 247
adjuvant, 8
Adler, Alfred, 2, 240
adolescence, *see* youth
adrenal(s), 5, 130
adrenalin, 107, 129, 130, 131
adrenergic, 131
adultery, 23, 98, 149, 266
Adventists, 284
advertising, 171, 265
Aeneas, 167
aerotherapy, 217
Aeschines, 103
Aesculapius (Asclepius), 109, 144, 186, 260
aestivation, 41
aetiology, *6*
Aga Khan, 247
agaric, 69

age-regression, 136
agoraphobia, 182
Agpaoa, Tony, 229
ague, 109, 226
Ahasuerus, 17
AID, 21
AIH, 21
Ainsworth, Lucy, 270
air, 217
Ajax, 167
akido, 155
Alans, 84
alchemy, 47, 172, 245
alcohol(ism), 15, 28, 29, 115, 169, 265, 283
alderman's nerve, 295
aldosterone, 130
Alexander, F. M., 155
Alexander the Great, 47, 91, 174
Alexander VI, 278, 279
Alexander of Tralles, 255
Alfieri, Vittorio, 77
algolagnia, 96, 206
alienation, 59
alienist, 59
allaesthesia, 209
allergen, 30, 95
allergy, 30, 95, 132
allocheiria, 209
allochiry, 59
allopathy, *8*, 128
allotriophagy, 37
aloes, 47
alternating personality, 185
aluminium, 173
ambergris, 18
ambidexterity, 57
Americans, 120, 265
Amerindians, 122, 127, 227, 277
ammonia, 251
amnesia, 294
amniocentesis, 179
amphetamines, 68, 131
amputation, 210
amulets, 172
anabiosis, 42
anaemia, 36, 95, 225
anaesthesia, 5, 41, 43, 136, 138, 210, 225

INDEX

anaesthetics, 205, 219, 229
analepsy (analeptic), 89
analgesia, 136
anal intercourse, 259
anal phase, 47, 48, 197, 200
Ananias, 289
anaphrodisiacs, *9*
anaphylaxis, 95
Anaxagoras, 167
ancestors, 6, 120
ancillarists, 142
Andrewes, Christopher, 153
androgen, 130
androgenesis, 23
andromania, 92
androsterone, 130, 251
angel, 18
angel (coin), 288
anger, 89, 123, 124
angor animi, 280
angst, 7, *10,* 12
anguish, 10
animal(s), 14, 29, 42, 56, 65, 90, 96,
    97, 121, 126, 133, 174, 218, 250
animal magnetism, 30, 159
animals, experiments on, *see*
    vivisection
animal spirits, 137
Anne, Queen, 289
anomie, 1
anorexia nervosa, 193
ANS (autonomic nervous system), 107,
    130
Antabuse, 28
Antaeus, 119
Antarctica, 174
ante-partum, 80
Anthony, St, 196
anthroposophy, 154
antiadrenergic, 131
antibiotics, 38, 71, 100, 141, 142, 146,
    250, 267
antibody, 5, 203
anticholinergics, 131
anticholinesterase, 132
antidepressant, 68
antidote, 8
antigen, 203
antihistamine, 95
antileptol, 156
antimony, 47, 244
antipsychotic, 68
antiseptic, 141, 225, 229, 244
antiserum, 203
antisocial behaviour, 237
antitoxins, 71, 203
Antoine (Antoinism), 270
anus, 46, 197
anxiety, 6, *11*

anxiolytics, 68
apathy, 1
aphairesis, 203
aphasia, 81
aphrodisiacs, *13,* 252
Aphrodite, *see* Venus
Apollo, 113, 144
Apollonius of Tyana, 245
apomorphine, 28
apoplexy, 89
apothecary, 17, 67, 69, 126
appendix, 141
apple, 16
apports (asports), 35, 96
Apuleius, 19
Arabs, 8, 187
Arcady, 66
arc-en-cercle, 50
archetypes, 241
arecoline, 131
Aretaeus, 6, 88
Arigo, 229
Ariosto, Ludovico, 95
Aristaeus, 245
Aristotle, 22, 45, 56, 90, 91, 116, 126,
    149, 166, 167, 171, 180, 188, 234,
    256
Ark, 83
Arnold, Thomas, 206
Arnold of Villanova, 110
aromatherapy, *15*
arousal, 273
ars moriendi, *18*
art(s), 58, 164, 165
Artephius, 219, 231, 245, 252
artery, 204
artificial aids (in sex), 34
artificial fertilization, 20, 102
artificial generation, *20,* 102
artificial insemination, 20
artificial limbs, 214
artificial organs, *see* transplantation
art therapy, *24*
asana, 253, 254
asceticism, 10, 45, 93, 253, 257, 283
Asclepiades, 187
Asclepidae, 144
Asclepius, *see* Aesculapius
Aslan, Ana, 247
asoma, 94, 200
aspirin, 226
asportation, *see* apports
asthma, 30, 89, 94, 95
astral body, 55, 59, 94, 195
astral chord, 55, 96
astral projection, 41, 96
astrology, 6, 36, 52, 62, 126, 127,
    150, 151, 165, 172, 232, 277
astronauts, 42

asylums, *25*, 208
ataractics, 68
ataraxia, 1
atavism, 56, 97
ataxia, 89
atheism, 282
Athenaeus, 187
atmospheric phenomena, 6, 77
atropine, 131
Atum, 253
Augustine, St, 257
aura, 7, 18, 97, 261, 270, 289
aura, epileptic, 87
aura, migrainous, 176
aura diagnosis, 62
aureomycin, 38
auroscopy, 97
Auschwitz, 2
autism, 81, 255
autoallergy, 95
autohaemic therapy, 202
autoimmunity, 95
automatism, 24, 233
autonomic nervous system, *see* ANS
autoscopy, 270
autotherapy, 202
Auxonne, 49, 210
aversion therapy, *28*
Avicenna, 8, 14, 243
axe, 120
ayurvedic, 226
Aztecs, 85, 227, 277, 278

Babylon, 143, 144
bacchantes, 162
Bach, Edward, 111
Bach, Johann Sebastian, 167
Bacon, Francis, 47, 63, 116, 119, 218, 224, 261
bacteria, *see* microbes
bacteriological warfare (BW), 181
baldness, 57, 149, 256
balneotherapy, 133
Balzac, Honoré de, 78, 115
bandaging, 225
banisterine, 9, 69
banya, 133
barbiturates, 71, 227
Bardo Thodol, 19
barrenness, 13, 148
Barry, Comtesse du, 17
basanotherapy, 208
bat, 42
bath, 133
Baudelaire, Charles, 78, 91, 117, 279
Beardsley, Aubrey, 292
Beatniks, 122, 163
Beauchamp, Miss, 185

Beaumarchais, 114
beauty, 44
Beddoes, Thomas, 219
Bedlam, 25
bedside manner, 142, 216
bees, 64
Beethoven, Ludwig van, 77, 114, 177, 279
Beggar Societies, 85
behaviour therapy, 9, *29*
beheading, 35, 53, 55
Bel, 144
belladonna, 13, 69
Bellerophon, 167
Benedict, St, 103
Bennett, Allan, 258
Bentham, Jeremy, 191
bergamot, 18
Bergerac, Cyrano de, 279
Bergson, Henri, 210
Berkeley, Bishop, 127
Berlioz, Hector, 91, 114
Bernard, Claude, 175
Berne, E., 122
Bernheim, Hippolyte, 32
berries, 14
berserker, 97, 113
Bertrand, Alexandre, 32
Bessemer, Henry, 247
bestiality, 96, 97
bhang, 69
Bible, 1, 17, 28, 83, 103, 157, 164, 186, 234, 251, 260, 289
bibliotherapy, 199
bilocation, 273
biochemistry, 129; *see also* tissue— salt therapy
bioelectricity, 79, 80
bioenergetics, 155
bioflux, 5, 30, 62, 231, 289
biogenic amines, 130, 132
biological engineering, 99
biomagnetic therapy, *30*
biomagnetism, 80, 231
bioplasma, 7, 55, 64, 97, 99, 222
biosignals, 33
biotelemetry, *33,* 63, 79
birds, 14, 42
birth, 82, 90
birth control, 81, 100
birth rate, 75, 76
birth trauma, 241
Bismarck, Otto von, 167, 216
bitters, 15
black box, 62
black death, 85, 153
black magic, *see* sorcery
black mass, 237
blackouts, 294

INDEX

Blake, William, 117
blastocyst, 21, 22, 75, 81
bleeding, *35*
blindness, 114
blood, 15, 35, 79, 81, 142, 156, 219
blood-brain barrier, 72, 129
blood-drinking, 90, 96, 251, 252, 261
blood-letting, 35, 128, 246
blood pressure, 130, 188
blood transfusion, 142, 202, 246, 252
Bloody Mary, 278
Boaz, 17
Bodin, Jean, 50
body, 190
Boece, Hector, 90, 157
Boerhaave, Hermann, 261
Boguet, Henri, 56
bokon, 96
bone(s), 203
bone-setting, 203
Bon sect, 191
Book of the Dead, 19
Booth, William, 247
borboric therapy, *36*
Borgia, Cesare, 278
Bossuet, Jacques, 91
botanotherapy, 215
Boucher, François, 47
boxed-in syndrome, 43
Boyesen, Gerda, 161
Boyle, Robert, 90
Brahe, Tycho, 95, 116
Brahms, Johannes, 78
Braid, James, 32, 268
brain, 130, 206
brain death, 54
brain surgery, 26
brain transplants, 99
brainwashing, 98, 170
brain waves, 34, 54
Brave New World, 22
breathing, 31, 50, 54, 154, 217
bregma, 139
Brethren of the Free Spirit, 162
Breuer, Josef, 259
bromides, 9, 68
Brontë, Charlotte, 292
Brontë, Emily, 292
Browne, Thomas, 195, 225, 254, 258
Browning, E. B., 78, 117, 292
Brown-Séquard, Charles, 246
Buber, Martin, 247
bubonic plague, *see* plague
Bucke, Richard, 198
Buckingham, Lord, 262
Buddha (Buddhism), 10, 66, 103
bufagin, 226
bufontenin, 69
bulimia, 139

Bunyan, John, 116
Buoninsegni, Domenico, 150
Burchard, Bishop, 253
bureaucracy, 140, 142, 213, 274
burial, 119
burial alive, 41, 43, 53, 54
Burnet, Gilbert, 235
Burnet, Macfarlane, 181
Burns, Robert, 114, 167
Burr, Harold, 79
Burton, Richard, 93
Burton, Robert, 261, 262
Butenandt, Dr, 251
buttocks, 13
BW, *see* bacteriological warfare
Byron, Lord, 91, 114, 167
Byzantine empire, 84

caapi, 9, 69
cactus, 69
Caesar, Caius Julius, 83, 91, 95
Caesarean section, 225
Caesar's world, 249
Caesonia, 13
Calabar bean, 132, 226
calcium, 130, 274
Caligula, 13, 91, 278
Callimachus, 91
calor, 207
Calvin, John, 292
Cambyses, 91
camphor, 9
Canaan, 46
cancer, *39*, 146, 247
cannabis, 13, 69
cannibalism, 96, 97, 191
Cannon, Walter B., 286
cantharides, 14
carbon-dioxide therapy, 220
carcinogen, 39
Cardan, Jerome, 95
cardiazol, 208
cardiotachometer, 33
Carlyle, Thomas, 114, 117, 164, 167,
    177, 247
carminative, 134
carotids, 41, 135, 210
Carrell, Alexis, 74, 202, 244
carriers, 174
Carroll, Lewis, 177
Carver, G. W., 111
Casanova, 92
cascara, 47
case history, 62
castor oil, 47
castration, 12, 90, 149, 157, 257
catalepsy, *41*, 48
cataplexy, *42*

catarrh, 88
catatonia, 41, 42, 201, 254
catecholamines, 130, 131
catharsis, 45, 123, 125, 187, 234
Catherine, St, 287
cattle, 218
causes of disease, *see* aetiology
cauterization, 90, 207
Cavendish, Ada, 54
Cavour, Count, 177
Cayce, Edgar, 270
celibacy, 93
cell(s), 22, 31, 39, 79, 179
Cellini, Benvenuto, 91, 279
cell therapy, 180
cellular biology, 179
cellular therapy, 247
Celsus, 148, 207, 255, 277
central nervous system, *see* CNS
cereals, 14
cerebral death, 54
cerebral palsy, 81
Cerletti, Ugo, 208
chamber pot, 47
chameleon, 14
chance, 86
chancroid, 277
change, 12
Chapman, George, 269
Charcot, Jean, 32, 159, 240, 259
charlatan, 242
Charles I, 289
Charles II, 163
Charles V, 86, 91
Charles VIII, 277, 278
Chateaubriand, François, 117
chaulmoogra, 156
cheese, 132
cheiropractic, *see* chiropractic
cheirothesy, *see* chirothesy
Chekhov, Anton, 292
chemical gases, 219
chemise cagoule, 257
chemotherapy, *see* drug therapy
Cheyne, Dr, 235
ch'i, 3, 4, 108
chicken-pox, 149
chilblains, 127
childbed fever, 141
childbirth, 119, 136
children, 2, 7, 24, 44, 146, 169, 266
China (Chinese), 3, 10, 19, 108, 156,
    245, 296
chiropractic, 204
chirothesy, 289
chloroform, 219
chlorpromazine, 68
chod, 191
cholera, 83

cholesterol, 158, 274
cholinergic, 131
cholinesterase, 132
Chopin, Frédéric, 78, 115, 292
Christ, 78, 103, 104, 157, 221, 272
Christians (Christianity), 20, 145, 157
Christian Science, 118, 178
Chrobak, Dr, 259
chromidrosis, 273
chromosomes, 74, 179, 238
chromotherapy, *44*
chronic, 206
chronoleptogenics, 69
Chrysostom, John, 157
Churchill, Randolph, 279
Churchill, Winston, 247, 279
chylification, 64
chymification, 64
chypre, 17
Cicero, 113
cinchona bark, 127, 227
circadian rhythm, 129
circular psychosis, *see* cyclothymia
circumcision, 46
clairvoyance, 16, 176
clairvoyant healing, 270
claustrophobia, 182
clavus hystericus, 139
Clemenceau, Georges, 247
Clement VI, 85
client-centred therapy, 122
climate, 6, 77, 120
clitoridectomy, 46
clitoris, 149
clones and cloning, 22
clonus, 89
clothes, 10, 80, 96, 120, 232
Clough, Arthur Hugh, 99
Clovis, 288
clyster, *see* enema
CNS (central nervous system), 130
cobwebs, 38, 109
cocaine, 9, 13, 69
coffee, 9
Cohausen, J. H., 246
coil, 81
coitophobia, 256
coitus, 90, 124, 125, 138, 256, 258,
    259
coitus reservatus, 253
cold, 285
cold, common, 65, 109
Coleridge, S. T., 219
collagen, 203
collective unconscious, 241
Collins, Wilkie, 54
colour, 44, 57
colour-hearing, 211
Columbus, Christopher, 277

INDEX

coma, 41, 53, 73, 89, 99, 139, 294
Combe, George, 198
Commodus, 252
compulsion, 196
computer diagnosis, 140, 190
Comte, Auguste, 117
concentration camps, 2, 26, 98, 170, 208
conception, 20, 80
concept therapy, 178
conditioned reflex, 29
conditioning, 29
confessions, 123, 125
confusants, 69
congressus subtilis, 96, 253
consciousness, 55, 59, 176, 205, 217, 294
consent for experiments, 106
Constantine, 156
constipation, *45*
consultants, 142
consumption, *see* tuberculosis
contortions, 48
contraceptives, 71
contract therapy, 122
convent hysteria, 48, 49, 91, 93, 137, 163
conversion, 123, 249
conversion hysteria, 138
convolvulus, 69
Convulsionaries, 139, 210, 270, 284
convulsions, *48,* 88
convulsive therapy, 208
co-operative therapy, 122
coprolalia, 58
coprophagy, 96
coprophilia, 47
Coptics, 41
Corday, Charlotte, 53
Cornwallis, Lord, 262
corpses, 191
correspondence, 112
cortical death, 54
cortico-steroids, 130, 274
cortico-tropin, see ACTH
cortisone, 130
corybantes, 162
Cos, 144
cosmetics, 16
cosmic rays, 40
cosmobiology, 6, 52, 82, 86, 118, 146, 169, 175
councils, church, 103
counselling, 249
counter-irritation, 207
Counter-Reformation, 164
couple therapy, 122
cow(s), 218, 291
Cowper, William, 116

cowpox, 225
crasis, 7
Crécy, 85
cremation, 55
crimes, 58, 238, 265
Cripps, Stafford, 155
crisis, 200
Croce, Benedetto, 247
Crookes, William, 247
crowd psychosis, 161
Crowley, Aleister, 17, 155, 279
Crusades, 85, 162
cryotherapy, 110, 246, 287
crystallography, 179
Cullen, William, 127, 192
culling, 126
Culpeper, Nicholas, 127
cupping, *51*
curare, 227
curses, 236
cuscus, 17
Cybele, 284
cyclothymia, 44, 52
Cyprian, St, 84
cytology, *see* cell

Dadd, Richard, 118
Daedalus, 22
dagga, 69
damiana, 13
Damien, St, 145
dance, 49, 85, 154, 155, 164
dancing mania, 91, 162, 284
danse macabre, 19, 85
dapsone, 147
Darnley, Lord, 278
Darwin, Charles, 25, 117, 177
Darwin, Erasmus, 25
datura, 13, 69
Daudet, Alphonse, 279
David, King, 186, 260, 262
Davis, A. J., 270
Davy, Humphry, 219
day and night, 6, 36, 77
deadly nightshade, 13
Dead Sea fruit, 2
deafness, 57, 114
death, 94, 280; *see also* dying
death, autosuggestive or suggested, 235
death, fear of, 280
death, love of, 191
death diagnostics, *53*
death instinct, 281
death wish, 281
decadence, 56, 266
decapitation, *see* beheading
deconditioning, 29
Defoe, Daniel, 86

deformity, 114
Degas, Edgar, 247
degeneration, 44, *56*, 188
déjàism, 88, 90, 176
dejection, 60
dejuvenation, 246
De la Mare, Walter, 247
Deleuze, J. P. F., 32
Delius, Frederick, 279
delusions of grandeur, 196, 201, 254
dementia, 1
dementia praecox, 89, 254
Demichov, Vladimir, 105
Democritus, 115, 187
demography, 75
demons, 6, 18, 25, 46, 50, 65, 96, 102, 103, 194, 221
demositis, 75, 100, 150
Demosthenes, 103, 114
dentists, 243
depersonalization, *58*, 61
depression, 1, *60*
depth psychology, 32, 231
dermography, 273
Descent into Hades, 19
desensitization, 29, 30
Desmoulins, Camille, 114
destructiveness, 57
destrudo, 282
DET, 69
Deutsch, Albert, 26
Deutsch, Felix, 67
devils, *see* demons
Dewey, John, 155
diabetes, 130, 149
diagnosis, 4, *61*, 285
Diana, 37
diaphoretic, 134
diathermy, 79, 214
diathesis, 6, 7
diazepam, 68
Dickens, Charles, 78, 115, 158
Diderot, Denis, 116
diet, *63*, 81
Digby, Kenelm, 219, 224
digestion, 64
Diodorus Siculus, 83
Dionysus, 113, 234, 284
Dioscorides, 126
diosgenin, 227
dipsomania, 183
dirt therapy, 36
discipline, 121
discoincidence, 294
disease, *65*
diseases of medical practice, 140
disinhibitors, 69
dissociation, 97, 137, 185
distant healing, 270

disulfiram, 28
diuretic, 134
divination, 144, 232
divine healing, 269
Divine Science, 177
DMT, 69
DNA, 74, 179, 180
doctor, 98, 140, 212
dolor, 207
DOM, 69
DOMP (diseases of medical practice), 140
Donizetti, Gaetano, 117
Don Juan, 92
doodles, 233
dopamine, 132
dose, 128
dosology, 285
Dostoevsky, Fyodor, 91, 117, 292
double blind, 217
dowsing, 40, 62
drama, 234
drawing, 24
dreams, 34, 143, 194, 224, 233, 263, 264
dropsy, 226
drug(s), 13, 19, 26, 57, 82, 93, 146
drug addiction, 265, 283
drugs and dreams, 264
drugs, excessive use of, 8, 9, 63, 68, 70, 142
drugs, manufacture of, 68, 70, 101, 228
drugs and the mind, 59, 68
drugs, origin of word, 69, 126
drugs, reduced effectiveness, 70, 146, 147
drugs, side-effects, 67, 70, 71, 82
drug therapy, *67*
Druids, 136
dual personality, 185
Duggar, Benjamin, 38
Dumas, Alexandre, 78
Duncan, Dr C., 202
dung, *see* faeces
Duns Scotus, 91
Dürer, Albrecht, 114, 167, 279, 292
Durkheim, Émile, 1
dyadic eye-fixation, 123
dying, 9, 18, 90
dyscolic, 205
dyscrasis, 7, 200
dysentery, 83
dysgenics, *72*
dyspeptic, 200
dysthymia, 201

earth, 37, 38, 40, 118, 133, 158, 171, 215, 216, 218

INDEX

earth-bound, 96, 102, 221, 222
eau-de-cologne, 18
Ebers papyrus, 31, 126, 176, 226, 251
eccentricity, 1, *76*
ecchymosis, 273
ECG (electrocardiograph), 33
echolalia, 160, 255
echopraxia, 255
ecology, 6
ecstasy, 48, 49, 59, 66, 90, 93, 219, 283
ECT (electroconvulsant therapy), 79, 209
ectogenesis, 20
ectoplasm, 96
Eddy, Mary Baker, 118, 178, 247
Edison, Thomas Alva, 247
educational therapy, 121
Edward the Confessor, 288
Edward III, 278
Edward IV, 278
Edwards, Harry, 39, 271
Edwin Smith papyrus, 204
EEG (electroencephalograph), 34, 54, 238
eggs, 14
ego, 55
Egypt (Egyptians), 10, 17, 19, 31, 35, 37, 41, 46, 143, 148, 191, 225, 253
Egypt, plagues of, 83
Ehrlich, Paul, 278, 292
Eiffel, Alexandre, 247
ejaculation, 9
elation, 160
El Dorado, 133
electrical energy, 79, 89, 124, 259
electrical stimulation of the brain, *see* ESB
electric girls, 80
electric shock treatment, *see* EST
electrocardiograph, *see* ECG
electroconvulsant therapy, *see* ECT
electroencephalograph, *see* EEG
electrolysis, 79
electromyograph, *see* EMG
electron microscope, 173, 179
electro-oculograph, *see* EOG
electrotherapy, *78*
elementals, 96, 102
elephantiasis graecorum, 156
Eleusinian mysteries, 284
Eleutherians, 85, 162
Elisha, 157
elixir, 69
Elizabeth I, 278
Elliotson, John, 32
Ellis, Havelock, 253
embalming, 192, 253
embryo, 81
embryology, 80
embryonics, *80*

emerods, 83
Emerson, 126, 247, 292
emetics, 28, 90, 217
EMG (electromyograph), 33
Emmerich, Anna Katherine, 272
emotions, *see* pathemia
empathy, 115
Empedocles, 167
empiric, 242
encounter therapy, 122
encratites, 253, 257
endocrine glands, 7, 129
endogenous, 6, 61
endrophonium, 132
enema, 46
energumen, 103, 221
entertainment, 265
enthusiasm, 162, 284
enuresis, 28
environment, 6, 65, 120, 265
enzymes, 131, 158, 250
EOG (electro-oculograph), 33
epena, 69
ephedrine, 226, 278
Epicurus, 103
Epidaurus, 144
epidemics, *83,* 111
epidemiology, 285
epigastrium, 88, 89, 176, 193, 211, 296
epilepsy, 1, 44, *87,* 109, 189, 252
epinephrin, *see* adrenalin
epiphysis, *see* pineal
episome, 146
Erasistratus, 36
Erasmus, Desiderius, 95
erection, 9, 13, 88, 148
erethism, 46
ergonomics, *see* work
Eros, 113, 200
erotomania, *92,* 97
eryngo, 13
erythema, 273
erythroblastosis, 81
Esalen, 122
ESB (electrical stimulation of the brain), 26, 228
Esdaile, James, 32, 136
ESP (extrasensory perception), 31, 34
Esquirol, Jean, 32
EST (electric shock treatment), 209
Establishment, 57
Esther, 17
estrogen, 130, 247
ether, 219
etheric body, 7, 16, 40, 55, 64, 71, 94, 99, 169, 188, 189, 205, 218, 256, 294, 295
etherosis, *94,* 175
ethical drugs, 69

ethics and healing, 23, 55, *98*, 193, 249
ethologists, 28
ethnopathology, 264
eucolic, 205
eucrasis, 7, 200
eugenics, *101*
eunuch, 246
eupeptic, 200
euphoriants, 68, 160
eurhythmy, 49, 154
euthanasia, 73, 99, 100
Evans, John Arthur, 247
Evans, William, 216
Eve, 257
Evelyn, John, 25
exchange transfusion, 82
exercise, 154, 155, 198
exhaustion, 155
exhibitionism, 57, 125, 237
existentialism, 2, 11, 281
existential neurosis, 2
exogenous, 6, 61
exorcism, 97, *102*
experimental medicine, 29, *104*
experimental psychology, 170
expersonation, 59, 96
extrasensory perception, *see* ESP
extreme unction, 19
eye(s), 57
eyeless sight, 211
Eysenck, H. J., 242

Fabre, Jean Henri, 247
face, 232
faeces, 46, 47, 90, 96, 250, 251
fainting, 89
faith healing, 145, 216, 270
fallopian tube, 80
family therapy, 122
fanatic, 284
Fancher, Mollie, 185
fantastics, 68
Faraday, Michael, 78, 158
Fareinists, 210
Farinelli, Carlo, 186
fart bottle, 219
fascia, 161
fashions, 265
fasting, 64, 103, 139
Faustina, 252
Fawkland, Anna, 262
fear, 11, 18, *107*
Fechner, Gustav, 247
feedbacks, 123, 190
Felstein, Ivor, 189
Ferdinand of Castile, 13
Ferenczi, Sandor, 48, 241, 290

ferita, 272
ferments, 37, 38, 174
fertility, 75, 100, 148
fertilization, 20, 80
fetishism, 28
fever, 90, *108*, 149
Ficino, Marsilio, 113, 167, 261
fight-training, 123
films, *see* media
filth, 37
finger-lopping, 35
fire-walking, 139, 210, 286
Fischer, Doris, 186
fish, 14, 156, 157
Fitzgerald, W. H., 296
Flach, F., 169
Flacht, F., 255
Flagellants, 85, 90, 162, 284
flagellation, 13, 206, 208
flatulence, 14
Flaubert, Gustave, 91, 115, 117
flea, 175
Fleming, Alexander, 38, 225
flexibilitas cerea, 41
flooding, *see* implosion
floritherapy, *111*
flowers, 14, 15, 16, 111
Fludd, Robert, 31
fly agaric, 69
focal sepsis, 141
foetus, 7, 20, 71, 75, 80, 81, 90, 179
folie-à-deux, 162
folie louvière, 97
folk medicine, *see* primitive medicine
fontanelle, 208
food, *see* diet
foot therapy, 297
Forgione, Francesco, *see* Pio, Padre
Forster, E. M., 247
fou, 3
fourth dimension, 94
Fox, George, 164
Fracastoro, Girolamo, 277
Francis, St, 272
Francis I, 85, 278
Frankl, Viktor, 2
Franklin, Benjamin, 79
Frazer, Sir James, 236
freak, 180
Frederick Barbarossa, 260
Frederick II (the Great), 36, 77
free association, 24, 233, 241
free love, 162
Free Thought, 177
freezing, 42, 110, 286, 287
Freitas, J. P. de, 229
French Revolution, 53, 86
frenzy, 49, 113
fresh-cell therapy, 246

INDEX

Freud, Sigmund (and Freudians), 2, 12, 32, 33, 46, 47, 56, 66, 118, 138, 159, 193, 195, 197, 240, 246, 249, 259, 281, 290
fright, 109
fright hypnosis, 42
frigidity, 256
frog, 226
fruits, 14, 15, 16, 215
fumigation, 90
functional disorder, 137, 193, 200, 255
furor, 88, *113*
furor uterinus, 93

galangal, 17
Galen, 1, 8, 15, 56, 84, 124, 126, 165, 207, 243, 255, 293
galenia, 15
galenicals, 126
Galgani, Gemma, 272
gall bladder, 141
gallstones, 206
Galton, Francis, 101, 247
galvanic skin response, *see* GSR
gambling, 28
gametes, 74, 179
Gandhi, Mohandas, 261
Garuda Purana, 19
gases, 219
Gauguin, Paul, 279, 292
gauss meters, 35
Ge, 119, 120
gelsemium, 97
gems, 171
gene(s), 74, 179, 180
geneosis, 74, 101
general paralysis of the insane, *see* GPI
general practitioner, 142, 213
generation gap, 267
gene therapy, 180
genetic crossing, 180
genetic diseases, 73, 180
genetic engineering, 179
Genghis Khan, 174
genius, 110, *114*
geology, 40, 118
geopolitics, 120
geotherapy, *118*
geriatrics, 99, 100
germ(s), *see* microbes
German measles, 81
gerocomy, 261
gerontology, 99
gestalt, 122
gestogen, 130
ghosts, 96
Gibbon, Edward, 177
giddiness, *see* vertigo

Gide, André, 247
ginseng, 13
Gladstone, William, 247
Glasser, William, 122
globus hystericus, 138
glossolalia, 139
glucagon, 130, 201
glue-sniffing, 220
glutamic acid, 132
glycerol, 21
gnostics, 257
goats, 90
God, 1, 67, 86, 88, 93, 157, 249, 258, 270, 287
Goethe, Johann Wolfgang von, 117, 164, 167, 247, 292
Gogh, Vincent van, 91, 118
goitre, 130
gold, 47, 156
gold rush, 163
gonad(s), 130
gonadotropin, 21
Goncourt, Edmond de, 91
Goncourt, Jules de, 91, 279
gonorrhoea, *see* venereal disease
Gorky, Maxim, 292
Goths, 84
Goya, Francisco, 114, 247, 279
GPI (general paralysis of the insane), 110, 169
grafting, 22
Graham, James, 119, 158
grains, 14
grand mal, 88
graphology, 232
graveyards, 191
Greatrakes, V., 289
Greeks, 17, 19, 31, 36, 38, 47, 69, 103, 111, 115, 137, 144
Gregory of Nazianzus, 157
Gregory of Nyssa, 257
group-grope, 124
group therapy, *121*
growth hormone, 130
GSR (galvanic skin response), 34
guaiacum, 226, 278
Guercino, Francesco, 114
guilt, 11, 28, 59, 61, 93, 138, 193, 196, 206, 238, 267
Gull, William, 72
Gurdjieff, George, 155, 218
Guthrie, C. C., 104
gymnastics, 154

Haddon, Alfred, 236
Hadrian, 288
haemetidrosis, 273
haemolagnia, 96

308

haemolytic anaemia, 95
haemophilic, 150
haemorrhage, 37
haemotherapy, 202
haemothymia, 97
Hahnemann, C. S., 8, 127, 128
Haig, J. G., 251
hair, 53, 57
Haldane, J. B. S., 22
Hall, Spencer, 32
Hallaj, Mansur al, 284
Hallet, James, 289
hallucinations, 45, 135, 255, 263
hallucinogenics, 16, 69
Hamilton, Lord, 159
hamster, 41
Handel, G. F., 91, 116
hanging, 253, 280
Hannibal, 83, 84
Hardy, Thomas, 247
harmine, 69
Hartmann, Franz, 53
hashish, 13, 69
Hastings, Warren, 91
hate-in, 123, 124
Hauffe, Frederica, 231
Haviland, Alfred, 40
hay fever, 95
headache, 89, 176
headshrinker, 242
headstand, 253
healing, 65
health, 65
Heape, Walter, 22
heart, 54
hearth, 46
heat, 285
hebephrenia, 89, 254
Hebrews, *see* Jews
Hector, 167
Hegel, G. W. F., 117
Heine, Heinrich, 279
Helicon, 116
Heliogabalus, 278
heliotherapy, 190, 225
hell, 157
Helmont, J. B. van, 31, 89, 277
Helsinki declaration, 105
hemispherectomy, 26
hemp, 69
henbane, 69
Henry III, 95
Henry VII, 288, 289
Henry VIII, 127, 243, 278, 293
heparin, 203
hepatitis, 142
herb(s), 14, 15
herbalism, *126*
Hercules, 87, 91, 119, 156, 167

heredity, 6, 7, 62, 102, 146
Hermippus, 245, 260
hermits, 1
Herodotus, 19, 46, 83, 133, 144, 192
heroin, 69
Herschel, William, 248
Hesiod, 187
Hezekiah, 83
hibernation, 41, 286, 287
hiccup, 200
Hildegard, St, 127, 177
Hindus (Hinduism), 19, 156, 277, 283
Hippies, 122, 163
hippocras, 15
Hippocrates, 10, 15, 17, 31, 39, 62, 87,
    90, 98, 109, 120, 127, 132, 144, 148,
    161, 190, 204, 207, 273, 277
Hippocratic oath, 212
hippomanes, 15
hippopotamus, 35
histamine, 95, 132, 208
Hitler, Adolf, 105, 174, 269, 278, 292
Hoffmann, Ernst Wilhelm, 77
Hogarth, William, 25
Hokusai, 248
Hölderlin, Johann, 117
holiness, 65
Holmes, O. W., 72, 244
Holophernes, 17
Holywell, 270
homeostasis, 108, 190, 286
Homer, 114, 160, 187
homoeopathy, 8, *127*
homosexuality, 28, 44, 57, 71, 93, 96,
    97, 98, 114, 123, 266
honey, 14
Hooker, Joseph, 248
Hoover, Herbert, 248
hormone(s), 7, 21, 71
hormone therapy, 81, *129*
horripilation, 108
horses (horse riding), 10, 194, 195
hospitals, 67, 140
hot seat, 123
Housman, Laurence, 248
Hoxley, John, 126
Hoyle, C., 216
Huang-ti, 3
Hubert, St, 145
Hugo, Victor, 118, 248
Humboldt, Alexander, 248
Hume, David, 167, 211
humours, 7, 36, 113, 154, 165, 188,
    207
humus, 119
Hun(s), 84
huna, 224
Hunter, John, 253, 279, 286
Hurst, Lulu, 80

Hutten, Ulrich von, 279
Huxley, Aldous, 22, 47, 155
hydropathy, *132*
hydrophobia, 183
hydrotherapy, 132
Hygeia, 144
hyoscine, 131
hyperacuity of the senses, 209
hyperaesthesia, 138, 209
hyperbaric, 220
hyperkinesis, 160
hypertension, 71, 239, 274
hypertherm, 109
hyperthermia, 110
hyperthymia, 160, 201
hyperthyroidism, 130, 201
hypnagogia, 294
hypnoanalysis, 136
hypnodontics, 136
hypnosis, 32, 41, *134,* 268
hypnotherapy, 136
hypnotics, 68
hypnotoxin, 263
hypochondria, 60, 77, 116, 137, 166,
    177, 193, 296
hypochondrium, 193, 296
hypogastric, 296
hypoglycaemia, 200, 208
hypomania, 160
hypophysis, *see* pituitary
hypothalamus, 130
hypothermia, 287
hypothymia, 60, 201
hypothyroidism, 130, 201
hysterectomy, 141
hysteria, 33, 37, 41, 49, 136, *137*

Iamblichus, 187
iatrochemistry, 67
iatrogenics, *140*
ibis, 46
Ibn Saud, 247
ibogaine, 69
Ichazo, Oscar, 155
ICT, *see* insulin coma therapy
idée fixe, 182
idiopathic, 89
idiosyncrasy, 7, 71, 115
idiot, 169
idleness, 13, 198
Ignatius, St, 164
iliac, 296
Iliad, 187
illness, 65
image experience, 242
imagogy, 233
imbecile, 169
imitation, 234

immunization, 66, 203
immunology, 70
immunosuppression, 70, 146
implantation, 20, 21, 80
implosion (implosive) therapy, 30
impotence, 9, 10, 28, 52, 69, 114, 148,
    149
impregnation, 20
impressionism, 165
imprinting, 29
Incas, 227
incendium amoris, 93, 287
incense, 16, 215
incubation, *143*
incubus, 96, 194
indifference, 1
indoctrination, 171
induced labour, 82
inductance therapy, 110
industrial psychology, 121
infancy, 294
infanticide, 100, 266
infantile paralysis, *see* polio
infant mortality, 75
infection, 7, *145*
inferiority, 241
infertility, 74, *148*
influenza, *150*
infrared rays, 79
Inge, W. R., 248
inguinal, 296
inhalation therapy, 219
initiation, 19, 28
Innocent VIII, 252, 260
inoculations, 146, 153, 203, 225
Inquisition, 170
insanity, 25, 115, 168
insects, 14, 42, 174
insemination, 20
insomnolence, 7, 59, 60, 139, 167, 170,
    263
inspiration, 66, 91, 116
institutional neurosis, 26, 140, 190, 198
insufflation, 135
insulin, 130, 201
insulin coma therapy (ICT), 26, 208
intelligence tests, 233
intensive care therapy, 55, 73, 99, 100
interrelation, 223
intra-uterine device, *see* IUD
invagination, 231
invalidism, 138
in vitro, 20
in vivo. 20
involutional melancholia, 60
IQ, 114
iridology, 296
iris, 296
Irving, Washington, 292

Isawa dervishes, 210
Isis, 143
iso-electric line, 54
Israelites, *see* Jews
IUD (intra-uterine device), 81
Ivan the Terrible, 278

Jackson, John Hughlings, 90
Jacó, Zuave, 270
Jains, 257
James I, 278, 289
James, William, 110, 164, 187, 222
Janet, Pierre, 33, 193, 240
Janus, Madame, 261
Japan (Japanese), 105
jaundice, 82
Jefferson, Thomas, 177, 248
Jekyll and Hyde, 185
Jenner, Edward, 225
Jesus, *see* Christ
Jews, 10, 17, 71, 83, 103, 120, 144, 157,
    198, 221
Joan of Arc, 164
Job, 108
John, St, 90
John XXIII, 248
John of Gaunt, 278
Johnson, Samuel, 77, 99, 196, 289, 292
Johnson, Virginia, 34
jokes, 232
Jones, Ernest, 116
Joneses, keeping up with, 239, 274
Judith, 17
Julian the Apostate, 161
Jung, C. G., 2, 121, 241, 248, 249
Justinian, 85, 153

Kafka, Franz, 292
kahuna, 224
Kant, Immanuel, 66, 114, 117, 166, 177,
    248
karma, 7
Kean, Edmund, 117
Keats, John, 164, 279, 292
Kemble, John, 117
Kennedy, John and Robert, 169
Kenny, Sister, 161
Kepler, Johann, 116
Kerin, Dorothy, 271
Khrushchev, Nikita, 247
khyphi, 17
kidneys, 293
Kierkegaard, Søren, 11, 258, 279
kif, 69
kinesiotherapy, *154*
king's evil, 288
Kircher, Athanasius, 43, 187

Kirchner, E. L., 292
kirlian photography, 62
Kleist, Heinrich von, 117
kleptomania, 183
knee-jerk, 136
Kneipp, S., 133
knotting, 148, 149
Korsakov's syndrome, 169
koumiss, 64
Kraepelin, Emil, 52
Kreisler, Fritz, 187
Kuleshova, Rosa, 211
kymograph, 34

Laban, Rudolf, 155
labour, 130, 136
labour, induced, 82
lactic acid, 64
Laennec, René, 291, 292
Laforgue, Jules, 292
Lakhovsky, Georges, 40
laliognomy, 232
lama(s), 251
Lamartine, Alphonse de, 116
Lamb, Charles, 117
Landor, Walter Savage, 117
Landseer, Edwin, 117
Lanier, Sidney, 292
lant, 251
Laodiceans, 1
laparoscopy, 21
laudanum, 69
laughing gas, 219
laughter, 160, 166, 232
Lawrence, D. H., 58, 279, 292
laxative, 46
laying on of hands, 269, 270, 271, 289
Lazarus, 157
Lebensraum, 120
Lee, Nathaniel, 116
leeches, 35, 110
lees, 37
left-handedness, 57
lemmings, 86
Lemnian earth, 37
Lenoble, Abbé, 159
leprosy, 147, *156*
lepsy, 89
lesbianism, 92
leucotomy, 26
Leverett, James, 231, 289
ley-lines, 158
liars, 57, 237
libido, 47
Liébeault, A. A., 32
lie detector, 34
ligature, 148, 149
lignum vitae, 226

INDEX

Linnaeus, Carl, 78
Lister, Joseph, 141, 248
lithium, 68
lithotomy, 225
Livingstone, David, 43
Livy, 84
lizard, 14, 90
loa, 37, 221
lobotomy, 26
logos, 2
logotherapy, 2
Lombroso, Cesare, 56, 89, 91
longevity, 245
loop, *see* IUD
Lorenz, Konrad, 171
Lothario, 10, 92
Louis XI, 90, 252
Louis XIII, 8
Louis XIV, 15, 288
Louis XV, 17
Lourdes, 270
Louviers, 49
love-in, 124, 125
Lowen, Alexander, 155
loyalty, 121
Loyola, Ignatius, 164
LSD, 9, 69, 82, 128, 131
Lucilia, 13
Lucretius, 13, 167
Lucullus, 13
lumbar region, 296
lunacy, 169
lupinomania, 97
lupus, 291
Lupus, St, 90
Luther, Martin, 164, 167
lycanthropy, 97
lycopodium, 14
lycorexia, 97
lye tea, 251
lying, 57, 237
Lyon, Emma, 159
lysis, 200
lysozyme, 250
Lytton, Edward Bulwer, 117

Machaon, 38
machine and body, 190
Macmillan, Harold, 276
macrobiotic diet, 64
madness, 25, 115, 168
Maeterlinck, Maurice, 248
magic, 98
magnale magnum, 31
magnetism, 30, 31, 33, 118, 135, 158, 178
magnetizers, 31, 119, 135, 172, 178, 240
magnetotherapy, *158*
Maillard, John, 271

Maimonides, 212
malaria, 109, 146, 147, 225, 226, 251
maleficia, 6
malingering, 57, 138, 193, 213, 283
Malleus Maleficarum, 26
Malthusians, 75
mana, 289
mandala, 25
mandrake, 14, 253
manes, 159
Manet, Edouard, 279
mania, *159, 182*
maniac, 159
manic depression, *see* cyclothymia
Mann, Thomas, 247, 248
Mansfield, Katherine, 218, 292
MAO and MAOIs, 68, 131, 132
Mao Tse-tung, 247
Marat, Jean-Paul, 53, 78
marathon group therapy, 122
Marcus Aurelius, 84, 252
marihuana, 69
Mars, 113
Marsii, 288
Martial, 14
Martians, 163
Martineau, Harriet, 32, 54
martyromania, 201, 283
Mary I (Mary Tudor), 278
Mary Magdalene of Pazzi, St, 287
Mary Queen of Scots, 278
masks, 234
masochism, 96, 206
massage, 90, *160*
mass hysteria, 48, *161*
Masters, William, 34
masturbation, 21, 37, 46, 123, 149, 253
materialism, 282
materialization, 96, 230, 231
materia medica, 72, 126, 226, 285
mathematics, 10
Matisse, Henri, 248
Maugham, Somerset, 247, 248
Maupassant, Guy de, 118, 279
Maurier, George du, 134
Mayas, 227
meaning, 2
measles, 146
media, 57, 171, 274
medical materialism, *164*
Medici, Marie de, 95
medicine, 285
medicine-men, 224, 225, 240, 269,
meditation, 122, 132, 154
mediums, 90, 96, 135, 220, 231, 269
Meduna, L. J., 208
Meerloo, Joost, 40
megalomania, 184, 201, 254
megrim, 175

Melampus, 120
melancholy, 1, 11, *165*
melatonin, 129, 132
Melissa, 192
Melville, Herman, 118
memento mori, 19
memory, 59, 89, 135, 176
menarche, 252
Mendelssohn, Felix, 91, 117
menopause, 60, 247
menstruation, 15, 37, 252
mental healing, 177
mental illness, 57, 95, 115, *168*
menthol, 9
menticide, *170*
menticulture, 177
meprobamate, 69
mercury, 146, 277, 278
merhu, 17
meridians, 3, 4
mescaline, 69, 131
Mesmer, Franz Anton, 31, 110, 136, 187, 210
mesmerism, 32, 136, 210, 244
Messianists, 284
metallotherapy, *171*
metal sensitivity, 172
Metamorphosis, 19
metanoia, 249
metasyncrisis, 8
Metchnikov, I., 64
Methodists, 284
metrazol, 208
Meyerbeer, G., 54
Michael, Archangel, 145
Michelangelo, 116, 177
microbes, 7, 39, 65, 70, 86, 145, 146, 147, 153, *173*, 181
microdose, 128
microsleep, 263
microwaves, 79
midriff, 113
midwife, 144
migraine, 89, *175*
milieu therapy, 121
milk, 15, 130
Mill, J. S., 77
Milton, John, 77, 114, 279
mimesis, 234
mind, 239
mind cure, *177*
mind-induced death, 235
minerals, 171, 226
Mirabeau, Comte de, 114, 116
Miriam, 157
misandry, 256
misanthropy, 166
miscarriage, 71, 74, 81, 82
misogyny, 256, 258

mistakes, 232
Mizraim, 253
Modigliani, A., 292
Mohammed, *see* Muhammad
molecular biology, *179*
Molière, 91, 292
money, 47, 48
mongolism, 81, 179
Moniz, Egas, 26
monkey-gland treatment, 246
monomania, *181*
monsters, 180
Montaigne, Michel de, 16
Montgomery, Bernard, 247
Montpellier, 252
moon, 6, 52, 88, 109, 169
mor, 17
morals, *see* ethics and healing
morbus comitialis, 87
morbus demoniacus, 87
morbus germanicus, 277
morbus maior, 88
morbus sacer, 87
More, Sir Thomas, 16, 25, 293
Morel, B. A., 57
Moreno, Jacob, 234
Moriscos, 274
morning glory, 69
morning sickness, 82
moron, 169
morphine, 69
mortido, 282
Morzine, 48
Moses, 83, 157
moss, 38
Motoyama, Hiroshi, 5
moulds, 37, 225
mountebank, 242
mourning, 18
mouth, 47, 65
movement, 154
movement meditation, 122
moxabustion, 4
Mozart, Wolfgang, 77, 91, 116, 167, 292
MS (multiple sclerosis), 73
mud, 37, 119
Muhammad (Muhammadans), 84, 91
muiracitin, 13
multiple births, 75
multiple personality, 90, *185*
multiple sclerosis, *see* MS
mummy, 19, 38, 225, 253
mumps, 149
murder, 98, 265, 276, 282
Murphy, M., 122
muscarine, 69, 131
muscle-twitch psychology, 30
Muses, 113, 116

INDEX

mushroom, 14, 69
music, 44, 57, 89, 237
music therapy, *186*
musk, 18
Musset, Alfred de, 91
Mussolini, Benito, 278
Mussorgsky, Modest, 91
mutation, 81, 102
mutilation, 81
myoclonus, 89, 90, 189
myristics, 9, 17, 69
myrobalan, 17
myropola, 17
myrrh, 17
mysteries, 19, 284
mysterium tremendum, 11
mysticism, 57, 90, 139, 176
mythomania, 139
myxoedema, 201

Naaman, 157
nadi, 5
Nambudri, 192
name, 103
Nanahuatl (Nanahuatzin), 277
Nancy school, 32
Napoleon, 83, 86, 91, 164, 174, 177, 278
narco-analysis, 233
narcolepsy, 89, 294
Nasamonians, 144
Nash, John, 248
national health, 212, 282
natural selection, 72, 75, 102
nature spirits, 96
naturopathy, 8, *190*
Nazis, 26, 98, 102, 105, 163, 170
necromancy, 96, 191
necrophagy, 96
necrophilia, 96, *191*
needle, 3, 4
Nefzawi, Sheikh, 259
Negovsky laboratory, 53
Negro, 71
N'ei Ching, 3
Nelson, Horatio, 159
neomorts, 55
neonates, 73
neoplatonism, 257
neostigmine, 132
nephritis, 95
Neptune, 119
Nero, 84, 278
Nerval, Gérard de, 117
nerve(s), 99, 204
nerve gas, 220
nerve poisons, 132
nervousness, 12

nervous system, 130
Nestor, 38
network therapy, 122
Neumann, Teresa, 272
neurasthenia, 193
neurohormone therapy, 130
neurosis, 25, 115, 169, *192*
Newman, John Henry, 248
New Thought, 177
Newton, Isaac, 114, 116, 167
Nichiren, 103
Nicolson, Harold, 116
nicotine, 131
Niehans, Paul, 246
Nietzsche, Friedrich, 66, 118, 279
night, *see* day
Nightingale, Florence, 118
nightmare, 96, *194*
Nijinsky, Vaslav, 118
nitrogen, 174
nitrous oxide, 219
Nobel Prize, 26
nodes, 3, 4
noise, 30, 57, 170, 265, 274
noradrenalin, 61, 130, 131
Nordau, Max, 56
norepinephrin, *see* noradrenalin
nosology, 285
nosophobia, 182
Novalis, 292
novocain, 247
nucleic acid, 173, 179
nudity, 124, 125, 162
Nuremberg code, 105
Nuremberg trials, 105
nurses, 141, 142, 220, 290
nut(s), 14, 215
nutmeg, 9, 69
nux vomica, 13, 226
nyctalopia, 210
nymphomania, 92, 164
nystagmus, 57

oak, 120
obeah, 96
obscenity, 58, 266
obsession, *196,* 221
occultism, 40, 55, 57, 62, 64, 65, 94, 96, 99, 119, 139, 142, 154, 160, 169, 195, 197, 212, 232. 262
occupational therapy, 121, *198*
ocelli, 211
odour, 15, 217
Oedipus complex, 241
Ogilvie, Heneage, 40
Ogilvie, William, 105
old age, 99
olfactory intoxication, 218

ololiuqui, 69
O'Neill, Eugene, 292
opium, 69
opotherapy, 202
oppilation, 88
opposites, *199*
oracles, 16, 113, 144
oral phase, 47
oral sex, 149, 259
orchitis, 149
organic disorder, 137
organogenesis, 81
organotherapy, 71, *202*
orgasm, 9, 13, 17, 79, 90, 93, 148, 258, 282
orgasmogenics, 69
Oribasius, 161
orificial surgery, 46, 141
Origen, 257
original sin, 257
Orphics, 19
orthopaedics, 214
Orwell, George, 292
Osanami, Tosi, 270
Osiris, 234
Osler, William, 36, 147
osphresiology, 15
osteopathy, 204
osteopractic, *203*
Oswald, L. H., 169
ova, *see* ovum
ovarie, 139
ovary, 21, 130, 139
ovulation, 21, 80, 130
ovum, 20, 21, 80, 148
oxygen, 81
oxytocin, 130
ozone, 218

Paderewski, Ignacy, 248
paean, 186
Paganini, Nicolò, 91, 279, 292
pain, 13, *205*
pain therapy, *207*
painting, 24, 164, 165
Paisiello, Giovanni, 77
Palmer, D. D., 204
palmistry, 62
Pan, 108
panacea, 133
pancreas, 130
panic, 108
Paracelsus, 8, 31, 65, 127, 128, 158, 172, 187, 219, 243
paraesthesia, 94, *209*
paralysants, 43
paramedicals, 142
paranoia, 44, 193, 201, 254

paraperception, 129
paraplegia, 73
parapraxis, 232
parasympathetic system, 131
parasympatholytic, 131
parasympathomimetic, 131
parathione, 132
parathyroid, 130
Paré, Ambroise, 67, 210, 215
parents, 6
paresis, 110, 279
parica, 69
Paris, Abbé François de, 270
Parkinson's law, 213
Parmenides, 110
paroptic sense, 210
paroxysm, 89
parthenogenesis, 23
Pascal, Blaise, 164, 168, 177
passes, hypnotic, 135
Pasteur, Louis, 175
Patagonians, 287
patchouli, 18
pathemia, 94, 95, 109, 112, 162, 239
pathogenic, 142, 174
pathology, 285
pathomimesis, 138
patient, *212,* 217
Patmos, 1
patriotism, 120, 283
Paul, St, 91, 104, 164, 272, 289
Paul V, 103
Pavlov, Ivan, 28, 29, 248
pavor, 108
Peczely, Ignatz, 296
Pelusium, 83
penetrance, 102
penicillin, 38, 128, 225
penilingus, 253
penis, 13, 34, 52, 88, 92, 215, 241, 250
penis, artificial, 34
penis aculeatus, 256
Pentecostalists, 90, 270, 284
Penthesilea, 192
Pepys, Samuel, 86
perfumes, 15, 16, 17, 111, 218
Periander, 192
Pericles, 83
Perkins, Elisha, 172
Perls, F., 122
permissiveness, 266, 267
persecution complex, 60, 183, 196, 201, 254
personality, 58
perspiration, *see* sweat
pessimism, 61
Pétain, Henri Philippe, 248
Peter, St, 245
Peter the Great, 91

INDEX

petit mal, 88
Petrarch, Francesco, 91
Petrucci, Daniele, 22
Petrus Hispanus, 243
peyote, 69
Pfeiffer, John, 39
Pfeiffer, Richard, 150
PGR (psychogalvanic reflex), 33
phalange therapy, 296
phallus, *see* penis
phantom limb, 206
pharmaceutics, 67, 69
pharmacist, 17, 69, 126
pharmacogenics, 67, 70
pharmacology, 67, 285
pharmacopathology, 70
pharmacopoeia, 37, 156
pharmacopsychopathology, 70
phentolamine, 131
philia, 182
Philip II, 278
Philip V, 186
Philip Neri, St, 287
Philistines, 83
philosopher's stone, 245
phlebotomy, 35
phlegmagogic, 134
phobias, 29, 95, 182
phocomelia, 82
phonognomy, 232
phosphorus, 130, 201
phrenology, 198, 232
phrensy, *see* frenzy
phthisis, 291
physicians, *see* doctor
physiognomy, 56, 232
physiotherapy, 154, *214*
physostigmine, 32, 226
phytotherapy, *215*
Picasso, Pablo, 248
picrotoxin, 226
Pied Piper, 85
pilgrims, 120, 145
pilocarpine, 131
pineal, 94, 129
Pinel, Philippe, 25, 32, 198, 228
Pio, Padre, 272
piss-prophet, 293
Pitt, William, 78, 116
pituitary, 5, 129
pituri, 69
Pius XII, 247
PK (psychokinesis), 31
placebo, *216*
placenta, crossing of, 71, 81, 82
plague, 16, 37, 83, 146, 175
Planck, Max, 248
planets, *see* astrology
plants, 13, 215

plasma, 203
plasmapheresis, 203
plastic surgery, 214
Plato, 16, 66, 113, 166, 167, 188,.205
Platonic love, 262
play-acting, 234
playing possum, 107, 274
Pleasanton, Augustus, 44
pleasure, 283
plethora, 35, 259
plethysmograph, 34
plexus, 94, 193
plexy, 89
Pliny, 9, 252
Plotinus, 156
plural personality, 185
Plutarch, 89
pneumatic medicine, 219
pneumograph, 33
pneumonia, 100
pneumopathy, *217*
pneumosphere, 217
podology, 297
Poe, Edgar Allan, 114, 115, 117, 167, 292
poet(ry), 113, 116, 199
poison(s), 285
poison gas, 220
polarity, 31, 79, 199
polio, 146, 161
politics, 57
pollution, 265
poltergeists, 222
polyaesthesia, 209
polyaetiology, 7
Polybius, 120
polycythaemia, 36
polygraph, 34
polylogia, 160
polypharmacy, 8, 128, 151
polypragmacy, 8
polysurgery, 283
Pompadour, Marquise de, 17
pop art and music, 58, 163, 189, 274
Pope, Alexander, 114, 177
Popish plot, 163
population, 75, 265
pornography, 58, 96, 237, 266
pornomania, 92
Porta, Giambattista della, 56
posology, 285
possession, 25, 37, 46, 48, 59, 90, 103, 115, 135, 139, 162, 185, *220*
posture, 154, 259
potassium, 202, 274
potentization, 128
powder of sympathy, 224
Powell, Eric, 142
Powys, John Cowper, 248
pox, 277

Poyen, Charles, 178
prayers, 97, 249, 269, 270, 283
praying to death, 236
prefrontal lobes, 26
Prehoda, Robert, 99
pregnancy, 7, 9, 81, 82, 139
premature birth, 74
premature burial, *see* burial alive
premature ejaculation, 148, 164
press, *see* media
preventive medicine, 203, 285
Priam, 167
priapism, 92
Priesnitz, Vincenz, 133
Priestley, Joseph, 219
priests, 98
primitive(s), 24, 44, 56, 65
primitive medicine, 37, 126, *223, 243*
primum non nocere, 70
Prince, Morton, 185
Prince, Walter Franklin, 186
procaine, 247
prodigy, 180
progenism, 56
progesterone, 71, 130, 227
prognosis, 285
progress, 2, 7, 11, 98, 282
projectivism, 233
promiscuity, 266
propaganda, 171
propanolol, 131
prophecy, 113
prophylaxis, 285
prostate, 39
prosthetics, 214
prostitute, 92
protoplasm, 31
Proust, Marcel, 116, 118
pseudaesthesia, 209
pseudocyesis, 139
pseudolism, 237
psi, *see* psychic
psilocybin, 69
psionics, 62
psora, 156
psychasthenia, 1, 193
psychedelics, 69
psychiatry, 27, 168, *227,* 240
psychic, 34, 66
psychic healing, 46, 270
psychic surgery, 34, *229,* 269
psychic vampirism, *230*
psychoanalysis, 48, 136, 165, 168, 233,
    240, 241, 290
psychochemotherapy, 72
psychodiagnostics, 24, *231*
psychodrama, *234*
psychodysleptics, 69
psychogalvanic reflex, *see* PGR

psychogenic, 280
psychogenic death, *235*
psychogram, 233
psychokinesis, *see* PK
psycholeptics, 68
psycholytics, 69
psychometry, 62, 270
psychomotor therapy, 123
psychopath(s), 58, 237
psychopathology, 168, 237
psychopathy, 29, 169, *237*
psychopharmacology, 68
psychosis, 25, 169, 193
psychosomatics, 7, *239*
psychosomatic sleep, 136
psychosurgery, 26
psychotherapy, 168, 227, *240*
psychotic, 169, 237, 254
psychotogenics, 69
psychotomimetics, 69
psychotropics, 68, 131
Psylli, 288
puberty, 79
public health, 285
puerperal death, 141
Pugin, Augustus, 117
pulse, 33, 51, 62, 108, 296
pun(s), 232
punishment, 28
pupils, 54, 108, 131, 188
Purcell, Henry, 292
purging and purgatives, 46
pus, 207
Puységur, Marquis de, 32
pyrethron, 14
pyrethrum, 226
pyretotherapy, 109
pyridostigmine, 132
Pyrrhus, 288
Pythagoras, 44, 66, 187

quackery, 216, 224, *242*
Quakers, 284
quebracho, 13
queer, *see* homosexuality
Quimby, P. P., 177
quinine, 9, 146, 147, 227

race, 6, 71, 102, 205
race improvement, 73, 101
radiation, 174
radiation (radio) therapy, 79
radiesthesia, 62, 97, 270
radionics, 62
rage, 89, 123, 124
Rank, Otto, 241
rape, 149

INDEX

Raphael, 292
rapport, 32, 134, 204, 224
rat(s), 146, 174
rat-race, 239
Rätzel, Friedrich, 120
rauwolfia, 226
Ravitz, Leonard, 79
Razi, 244
reality therapy, 122
recidivism, 238
referred pain, 206
reflexology, 29
Reformation, 164
rehabilitation, 214
Reich, Wilhelm, 79, 155, 241
reincarnation, 7, 222
rejuvenation, 36, *245*
relaxation, 154, 178
relics, 191
Religio Medici, 258
religion, 66, 90, 93, 98, 113, 283
religious therapy, 97, *249*
Rembrandt, 279
REM-sleep, 71, 268
repression, 195
reptiles, 14
research, 106
reserpine, 68, 226
resin, 127
resistance, 70
revenant, 191
reverence, 11
reverie, 294
revivals, 91, 163, 284
revulsion therapy, 28, 29
Rhazes, 243
Rh (rhesus) factor, 81
rhizotomoi, 126
Rhodes, Cecil, 292
Richelieu, Cardinal, 91, 292
Richet, Charles, 269
rickets, 225
riding, 10
ritual(s), 223, 224
RNA, 179
Robespierre, Maximilien, 116
rock music, 189
Rodocanachi, 261
Rogers, Carl, 122
Rogers, Dr L., 202
role-playing, 234
Rolf, Ida, 155, 161
Rome (Romans), 17, 19, 84, 87, 111,
    133, 167
Ronsard, Pierre de, 114
Roosevelt, Franklin, 269
Rorschach test, 233
Rosa, Salvator, 116
Rose, Miss, 269

Rosicrucians, 64, 245
Rousseau, Jean-Jacques, 10, 77, 116,
    167, 292
royal jelly, 64
royal touch, 288
Rubinstein, Artur, 248
rubor, 207
Rudolf I, 260
Rufus of Ephesus, 109
Rush, Benjamin, 36
Ruskin, John, 114, 118, 248
Russell, Bertrand, 248
Russia (Russians), 53
Ruth, 17

sabal, 13
Sacks, Oliver, 176
sacred disease, 87, 157
sacrifice, 35
sadism, 96, 97, 206
saint(s), 18, 93, 106, 115, 249, 270, 287
Saint-Germain, Count de, 245
Sakel, Manfred, 208
Salem, 163
Salerno, 252
salicylic acid, 9, 226
saliva, 50, 64, 250, 278
salivation, 278
Salpêtrière, 32
salvarsan, 278
Samuel, Herbert, 248
sand-painting, 224
Sandwich, Earl of, 270
Sanitas, 260
Satan (Satanism), 47, 96, 103, 124, 237,
    257
Saturn, 113, 165, 167
satyriasis, 92
satyrion, 14
Saul, 91, 186, 221
sauna, 133
Savage, Richard, 116
sawbones, 242
Scaliger, Joseph, 95
scarification, 90, 207
Scarron, Paul, 292
scatology, 9, 15, 46
scatotherapy, *250*
scents, 217
Schiller, Friedrich von, 77, 292
schizophrenia, 24, 41, 44, 52, 89, *254*
Schopenhauer, Arthur, 114, 116, 117,
    167, 258, 279
Schubert, Franz, 279
Schumann, Robert, 117, 167, 279
Schüssler, W. H., 128
science and scientists, 98, 282
scopolamine, 131

scotoma, 165
Scott, Walter, 177, 292
scrofula, 288, 291
sculpture, 24
Scythians, 10, 133
séances, 96, 139, 231
seasons, 6, 36, 52, 63, 77, 78, 88, 112,
  119, 126, 218, 259
second body, *see* astral body *and*
  etheric body
second sight, 94
secundines, 15
sedatives, 68
seeds, 14
Selade, Albert, 110
Selye, Hans, 274
semeiology, 285
semen, *see* sperm
Semmelweiss, Ignaz, 141
Seneca, 63, 116
senile dementia, 169
senility, 94, 99, 263, 294
Sennacherib, 83
senses and sensations, 209
sensitivity-training, 123, 124
sensory awareness, 123
sensory deprivation, 59, 170
seplasium, 17
Serafino of Dio, 287
Serapis, 143
serotherapy, 203
serotonin, 129, 132
serpent, 144
serum, 71, 203
serum sickness, 95
serum therapy, 203
setonation, 90, 207
seven deadly sins, 1
seven virtues, 1
sex, 17, 34, 39, 44, 58, 92, 96, 138,
  266
sex hormones, 39
sex-in, 125
sex madness, *see* erotomania
sex magic, 3
sexophilia, 92
sexophobia, *256*
sex perversions, 57, 93, 179
sex postures, 259
sex therapy, *258*
sexual intercourse, *see* coitus
Shakers, 284
Shakespeare, William, 91
shamans, 224, 225, 240, 269
shame, 28, 93, 238, 267
shampoo, 160
shape-shifting, 97
Shaw, G. B., 155, 248
Shelley, Percy Bysshe, 117, 292

Shen Nung, 156
Sherrington, Charles, 248
Shiva, 277
shock therapy, 9, 28, 79, 208
shoes, rubber, 120
shorinji kempo, 5
shortevity, 246
short-waves, 79
shunamism, *260*
Sibelius, Jean, 248
sickle-cell anaemia, 71
sickness, *see* disease
sick society, 264
Siddons, Sarah, 117
side effects of drugs, *see* drugs
signature, 13, 44, 112, 223
silk, 10
simillimum, 128
Simon the leper, 157
Simon Magus, 245
simples, 127, 128
sin and sinners, 18, 59, 103
Sirhan Sirhan, 169
sitting, 10, 154
situation therapy, 121
Sitwell, Edith, 117
sixth sense, 94
Sixtus IV, 279
skin, 34
skink, 14
Skinner, Burrhus, 29
skinsight, 211
skin writing, 273
skull, 90
sleep, 66, 90, 136, 268
sleeping sickness, 174
sleeplessness, *see* insomnolence
sleep therapy, 143, *262*
sleep-walking, 268
slipped disc, 154, 204
sloth, 1
smallpox, 81, 85, 146, 225
Smedley, John, 134
smell, 15, 217
smoking, 10, 28
snakes, 14, 25, 42, 43, 288
sneeze, 66, 90, 151, 200, 232
snuff, 9, 16, 251
soap, 16
socialism, 282
socialized medicine, 212
social psychology, 121
sociatry, 264
sociology, 57
socioneurosis, 264
sociopath, 238, 264
sociopathology, 264
sociopsychosis, 7, 11, 12, 175, *264*
Socotra, 47

INDEX

Socrates, 1, 56, 91, 115, 167, 279
soda water, 9, 10
sodium, 202, 274
sodomy, *see* homosexuality
soft-touch therapy, 161
soil, *see* earth
solanaceous drugs, 9, 69
soles of feet, 297
Solomon, 103
somatherapy, 154
somatotropin, 130
somnambulism, 32, 136, *268*
Soranus of Ephesus, 188
sorcery, 6, 96, 172, 192, 231
soul, 6, 11
sound, 188
Southey, Robert, 117
South Sea Bubble, 163
spa, 133
Spanish fly, 14
Spanish Inquisition, 26
sparagmos, 284
spare-part surgery, 99
spasticism, 81
speaking in tongues, 90, 139, 283, 284
specialists, 142
spectacles, 57
spectinomycin, 267
speech therapy, 199
Spencer, Herbert, 248
sperm, 15, 20, 48, 80, 96, 149, 219,
    250, 259
sperm banks, 21
spermepotation, 96, 253
spes phthisica, 291
Speusippus, 205
sphygmograph, 33
sphygmomanometer, 33
spices, 14, 15, 16, 63
spider, 162
spinal cord, 130
spine, 204
Spinoza, Baruch, 198, 292
spirit healing, 269
Spiritism, 229, 230
spiritual healing, 139, 229, *269*
spiritualism, 96
spleen, 166
split personality, 185
spontaneous generation, 22
springs, 133
Spurzheim, Johann, 198
squint-eyes, 114
stage-fright, 12
stale, 251
Stalin, Joseph, 36
stammering, 57
Stanhope, Lady Hester, 78
stars, *see* astrology *and* cosmobiology

starvation, 294
station fears, 12
status lymphaticus, 62
Stead, W. T., 258
Steinach, Eugen, 246
Steiner, Rudolf, 154
sterility, 9, 13, 20, 148, 149
sterilization, 73, 75, 100, 102
Sterne, Laurence, 292
steroids and steroid therapy, 71, 130
stethoscope, 291
Stevenson, R. L., 185, 292
stigmata, 56, 138, 139, *272*
Still, A. T., 204
stimulants, 68
stimulus and response, 29, 30
Stoics, 1, 89, 103
Stone, Edmund, 225
STP, 69
stramonium, 69
Strauss, Richard, 248
Stravinsky, Igor, 248
streptomycin, 38
stress, 6, *273*
stressors, 274
stridor, 50
Strindberg, August, 118, 164, 279
stroke, 54
strophanthin, 226
struma, 288
sfrychnine, 13, 226
stupor, 48, 61, 254
stuttering, 114
subego, 55
subluxation, 204
subtle arteries, 295
succubus, 96, 253
succussation, 154
sucking, 6, 52
suffering, 2, 66, 167, 206, 249
sufis, 20, 155, 284
sugar, 108, 130
suggestion, 32, 110, 134, 135, 137, 145,
    216, 235, 270
suicide, 37, 60, 61, 149, 166, 266, *275,*
sulphonamides, 100, 147
sulphuric, 201
sun and sunspots, 6, 52, 77, 156, 169
Superman, 66
superovulation, 22
suppository, 16, 148
surgery, 9, 141, 210, 224, 229, 243
surrealism, 165
survival of the fittest, 73, 100
suspended animation, 41, 53, 96, 139,
    235, 286, 287
Svengali, 134
sweat, 15, 109, 188, 250, 286
sweatbox, 109

sweating sickness, 85
Swift, Jonathan, 91, 114, 116, 167, 279
Swinburne, Algernon Charles, 91
Sydenham, Thomas, 190, 224, 261
Sylva Sylvarum, 119, 261
Symonds, J. A., 292
sympathetic nervous system, 131
sympatholytic, 131
sympathomimetic, 131
sympathy, *see* pathemia
symptoms, 6, 61, 62, 285
synaesthesia, 211
Synanon, 122
syncope, 89
syncrisis, 8
syndrome, 89
syphilis, 109, 266, 267, *277*
syringomyelia, 212
Szasz, Thomas, 26, 255

taboo, 6, 28, 236
tabune, 132
Tacitus, 84
Tagliacozza, Gaspare, 215
Taine, Henri, 120
talismans, *see* amulets
Tamisier, Rosette, 272
tantric, 190, 253
tao (taoism), 3, 160, 190, 245
tarantism, 162
tar-water, 127
Tasso, Torquato, 91, 116
tattoo, 57
Tay-Sachs disease, 71
Tchaikovsky, Piotr, 167
tchet oil, 17
tea, 9
teaching, 231
tears, 250
technology, 7, 30, 34, 142
teeth, 57
telepathic healing, 270
telestic, 284
teletherapy, 270
television, *see* media
telluric force, 119
temperature, 62, 108, 285
Temple, William, 155
temple-sleep, 143
Tennyson, Alfred Lord, 78, 118
teonanactl, 68
teratogenesis, 82, 180
Teresa, St, of Avila, 91, 164
Teresa, St, of Lisieux, 91
terra sigillata, 37
testes (testicles), 130, 149
testosterone, 130, 247

test-tube babies, 20, 21, 101
tetany, 48, 89
tetraplegia, 73
Teucer, 109
Teutonic zone therapy, 295
T-Groups, 121
Thackeray, W. M., 78
thalamus, 130
Thales, 167
Thaletas, 187
thalidomide, 71, 82
thanatomania, *280*
thanatophilia, *281*
thanatophobia, 280
THC, 69
thematic apperception test, 233
theolepsy, 284
theomania, *283*
Theophrastus, 126
therapy, *285*
therianthropy, 97, 191
theriomimicry, 50
thermosomatics, *285*
third eye, 94, 129
Thompson, Francis, 292
Thoreau, Henry, 292
thorn apple, *see* datura
Thrale, Hester, 77
three wise men, 90
Thucydides, 83
thymus, 62, 130
thyroid, 51, 130
thyrotoxicosis, 201
thyrotropin, 130
Tibet (Tibetans), 19, 191, 257, 287, 296
tic, 166
Timaeus, 66
time, 69, 176
Timothy, 289
Tinbergen, Professor, 155
tinnitus, 164
tissue-salt therapy, 129
toady or toad-eater, 242
tobacco, 9, 10, 16, 227
tobiscope, 5
toilet training, 47, 164, 197
tolazoline, 131
Tolstoy, Leo, 59, 167
tonsils, 141
topology, 6, 120
torture, 170, 208, 263
totalitarianism, 30, 170
touch, 123, 124, 205, 257
touch healing, *288*
touch-piece, 288
Toulouse-Lautrec, Henri, 114, 279
Tourette's syndrome, 58
Townshend, Colonel, 235

toxaemia, 45
toxicology, 285
toxins, 203
toxoids, 71
trachoma, 226
tractors, 172
tragedy, 234
trance, 41, 53, 88, 123, 134, 136, 233
trance healing, 269
tranquillizers, 68
transactional analysis, 122
transferation, 224
transference, *289*
transfiguration, 139
transits, 12, 18
transmitter substances, 130
transplantation, 55, 70, 99, 142
transposition of the senses, 211
transsexualism, 96
transvestism, 28, 96
trauma, 138, 193, 241
trees, 32, 215
Tremblers, 48
trepanning, 90, 222, 225
Trevelyan, George, 248
tribal medicine, *see* primitive medicine
tricyclics, 68
Trilby, 134
triumph, Roman, 19
truancy, 238
truffle, 14
Truman, Henry, 248
truth labs, 123
tsang, 3
tuberculosis, 38, 146, 218, *291*
tulipomania, 163
tummo, 287
tumor, 207
Turenne, Henri de, 91
Turgenev, Ivan, 78
Turner, J. M. W., 78, 117
turnera, 13
typhoid, 83, 147
typhus, 83
tyramine, 132

ugliness, 44, 114
ultrasonics, 79
ultraviolet rays, 79, 191, 246
umbilical zone, 296
unconscious, 24, 32, 56, 218, 268
unfit, 73, 74, 75, 102
unguents, 16
unio mystica, 93, 287
United Nations, 75, 102
Upanishads, 283
Urban VI, 279
urine, 15, 96, 130, 151, 250, 251

urinoscopy, *293*
urodipsia, 96
use, 155
usnea, 226
Utopia, 101

vaccines (vaccination), 71, 127, 146, 203
vacuum neurosis, 2
vagina, 17, 206, 215, 241
vagina dentata, 256
vaginismus, 256
vagus, 295
Valentine, St, 90
Valentine Basil, 47
valerian, 9
valetudinarian, 193
values, 2
vampire, 96, 139, 191, 253
Vandals, 84
Vannier, Léon, 175
vapours, 137
variolation, 225
vasectomy, 21
vasoligation, 246
vasopressin, 130
vaticination, 113
Vaughan Williams, Ralph, 248
vectors, 174
vegetables, 14, 167
vegetotherapy, 215
vena cava, 293
venereal disease, 83, 101, 109, 147, 189,
    266, 267
venesection, 35
ventricles, 88, 89
Venus (Aphrodite), 13, 113
Verdi, Giuseppe, 248
Veronica Giuliani, St, 164
vertigo, 89
Verus, 84
vesication, 207
Vespasian, 288
villi, 64
Villon, François, 114
violence, 57, 189, 237, 265, 282
Virchow, Rudolf, 175
virgin(s), 231, 252, 260, 261, 278
virgin birth, 23
virola, 69
virus, *see* microbes
visions, 59, 139
vis medicatrix naturae, 67, 190
vital spirits, 62
vitamins, 64, 81
Vitus, St, 85, 90
vivisection, 101, 104, 105
Vollum, E. P., 54
Voltaire, 72, 292

Voodoo, 37, 49, 96, 221
voodoo death, 236
Voronoff, S., 246

Wagner, Richard, 78, 114
Wagner-Jauregg, Julius, 110
wakathons, 263
Waksman, Selman A., 38
walking, 10
Wallace, John, 142
Walshe, Francis, 139
Wandering Jew, 245
wanga, 96
war, 282
wart-charmers, 269
Washington, George, 36, 172
water, 132
water-caster, 293
water closet, 45, 46, 47
Watson, J. B., 28, 29
Watson, Lyall, 54, 230
Watt, James, 248
Watteau, Antoine, 292
weapon salve, 224
weather, 6, 77, 94
Weber, C. E. von, 292
Webster, Noah, 248
weeds, 126
Weil, Simone, 292
welfare medicine, 212
Welles, Orson, 163
Wellington, Duke of, 91
Wells, H. G., 163, 248
Weltschmerz, 11
were-animal, 97
werewolf, 97, 139
Wesley, John, 40, 224
Wickland, Carl, 222
wife-swapping, 266
Wilde, Oscar, 279
William III, 289
willow bark, 226
Windsor, William, 37
witch-doctor, 224, 225, 240, 269
witches and witchcraft, 6, 26, 37, 45,
    96, 149, 163, 253, 254
witch-hunting, 241
Withering, William, 226
wolf, 97
Wolf, Hugo, 118, 279
Wolsey, Cardinal, 279
woman, 256, 257, 259
womanizers, 114

womb, 137
Woolf, Virginia, 167
word association, 233
Wordsworth, William, 117, 177, 248
work, 265
work therapy, 198
World Health Organisation, see United
    Nations
worms, 93, 146, 225
wort, 126
wraiths, 96
Wright, Frank Lloyd, 248

Xante, 50
Xanthippe, 1
X-chromosome, 238
xenoanalysis, 232
xenoglossis, see speaking in tongues
xenophrenia, 59, 113, 219, 294
Xerxes, 83
X-ray, 79, 81
X-ray diffraction, 179

yagé, 69
Yang-Yin, 3, 4
Yates, Edmund, 54
yaws, 277
yellow babies, 82
Yellow Emperor, 3
yoga, 5, 49, 155, 253, 255, 286
yogurt, 64
yohimbe, 13
Young, Brigham, 278
youth (adolescence and adolescents), 2,
    37, 46, 79, 89, 115, 149, 169, 189,
    221, 231, 254, 266
youth, recovery of, 245
youth gland, 130
youth pills, 68, 247

Zen, 64
Zeus, 120
Zilboorg, Gregory, 26
Zinsser, H., 83
zoanthropy, 97
Zola, Emile, 78
zombie, 96, 191
zone therapy, 295
zoonoses, 174
Zoroastrianism, 256